AF413093

ISOLATED CORONARY ANOMALIES
(Unassociated with Another Congenital Heart Disease)

Collected Reprints
(1962-1993)

By

WILLIAM C. ROBERTS, MD

and

COLLEAGUES

ISBN: 979-8-88680-092-0
Printed in the United States of America on acid-free paper.

Preface

For decades an occasional coronary anomaly was observed at necropsy. I suspect that most were missed at autopsy. Origin of the left circumflex coronary artery from the right coronary artery or from the right sinus of Valsalva with retroaortic coursing to the left atrioventricular sulcus can easily be overlooked at autopsy without careful examination of the aortic-root area. Likewise, origin of both right and left coronary arteries from the same sinus of Valsalva is probably overlooked more often at necropsy than diagnosed. Coronary anomalies came to the forefront with coronary angiography in the 1970s when this procedure was required before coronary bypass could be performed. Today, it is essential that cardiologists be familiar with the many varieties of coronary anomalies so that corrective procedures can be performed in the right patients and not in the patients where corrective procedures would not be useful. To transfer a right coronary ostium arising from the left sinus of Valsalva to the right sinus is an unnecessary procedure, whereas transferring a left main coronary ostium to the left sinus may be lifesaving. These procedures are difficult and potentially hazardous, and no surgeon has extensive expertise in these operations.

—*William C. Roberts, MD*

Table of Contents

*Articles are numbered based on WCR's CV.

Anomalous Origin of Both Coronary Arteries from the Pulmonary Artery[*]

William C. Roberts, M.D.[†]

Bethesda, Maryland

Anomalous origin of either one or both coronary arteries from the pulmonary artery is rare. Less than 70 cases involving the left coronary artery have been reported. About 15 per cent of the patients lived to adulthood and had no recognizable clinical abnormalities;[1] the other 85 per cent had clinical and electrocardiographic features characteristic of this condition (Bland-White-Garland syndrome[2]) and died in infancy. Recognition of this anomaly is important because surgical treatment appears beneficial.[3,4] Anomalous origin of the right coronary is even less common, about 20 patients having been reported. These patients characteristically have no clinical symptoms referable to the anomaly, which is usually only an incidental finding at autopsy. Origin of both coronary arteries from the pulmonary artery is exceedingly rare, only seven patients having previously been reported.[5-11] This report describes another patient who died of this anomaly.

Case Report

N. M., a male Indian born of a normal pregnancy and delivery, died on his seventh day of life in the Turtle Mountain Indian Hospital, Belcourt, North Dakota. He had cyanosis and labored respirations at birth, and these symptoms progressively worsened until his death. No heart murmur was ever heard. The heart was normal in size by chest roentgenogram. He was treated with oxygen and digitalis without benefit.

Autopsy was performed at the Indian Hospital, and subsequently the heart and other tissues were submitted to the National Institutes of Health for examination. The heart (Fig. 1) weighed 27 gm., and the right atrium, right ventricle and left ventricle were dilated and hypertrophied. The wall of each ventricle measured up to 0.4 cm. in thickness. The endocardium of the outflow tract of the left ventricle was mildly but uniformly opaque. The four cardiac valves were normal. The foramen ovale was closed. Both coronary arteries originated from the pulmonary artery. The ostium of the right coronary artery was located in the right posterior sinus, and the left one in the left posterior pulmonic sinus. No coronary arteries arose from the aortic valve sinuses (Fig. 2); the course of distribution of the coronary arteries, which were of equal size, from there on was normal. The lungs were dark purple, virtually solid and without crepitation.

Histologically, the coronary arteries had the structure of arterial channels (Fig. 3A), although they carried only venous blood. Sections through both ventricles (Fig. 3B) disclosed minimal interstitial myocardial edema but no myocardial fibrosis nor inflammation. Myocardial fibers were fragmented, and cross-striations (phosphotungstic acid-hematoxylin stain) were poorly preserved. Some of the myocardial nuclei appeared enlarged, but most were normal. There was no periodic acid-Schiff-positive material in the myocardium. Fat stain (Oil red O) on the frozen-sectioned myocardium was negative (Fig. 3C). Cross-striations in the myocardial fibers were easily discernible in the frozen section. Section of the main pulmonary artery stained for elastic fibers (Verhoeff-Van Giesen method) disclosed a fetal, i.e., aortic-like, configuration of the elastica of this vessel. In the sections from the lungs there were extensive atelectasis and congestion.

Comment

Clinical Features: In contrast to the diagnosis of anomalous origin of the left coronary artery from the pulmonary artery, the antemortem diagnosis of anomalous origin of both coronary arteries from the pulmonary artery has not been reported. The probable reason is that this latter condition has not been considered clinically, and thus remains only a postmortem curiosity. However, the clinical features in both conditions are similar (Table I) and sufficiently characteristic so that the diagnosis might be suggested before death. The newborn is cyanotic and dyspneic from birth or shortly

* From the Pathologic Anatomy Department, Clinical Center, National Institutes of Health, Bethesda, Maryland.
† Present address: Department of Medicine, The Johns Hopkins Hospital, Baltimore 5, Maryland.

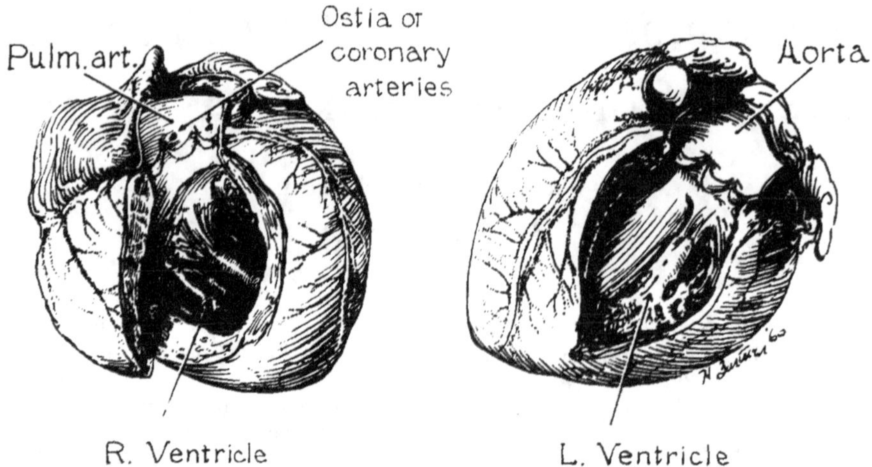

FIG. 1. *Drawing of heart. Left*, the right ventricle, pulmonary valve and pulmonary trunk are opened. Both coronary arteries arise from the base of the main pulmonary artery. *Right*, the left ventricle, aortic valve and ascending aorta are opened. No coronary arterial ostia are present.

thereafter. On the other hand, patients with only the left coronary artery originating from the pulmonary artery are normal at birth and usually remain so for one to three months when

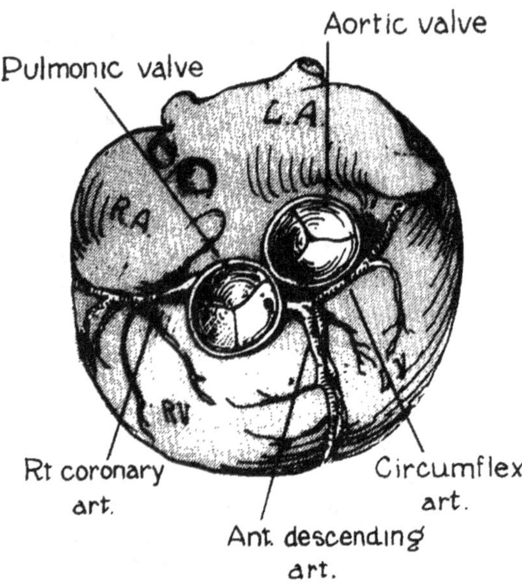

FIG. 2. *Sketch of heart showing both coronary arteries arising from the pulmonic valve sinuses.* The left coronary artery arises from the left posterior sinus and is composed of a circumflex branch which courses anterior to the aortic valve to lie in the left atrioventricular sulcus, and an anterior descending branch which descends in the anterior interventricular sulcus. The right main coronary artery arises in the right posterior pulmonic sinus and lies in the right atrioventricular sulcus, giving off several small branches, and at the base of the posterior interventricular sulcus becomes the posterior descending coronary artery.

evidence of heart failure, irritability or discomfort, and respiratory infection appears. The heart in children with two anomalous coronary arteries is usually enlarged (as it is in those with anomalous left coronary artery), sometimes reaching huge proportions, as in the patient reported by Swann and Werthammer.[9] No precordial murmurs are heard unless there is an associated defect of the heart or great vessels. Frank signs of heart failure are usually apparent, and these progressively worsen. Feedings are poorly tolerated. The electrocardiogram is virtually pathognomonic in the symptomatic infant with anomalous left coronary artery,[2,12] but no tracing has been made in reported cases of anomalous origin of both coronary arteries from the pulmonary artery. Findings of left ventricular ischemia would be expected. Breathing gradually becomes more labored, and life ends before two weeks have elapsed.

Pathologic Features: At autopsy, the ventricles, particularly the left one, are typically dilated and hypertrophied, and the endocardium of the left ventricle may be thickened. The coronary arteries, which arise from the right and left sinuses of the pulmonic valve (the anterior sinus being the noncoronary one), are normally distributed. Histologically, they may have the same morphologic features herein described; the vein-like structure reported by Schulze and Rodin[11] or the intimal fibrous proliferation observed by Tedeschi and Helpern.[8] Although there may be some focal degenerative changes of the myocardial fibers

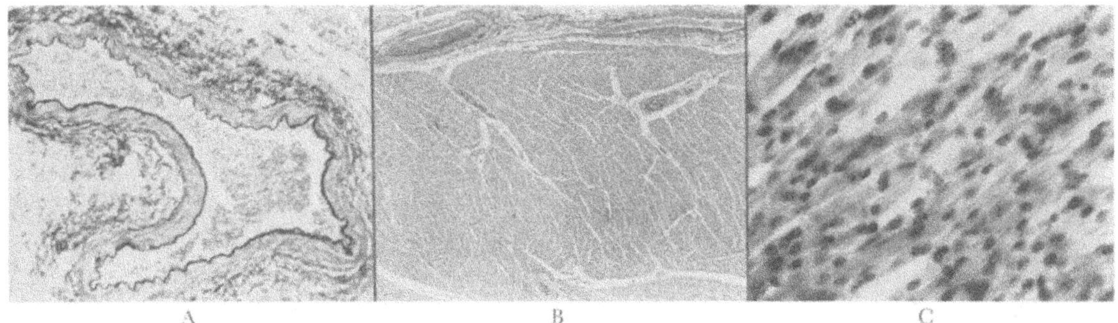

Fig. 3. Histologic sections. A, *photomicrograph of the anterior descending branch of the left coronary artery* 1.5 cm. from its ostium. This vessel has the histologic features of a muscular artery. Verhoeff-Van Gieson elastic tissue stain, original magnification, ×155. B, *photomicrograph of left ventricle.* The epicardial surface is at the top of the figure. Hematoxylin and eosin stain, original magnification, ×30. C, *fat stain of left ventricular myocardium.* Cross striations are apparent. Oil red O stain on frozen section, original magnification, ×480.

TABLE I
Anomalous Origin of Both Coronary Arteries from the Pulmonary Artery

Author Year	Sex	Age at Death	Condition at Birth	Weight of Heart (gm.)	Associated Cardiovascular Anomalies	Distribution of Coronary Arteries	Histologic Structure of Coronary Arteries	Histologic Structure of Myocardium	Other Findings
1. Grayzel & Tennant[5] 1934	F	9 hours	Cyanosis	19*	Atresia, tricuspid valve; VSD (2). Origin rt. PA from As.Ao; CS → LA & RA; PDA; PFO; hypoplasia, RV, PV, PA	Normal			Atelectasis, lungs. Hemorrhage, cerebellum
2. Limbourg[6] 1937	M	10 days	Cyanosis Unconsciousness	15	PDA	Normal		Fat droplets, focal, in myocardial fibers	Hemorrhage, subarachnoid, from tentorial tear
3. Williams, Johnson, Boulware[7] 1951	F	4 days	"Normal" Cyanosis on 2nd day, Systolic murmur	36	VSD, PS, PDA, PFO	Normal			Atelectasis, lungs
5. Tedeschi & Helpern[3] 1954	F	13 days	Cyanosis Dyspnea	39	PDA	Normal	Thickening of walls due to intimal fibrous proliferation & focal edema of media & adventitia	Norma	0
4. Swann & Werthammer[9] (Case 3) 1955	M	2 days	Cyanosis Dyspnea	56	PDA, PFO			Hypertrophy of myocardial fibers of both RV & LV. Fat positive vacuoles in myocardial fibers	Congestive heart failure
6. Alexander & Griffith[10] 1956	M	2 days	Cyanosis		PDA, PFO				Atelectasis, lungs
7. Schulze & Rodin[11] 1961	F	8 hours	Cyanosis	18	PDA	Normal	Vein-like	Nuclear pyknosis, loss of cross-striations, & interstitial edema with inflammatory cell infiltration	Congestive heart failure. Hyaline membrane disease, lungs
8. Present Author 1961	M	7 days	Cyanosis Dyspnea	27	0	Normal	Arterial	Normal	Atelectasis, lungs. Congestive heart failure

* Average normal heart weight for full-term newborn = 17 gms.
VSD = ventricular septal defect; PV = pulmonic valve; RV = right ventricle; CS = coronary sinus; LA = left atrium; RA = right atrium; PDA = patent ductus arteriosus; PS = pulmonic stenosis; PFO = patent foramen ovale; PA = pulmonary artery; As.Ao. = ascending aorta.

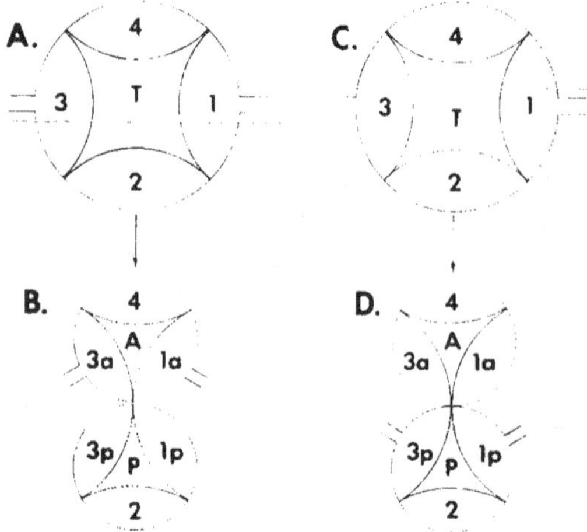

FIG. 4. *Illustration to demonstrate Abrikossoff's theory of normal and abnormal development of the coronary arteries. A and B, normal division of the truncus arteriosus by a septum (dotted line) so that two coronary anlagen are included with the aorta. C and D, abnormal division of the truncus arteriosus by a deviated septum so that the two coronary anlagen are included with the pulmonary artery. T = truncus arteriosus; A = aorta; P = pulmonary artery; 1a = left aortic valve cusp; 3a = right aortic valve cusp; 1p = left pulmonic valve cusp; 3p = right pulmonic valve cusp; 2 = anterior pulmonic valve cusp; 4 = posterior aortic valve cusp.*

suggestive of ischemia, there is no fibrous scarring nor other evidence of myocardial infarction. Major associated congenital cardiac defects have been recorded twice. The patient reported by Grayzel and Tennant[5] had tricuspid atresia, two ventricular septal defects, anomalous drainage of the coronary sinus into the left atrium, and origin of the right pulmonary artery from the ascending aorta. An anatomic tetralogy of Fallot was present in the patient described by Williams et al.[7] The lungs are usually collapsed and congested.

Mechanism for Heart Failure: The clinical manifestations of double anomalous coronary arteries appear to be attributable to left ventricular failure. It is now well established[3,4,13] that when only the left coronary artery arises anomalously from the pulmonary artery, the blood contained in the aberrant vessel is fully saturated and flows away from the left ventricle in a retrograde fashion toward the pulmonary artery. When both coronary arteries arise from the pulmonary artery, however, blood in the anomalous vessels is poorly saturated and flows from the pulmonary artery toward the myocardium.

The lowered oxygen content of the blood in

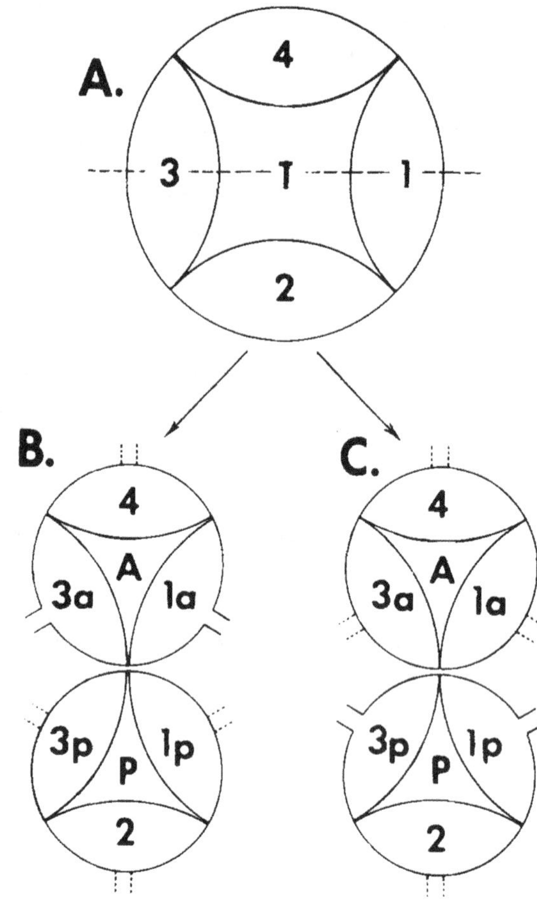

FIG. 5. *Illustration to demonstrate Hackensellner's theory of normal and abnormal development of the coronary arteries. A, normal division of the truncus arteriosus before formation of coronary anlagen. B, normal involution of all coronary anlagen (dotted lines) except the two that arise from the right and left aortic valve sinuses. C, involution of the two normally persisting aortic coronary anlagen (at 3a and 1a), with persistence of two normally involuted pulmonary coronary anlagen (at 3p and 1p). The result is anomalous origin of both coronary arteries from the pulmonary artery.*

the anomalous coronary arteries is certainly not the cause of the left ventricular failure. Some patients with congenital cyanotic heart disease and normally arising coronary arteries have an arterial oxygen saturation below that of venous blood and live for a number of years. The heart failure appears to be the result of low perfusion pressure in the two anomalous coronary arteries. At birth, the pressures in the right ventricle and in the pulmonary trunk are at or near normal systemic levels. Within a matter of hours or days after birth, however, the pressure in the pulmonary artery falls, and consequently, in patients with both coronary arteries arising from the pulmonary artery, the coronary arterial perfusion pressure diminishes. Finally, about two weeks following birth, the perfusion pressure apparently is completely inadequate to supply the nutritional requirements of the left ventricle, and life ends.

Surgical therapy in this condition would necessarily be directed toward increasing the coronary arterial perfusion pressure. Theoretically, this could be done by either transplanting or connecting the ostia of the coronary arteries with a systemic artery, or by constricting the pulmonary trunk above the anomalous coronary arterial ostia. Obviously, neither of these procedures has been performed in a patient with double anomalous coronary arteries. However, each procedure has been carried out in patients with an aberrant left coronary artery arising from the pulmonary artery. Mustard[14] ligated the anomalous left coronary artery in his patient and anastomosed it to a systemic artery. He demonstrated that this procedure was technically feasible, but his patient died eight hours following operation. An operating dissecting microscope may be of real use in this procedure. Morrow[3] constricted the pulmonary trunk in a patient with an aberrant left coronary artery, but ventricular fibrillation occurred after completion of the supravalvular pulmonic stenosis, and the patient died.

Embryology: The embryologic basis for anomalous development of both coronary arteries from the pulmonary artery has recently been thoroughly reviewed by Schulze and Rodin.[11] Briefly, two theories, septal deviation and involution-persistence, have received considerable attention. Abrikossoff[14] suggested that either the truncus arteriosus is abnormally divided so that the two coronary anlagen are included with the pulmonary artery (Fig. 4), or that a coronary bud arises anomalously from a part of the truncus destined to become the pulmonary artery. The involution-persistence theory suggested recently by Hackensellner[15] provides explanations for several anomalies of the coronary arteries which the former theories failed to do, and it appears more acceptable. He described the occurrence of an anlage of a coronary artery in each of the six regions of the semilunar valves of the aorta and pulmonary trunk. Normally, permanent coronary arteries arise from anlagen in two aortic sinuses, and the anlagen in the other aortic and in all three pulmonic valvular sinuses either are not formed or are rapidly involuted (Fig. 5). Thus, the combination of persistence of two normally involuted pulmonary coronary buds and involution of two normally persistent aortic coronary buds would result in anomalous origin of both coronary arteries.

SUMMARY

The clinical and pathologic features of a 7 day old infant in whom both coronary arteries arose from the pulmonary artery is presented, and information derived from the 7 previously reported patients with this anomaly is summarized. Characteristically, these infants have cyanosis and dyspnea at birth or shortly thereafter, cardiac enlargement and no heart murmur, and rapidly progress to heart failure. All reported patients with this condition have died within two weeks after birth. None of the reported patients with double anomalous coronary arteries has been diagnosed ante mortem.

ACKNOWLEDGMENTS

I wish to thank Dr. Benjamin Highman, Chief, Section of Pathology Anatomy, Laboratory of Experimental Pathology, National Institute of Arthritis and Metabolic Diseases, for his kindness in referring this case and for allowing me to publish it. Also, I am grateful to Dr. Louis B. Thomas, Chief of the Surgical and Post-mortem Service, National Cancer Institute, and to Dr. Ross C. MacCardle, Laboratory of Pathology, National Cancer Institute, for reviewing the manuscript.

REFERENCES

1. KEITH, J. D. The anomalous origin of the left coronary artery from the pulmonary artery. *Brit. Heart J.*, 21: 149, 1959.
2. BLAND, E. F., WHITE, P. D. and GARLAND, J. Congenital anomalies of coronary arteries. Report of an unusual case associated with cardiac hypertrophy. *Am. Heart J.*, 8: 787, 1933.
3. CASE, R. B., MORROW, A. G., STAINSBY, W. and NESTOR, J. O. Anomalous origin of the left coronary artery. The physiologic defect and suggested surgical treatment. *Circulation*, 17: 1062, 1958.
4. SABISTON, D. C., JR., NEILL, C. A. and TAUSSIG, H. B. The direction of blood flow in anomalous left coronary artery arising from the pulmonary artery. *Circulation*, 22: 591, 1960.
5. GRAYZEL, D. and TENNANT, R. Congenital atresia of tricuspid orifice and anomalous origin of coronary arteries from pulmonary artery. *Am. J. Path.*, 10: 791, 1934.
6. LIMBOURG, M. Uber den Ursprung der Kranzarterien des Herzens aus der Arteria pulmonalis. *Beitr. path. Anat.*, 100: 191, 1937.
7. WILLIAMS, J. W., JOHNSON, W. S. and BOULWARE, J. R. A case of tetralogy of Fallot with both coronary arteries arising from the pulmonary artery. *J. Florida M. A.*, 37: 561, 1951.

8. TEDESCHI, C. G. and HELPERN, M. M. Heterotopic origin of both coronary arteries from the pulmonary artery. Review of literature and report of a case not complicated by associated defects. *Pediatrics*, 14: 53, 1954.

9. SWANN, W. C. and WERTHAMMER, S. Aberrant coronary arteries. Experiences in diagnosis with report of three cases. *Ann. Int. Med.*, 42: 873, 1955.

10. ALEXANDER, R. W. and GRIFFITH, G. C. Anomalies of the coronary arteries and their clinical significance. *Circulation*, 14: 800, 1956.

11. SCHULZE, W. B. and RODIN, A. E. Anomalous origin of both coronary arteries. Report of a case with discussion of teratogenic theories. *Arch. Path.*, 72: 36, 1961.

12. TAUSSIG, H. B. Congenital Malformations of the Heart, p. 324. New York, 1947. The Commonwealth Fund.

13. EDWARDS, J. E. Symposium on cardiovascular diseases. Functional pathology of congenital cardiac disease. *Pediat. Clin. North America*, 1: 13, 1954.

14. ABRIKOSSOFF, A. Aneurysma des linken Herzventrikels mit abnormer Abgangsstelle der linken Koronararterie von der Pulmonalis bei einem fünfmonatlichen Kinde. *Arch. path. Anat.*, 203: 413, 1911.

15. HACKENSELLNER, H. A. Akzessorsiche Kranzgefässanlagen der Arteria pulmonalis under 63 menschlichen Embryonenserien mit einer grössten Länge von 12 bis 36 mm. *Ztschr. Mikroscopischanat. Forsch.*, 62: 153, 1956.

Compression of anomalous left circumflex coronary arteries by prosthetic valve fixation rings

William C. Roberts, M.D., and Andrew G. Morrow, M.D., Bethesda, Md.

Damage to a coronary artery is a rare but recognized complication of cardiac valve replacement. Thus, the ostium of a coronary artery may be occluded by the fixation ring of an aortic valve prosthesis, or the proximal portion of the artery may be lacerated or dissected during cannulation.[1, 2] The left circumflex coronary artery, located in the atrioventricular sulcus in close proximity to the mitral annulus, may be damaged during mitral valve replacement.[3] A more unusual complication of valve replacement has recently been observed in 2 patients with severe valvular heart disease in whom the left circumflex coronary artery arose from the right coronary artery. In each patient the anomalous coronary artery was compressed by the fixation rings of mitral and/or aortic valvular prostheses; in 1 patient, obstruction of the vessel led to fatal myocardial infarction. A brief description of the clinical and necropsy findings in these 2 patients is the subject of this report.

Descriptions of patients

CASE 1. W. R. (06-83-61), a 45-year-old man, was severely incapacitated, and severe mitral and aortic regurgitation were demonstrated at preoperative hemodynamic and angiographic assess-

From the Section of Pathology and the Clinic of Surgery, National Heart Institute, National Institutes of Health, Bethesda, Md. 20014.

Received for publication Oct. 7, 1968.

ments. At operation, the ascending aorta and aortic "annulus" were both relatively small, and the aortic valve was replaced with a size 8A Starr-Edwards prosthesis. The incompetent mitral valve was replaced with a 3M Starr-Edwards prosthesis. During the entire postoperative period the patient evidenced signs of inadequate cardiac output, and administration of isoproterenol was required to maintain an adequate systemic arterial pressure. Urine output initially was adequate, but oliguria appeared and the blood urea nitrogen rose to 200 mg. per 100 ml. Progressive hypoxia was treated by tracheostomy and assisted resuscitation; circulatory depression persisted and the patient died on the tenth postoperative day.

At autopsy (A68-22), the heart weighed 1,040 grams; the left ventricle and left atrium were greatly dilated. No thrombus was present on either prosthetic valve, but the aortic valve appeared large in proportion to size of the aorta into which it had been inserted. The left circumflex coronary artery arose from the right coronary artery immediately after its origin from the aorta. The left circumflex branch passed behind the aorta in the groove between both prosthetic valve rings (Fig. 1). The rings of the prostheses compressed the anomalous left circumflex branch, probably totally obstructing its lumen. After the left circumflex branch passed behind the aorta and pulmonary trunk it coursed normally in the left atrioventricular sulcus. The lateral wall of the left ventricle was focally hemorrhagic and acutely infarcted (Fig. 1).

CASE 2. M. G. (01-72-82), a 53-year-old woman, developed signs of cardiac dysfunction at the age of 37 years. When she had been studied at the age of 47, the pulmonary arterial pressure was 90/36, right ventricle 90/12, right atrial mean pressure 10 and v wave 13, and left atrial mean pressure 20 and v wave 50 mm. Hg;

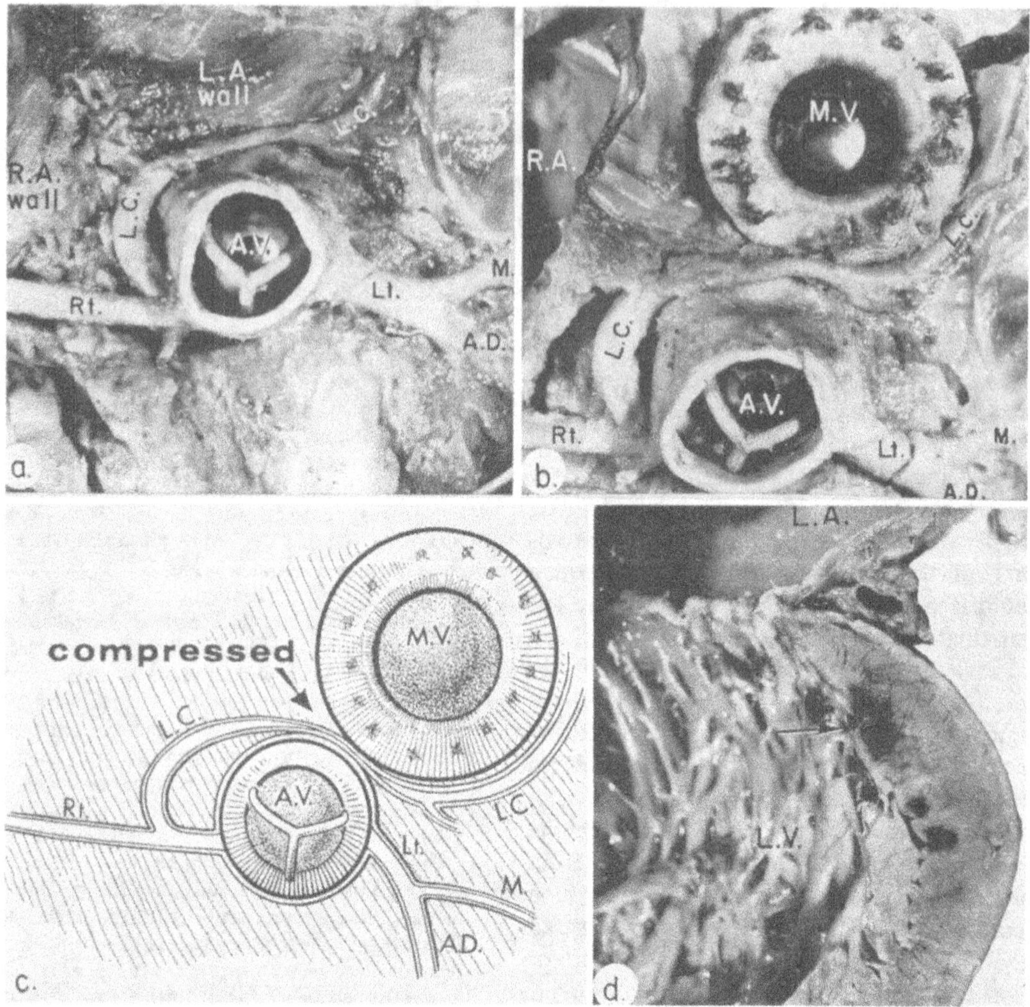

Fig. 1. Patient 1. *a,* Aortic root viewed from above shows the Starr-Edwards aortic valve *(A.V.)* prosthesis and the origins of the coronary arteries. The left circumflex *(L.C.)* arises from the right *(Rt.)* coronary artery immediately after the latter's origin from the aorta. The left circumflex coronary artery passes posteriorly, between the aortic root and base of the left atrium *(L.A.).* Its course thereafter is normal. The origin and distribution of the left *(Lt.)* coronary artery and its branches, anterior descending *(A.D.)* and marginal *(M.),* are normal. *R.A.,* Right atrium. *b,* The wall of the left atrium has now been excised, better demonstrating compression of the left circumflex coronary artery between the fixation rings of the mitral and aortic prostheses, shown diagrammatically in *c. d,* Cut surface of lateral walls of left atrium *(L.A.)* and left ventricle *(L.V.)* demonstrates focal hemorrhagic infarction *(arrow)* of the ventricular wall.

simultaneous left ventricular and brachial arterial pressures were 125/10 and 125/70 mm. Hg, respectively, and the left atrial and left ventricular mean diastolic pressure gradient was 8 mm. Hg. At operation, the mitral valve was replaced with a 4M Starr-Edwards prosthesis. The early course after operation was uneventful, but review of electrocardiograms 3 years postoperatively showed evidence of anterior myocardial infarction in the past and an intraventricular conduction defect, neither of which had been present before operation. At cardiac catheterization, 4½ years after mitral valve replacement, the pulmonary arterial pressure was 44/21 mm. Hg, the pulmonary arterial wedge mean pressure was 17 with v waves 20, and simultaneous left ventricular and brachial arterial pressures were 152/20 and 130/70 mm. Hg, respectively. A sudden cerebrovascular accident occurred 5⅔ years after valve replacement, and she died.

At autopsy (A68-141), the heart weighed 800 grams, and thrombus was present on the prosthetic valve. The left circumflex coronary artery arose from the right coronary artery, and passed behind the aorta in the groove between the prosthetic mitral ring and the base of the aorta (Fig. 2). The lumen of this artery was compressed by the prosthetic valve ring but sections of the vessel showed that it was patent (Fig. 3). The left circumflex coronary artery thereafter coursed normally in the left atrioventricular sulcus. Extensive scarring was present in the lateral wall of the left ventricle and in the free wall beneath the anterolateral papillary muscle (Fig. 3).

Comment

Origin of the left circumflex coronary artery from the right coronary artery is noted in about 0.3 per cent of autopsied subjects.[4] It originates just after the origin of the right coronary artery, and courses posteriorly around and between the root of the aorta and the left atrial wall, nearly at the level of the mitral annulus. Normally, the aortic and mitral annuli are pliable structures, but when either or both valves are replaced with caged-ball prostheses the valve rings become rigid. Consequently, if both mitral and aortic valves are replaced with rigid ring-type prostheses, and if the left circumflex coronary artery arises anomalously, the lumen of this vessel can be compressed between the two prosthetic annuli. In Patient 1, the anomalous left circumflex coronary artery was almost certainly occluded in this manner, as evidenced by the acute infarct of the lateral free wall of the left ventricle, the area normally supplied by the left circumflex coronary artery. In Patient 2, the mitral valve only was replaced, but the anomalous left circumflex coronary was nevertheless caught between the rigid mitral prosthetic annulus and the aortic root, which, of course, was distended by systemic arterial pressure. Although the anomalous coronary artery in this patient was not occluded, its lumen was much smaller than normal and the lateral and anterior walls of the left ventricle were focally scarred.

Antemortem diagnosis of anomalous origin of the left circumflex coronary artery from the right coronary artery was not accomplished in either patient. Even had the anomaly been appreciated at operation, it is unlikely that correction of the anomaly would have been warranted. External compression of the anomalous left circumflex coronary arteries may have been lessened or prevented in each patient, however, by use of smaller-sized mitral prostheses.

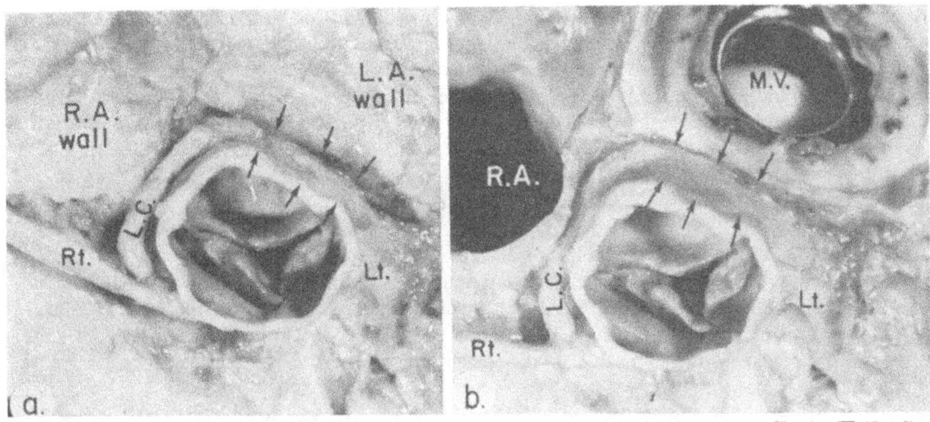

Fig. 2. Aortic root in Patient 2. *a,* The left circumflex (*L.C.*) coronary artery arises anomalously from the right (*Rt.*) coronary artery and is narrowed between the fixation ring of the mitral prosthesis and the base of the aorta. The site of compression of the anomalously arising vessel is shown by the *arrows. b,* The atrial walls have now been excised, demonstrating the mitral valve (*M.V.*) prosthesis. *R.A.,* Right atrium. *Lt.,* Left main coronary artery.

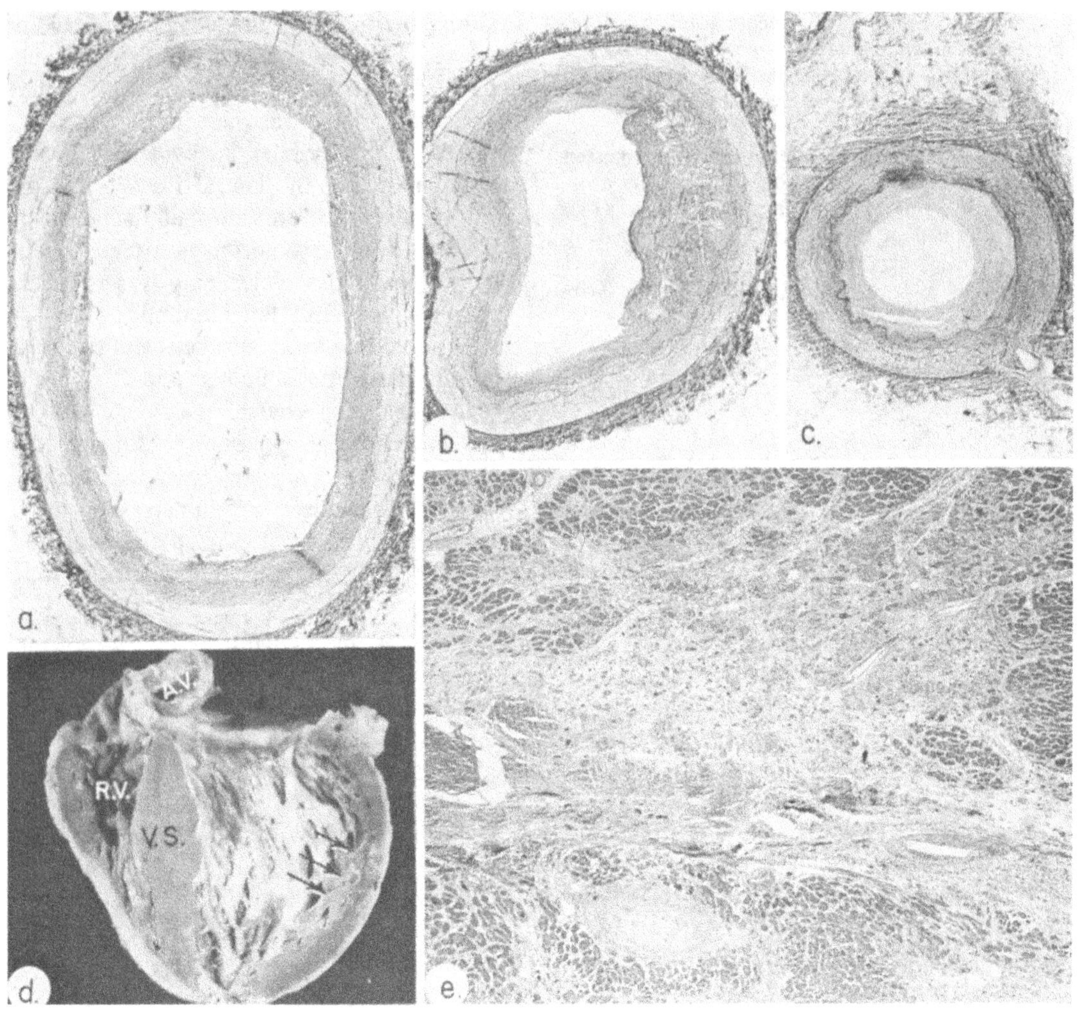

Fig. 3. Coronary arteries and cardiac ventricles in Patient 2. *a,* Cross-section of right main coronary artery 2 cm. from its origin from the aorta is shown for comparison with *b* and *c. b,* Left circumflex coronary artery 1 cm. after its origin from the right coronary artery. *c,* Left circumflex coronary artery more distal to *b* at the site of its being squeezed between the mitral prosthetic ring and the aortic root (see Fig. 2, between the *arrows*). The photomicrographs shown in *a, b,* and *c* were each taken at the same magnification (× 22) and demonstrate the degree of narrowing of the anomalously arising left circumflex coronary artery. The narrowing of this vessel clearly resulted from external compression to it by the fixation ring of the mitral prosthesis. Elastic van Gieson stains were used in the sections in each of the 3 photomicrographs. *d,* Posterior one half of the cardiac ventricles demonstrates thinning and fibrosis *(arrows)* of the left ventricular free wall at a site normally supplied by the left circumflex coronary artery. The left ventricular endocardial thickening is a late anatomic observation after replacement of the mitral valve with a Starr-Edwards prosthesis.[5] *R.V.,* Right ventricle. *V.S.,* Ventricular septum. *A.V.,* Aortic valve cusp. *e,* Section of portion of lateral wall of left ventricle shows extensive myocardial replacement and interstitial fibrosis. (Hematoxylin and eosin stain; × 16.)

REFERENCES

1 Roberts, W. C., and Morrow, A. G.: Causes of Early Postoperative Death Following Cardiac Valve Replacement. Clinico-pathologic Correlations in 64 Patients Studied at Necropsy, J. THORACIC & CARDIOVAS. SURG. **54:** 422, 1967.

2 Roberts, W. C., and Morrow, A. G.: Anatomic Studies of Hearts Containing Caged-Ball Prosthetic Valves, Johns Hopkins M. J. **121:** 271, 1967.

3 Danielson, G. K., Cooper, E., and Tweeddale, D. N.: Circumflex Coronary Artery Injury During Mitral Valve Replacement, Ann. Thoracic Surg. **4:** 53, 1967.

4 White, N. K., and Edwards, J. E.: Anomalies of the Coronary Arteries; Report of Four Cases, Arch. Path. **45:** 766, 1948.

5 Roberts, W. C., and Morrow, A. G.: Secondary Left Ventricular Endocardial Fibroelastosis Following Mitral Valve Replacement. Cause of Cardiac Failure in the Late Postoperative Period, Suppl. to Circulation *37* and *38:* II-101, 1968.

Origin of the Right Coronary Artery From the Left Sinus of Valsalva and Its Functional Consequences: Analysis of 10 Necropsy Patients

WILLIAM C. ROBERTS, MD, FACC*
ROBERT J. SIEGEL, MD*
DOUGLAS P. ZIPES, MD, FACC†

Bethesda, Maryland

Clinical and necropsy findings are described in 10 patients in whom the right coronary artery arose from the left coronary sinus and then passed to the right atrioventricular (A-V) sulcus by coursing between the aorta and the pulmonary trunk. In 7 of the 10 patients, the coronary anomaly never caused symptoms of cardiac dysfunction. In the other three, all of whom died suddenly, the coronary anomaly was the only significant abnormality found at necropsy: One patient had recurring ventricular tachycardia, one had typical angina pectoris and, in one, sudden death was the initial manifestation of cardiac dysfunction. Review of previous angiographic studies during life of 31 patients reported to have origin of the right coronary artery from the left sinus of Valsalva indicated that 9 had symptoms of cardiac dysfunction in the absence of intraluminal coronary narrowing or associated noncoronary cardiac disease. Thus, origin of the right coronary artery from the left sinus may produce cardiac dysfunction that can be fatal.

It is well established that the congenital coronary anomaly—origin of the *left main* coronary artery from the *right sinus* of Valsalva with subsequent coursing between the aorta and pulmonary trunk—may produce cardiac dysfunction, indeed, usually sudden death[1-4] (Fig. 1). Origin of the *right* coronary artery from the *left sinus* of Valsalva, in contrast, has been considered a minor congenital anomaly of no clinical significance (Fig. 1). Recently, however, we studied at necropsy three patients who died suddenly and had this anomaly as the only significant anatomic abnormality observed at necropsy. This report describes certain clinical and necropsy findings in these three patients, summarizes findings in seven other necropsy patients we studied in whom the anomaly caused no cardiac dysfunction, and reviews previous reports of others to determine if cardiac dysfunction has been observed in other patients with this coronary anomaly.

Results

Clinical features: Certain clinical and necropsy findings in the 10 patients are summarized in Table I. Their ages ranged from 17 to 51 years (mean 34); four were white, six, black; two were women, and eight, men. Of the three with evidence of cardiac dysfunction, one (Patient 1, Table I) died suddenly while playing basketball, and sudden death was his initial manifestation of illness. Patient 2 presented initially with syncope provoked while running and ventricular tachycardia was documented in her on many occasions thereafter. She was described previously by Pedersen et al.[5] as their Case 7 among 18 young patients who had ventricular tachycardia or ventricular fibrillation, or both. After that report we had an opportunity to examine the patient's heart and found the congenital coronary anomaly. Patient 3 had angina pectoris for 12 months and he died suddenly during coitus.

From the Pathology Branch, National Heart, Lung, and Blood Institute, National Institutes of Health, Bethesda, Maryland* and the Krannert Institute of Cardiology, the Department of Medicine, Indiana University School of Medicine, Indianapolis, Indiana.† Manuscript received August 11, 1981; revised manuscript received October 6, 1981, accepted October 16, 1981.

Address for reprints: William C. Roberts, MD, Building 10A, Room 3E30, National Institutes of Health, Bethesda, Maryland 20205.

The seven patients without evidence of cardiac dysfunction resulting from the coronary anomaly ranged in age from 19 to 51 years (mean 37). One (Patient 10) died from consequences of extensive coronary atherosclerosis; the other six died from noncardiac conditions.

Pathologic findings: The ostium of the right coronary artery arose either directly behind the commissure between the right and left coronary cusps or just to the left of that commissure (Fig. 2 and 3). In all 10 patients the ostium of the right coronary artery was *slit-like*, with the largest diameter located in a superior-inferior axis (Fig. 2 and 3). This ostium (Fig. 2 and 4) could easily be missed. In contrast, the ostium of the left main coronary artery in all 10 patients was round or nearly so. In 9 patients the lumens of the major epicardial coronary arteries were free of significant atherosclerotic plaques; in 1 (Patient 10), coronary atherosclerotic plaques were severe and the lumens of each of the major epicardial coronary arteries were severely narrowed by this process.

Grossly visible left ventricular scars were present in two of the three patients in whom the coronary arterial anomaly was of functional importance. The scarring in Patient 2 was transmural (> inner one half of wall), and this patient also had associated right ventricular scarring; in Patient 3, the scarring was subendocardial (< inner one half of wall). Among the seven patients

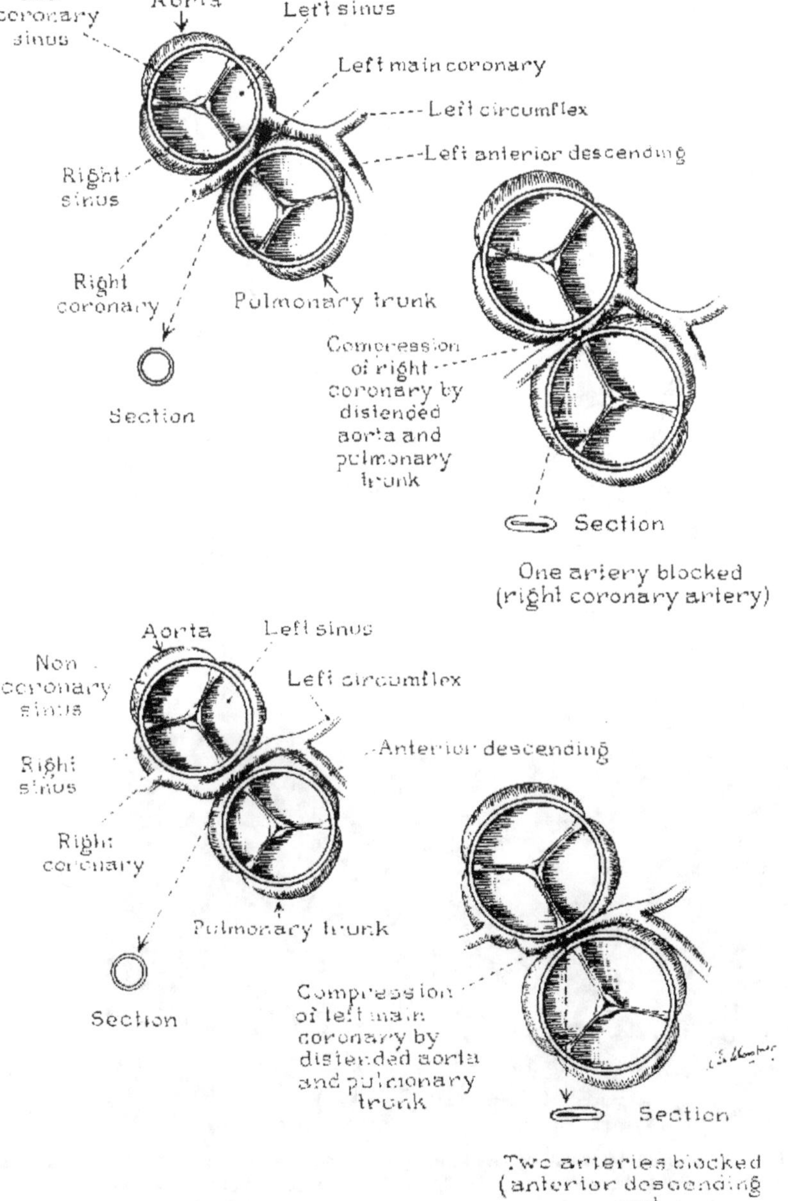

FIGURE 1. Diagram showing a proposed mechanism by which origin of the left main coronary artery (**lower**) can cause fatal or nonfatal cardiac dysfunction and an earlier view (**upper**) by which origin of the right coronary artery from the left sinus does not cause fatal or nonfatal cardiac dysfunction.

whose coronary anomaly was of no functional importance, only one (Patient 10) had grossly visible left ventricular scarring, and this patient had severe coronary atherosclerosis.

Histologic sections (one to seven per patient [average four]) of left ventricular wall additionally disclosed interstitial myocardial fibrosis in Patients 1 to 3 and in Patient 10.

Comments

Analysis of the findings in these 10 patients indicates that 3 had evidence of cardiac dysfunction (ventricular tachycardia in 1, angina pectoris in 1 and sudden death in all 3) during life, and necropsy disclosed that origin of the right coronary artery from the left sinus of Valsalva was the only anatomic explanation for the symptoms. The lumens of their major coronary arteries were devoid of significant coronary atherosclerotic plaques, and other types of cardiac disease and noncardiac conditions were absent.

Previously reported cases: In contrast to the occurrence of cardiac dysfunction in 3 of our 10 patients in whom the right coronary artery arose from the left sinus of Valsalva, analysis of previously reported data in 26 necropsy patients with this anomaly (Table

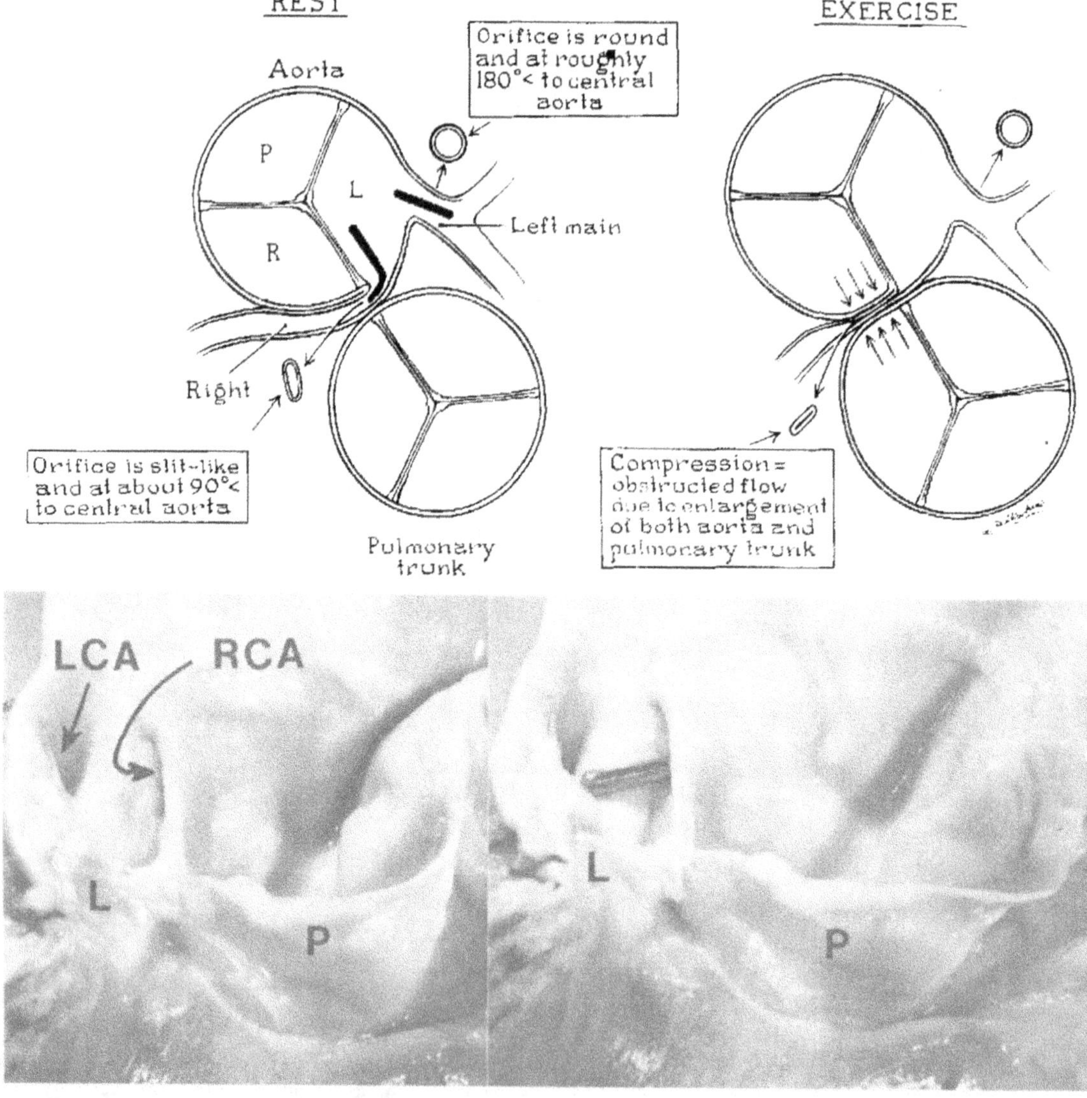

FIGURE 2. Case 3 (Table I). **Upper,** diagram showing possible mechanism by which origin of the right coronary artery from the left sinus causes cardiac dysfunction. **Lower,** opened aorta showing round ostium of the left coronary artery (LCA) and slit-like ostium of the right coronary artery (RCA) located directly behind the commissure between the left (L) and posterior (R) aortic valve cusps. In the **lower right view,** a probe protrudes from the ostium of the right coronary artery.

TABLE I

Clinical and Necropsy Observations in 10 Patients With Origin of Right Coronary Artery From the Left Sinus of Valsalva

Case	Age (yr)	Race	Sex	Duration (mo) Cardiac Dysfunction	AP	AMI	CHF	VT	S	SD	Activity Associated With SD	Cause of Death	Heart Weight (g)	Gross LV Scarring
											Symptoms of Cardiac Dysfunction and Insignificant Coronary Narrowing			
1	17	B	M	0	0	0	0	0	0	+	Basketball	VF	440	0
2	23	W	F	5	0	0	0	+	+	+	—	VF	340	+ (T)
3	49	B	M	12	+	0	0	0	0	+	Coitus	VF	490	+ (Su)
											No Symptoms of Cardiac Dysfunction or Significant Coronary Narrowing, or Both			
4	19	W	M	0	0	0	0	0	0	0	—	Leukemia	260	0
5	29	B	F	0	0	0	0	0	0	0	—	Opiate overdose	260	0
6	33	W	M	0	0	0	0	0	0	0	—	Melanoma	260	0
7	40	B	M	0	0	0	0	0	0	0	—	Alcoholism	410	0
8	41	B	M	0	0	0	0	0	0	0	—	Renal disease	540	0
9	41	B	M	0	0	0	0	0	0	0	—	Trauma	380	0
10	51	W	M	72	+	+	0	+	0	0	—	Atherosclerotic CA disease	540	+ (T)

AMI = acute myocardial infarction; AP = angina pectoris; CA = coronary artery; CHF = chronic congestive heart failure; LV = left ventricular; S = syncope; SD = sudden death; Su = subendocardial; T = transmural; VF = ventricular fibrillation; VT = ventricular tachycardia. 0 = absent; + = present.

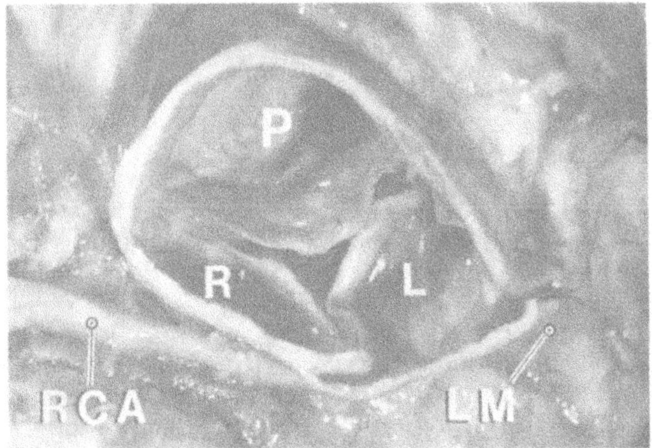

FIGURE 3. Case 9. View of aortic valve and proximal right (RCA) and left main (LM) coronary arteries from above with origin of the right coronary artery from the left aortic sinus. L = left, P = posterior and R = right sinuses of Valsalva, respectively.

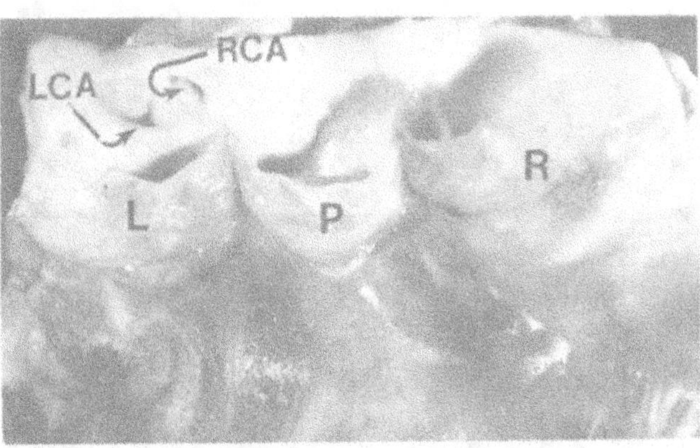

FIGURE 4. Case 4. Opened aorta showing the right ostium of the left main (LCA) and slit-like ostium of the right (RCA) coronary artery, both located above the left (L) aortic valve cusp. P = posterior and R = right aortic valve cusps, respectively.

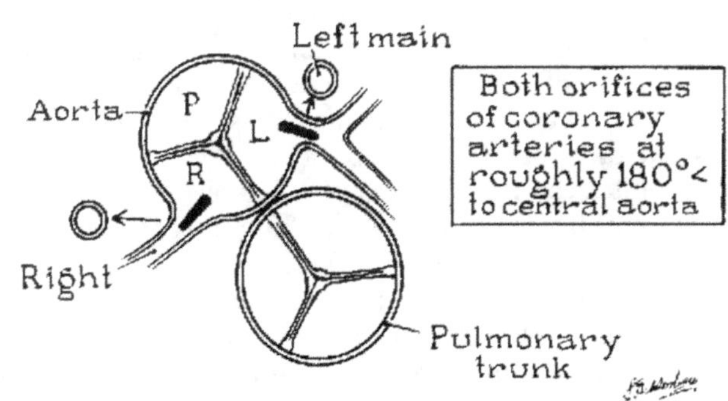

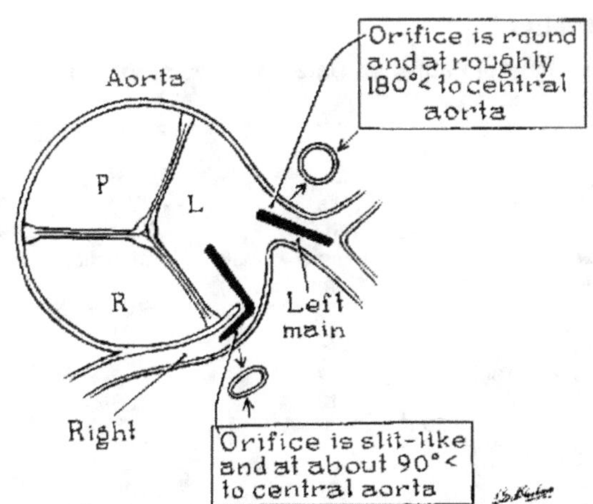

FIGURE 5. Diagram showing origin of the right coronary artery from the left (L) sinus (**lower**) compared to its normal origin from the right (R) sinus (**upper**). P = posterior sinus.

Summary of Published Data on 26 Necropsy Patients Whose Right Coronary Artery Arose From the Left Sinus of Valsalva

Case	Year of Report	First Author	Age (yr)	Sex	Symptoms of Cardiac Dysfunction	Significant CA Narrowing	Associated Noncoronary Cardiac Disease	Insignificant CA Narrowing	Noncoronary Cause of Death	Coronary Cause of Death (CA atherosclerosis)
1	1948	White[6]	77	M	0	...	0	...	+	0
2	1956	Alexander[7]	1	F	0	0	0	+	+	0
3			23	F	0	0	+	+	+	0
4			38	M	+	+	0	0	0	+
5			42	M	0	0	0	+	+	0
6			48	F	0	+	0	0	+	0
7	1974	Cheitlin[1]	25	M	...	0	+	+	+	0
8			28	M	...	0	0	+	+	0
9			28	M	...	+	0	0	0	+
10			45	M	...	+	0	0	0	+
11			53	F	...	0	0	+	+	0
12			59	M	...	0	0	+	+	0
13			59	M	...	0	0	+	+	0
14			61	M	...	+	0	0	0	+
15			61	M	...	+	0	0	0	+
16			63	F	...	0	+	+	+	0
17			65	M	...	0	0	+	+	0
18			68	M	...	0	0	+	+	0
19			69	M	...	0	0	+	+	0
20			70	M	...	0	0	+	+	0
21			72	M	...	0	0	+	+	0
22			76	M	...	+	0	0	0	+
23			77	F	...	+	0	0	0	+
24			80	F	...	+	0	0	0	+
25	1979	Liberthson[4]	25	...	0	0	0	+	+	0
26			60	...	+	+	0	0	0	+

CA = coronary artery; ... = not available.

II)[1,4,6,7] failed to reveal a single patient in whom symptoms of cardiac dysfunction or death could be attributed to the anomaly. In contrast, analysis of published data on 31 other patients[1–4,8,9] in whom this congenital coronary anomaly was detected by coronary angiography disclosed that 9 (29 percent) had symptoms of cardiac dysfunction unassociated with significant coronary atherosclerosis or a noncoronary cardiac condition (Table III). Of the nine, two had acute myocardial infarction, five had angina pectoris, one had

syncope and one had nonfatal ventricular fibrillation. Thus, in addition to our three patients whose coronary anomaly was confirmed at necropsy, the data in these nine patients whose anomaly was confirmed by coronary angiography indicate that origin of the right coronary artery from the left sinus of Valsalva can produce symptoms of cardiac dysfunction that may be fatal.

Mechanism of cardiac dysfunction: The mechanism by which origin of the right coronary artery from the left sinus may cause cardiac dysfunction is unclear.

Summary of Published Data on Patients With Angiographic Diagnosis of Origin of the Right Coronary Artery From the Left Sinus

Year of Report	First Author	Pts. With CA Angio (n)	Males (n)	Pts. With Cardiac Dysfunction (n)	Pts. With Significant CA Narrowing (n)	Pts. With CA Narrowing and Cardiac Dysfunction (n)	Pts. With Insignificant CA Narrowing (n)	Pts. With Insignificant CA Narrowing But Cardiac Dysfunction (n)	Type of Cardiac Dysfunction AP	AMI	VF	S
1974	Cheitlin[1]	1	1	1	0	0	1	1	0	1	0	0
1976	Chaitman[2]	7	...	7*	4†	4	3	1	1	0	0	0
1976	Thompson[8]	2	2	2	0	0	2	2	2	0	0	0
1978	Kimbris[3]	12	...	9‡	2	2	10	3	1	0	1	1
1979	Liberthson[4]	8	7	8§	6	6	2	1	1	0	0	0
1980	Benge[9]	1	1	1	0	0	1	1	0	1	0	1
Totals		31	...	28	12	12	19	9	5	2	1	2

* From associated valve disease or ventricular septal defect in two patients. † One also had associated cardiac valve disease or ventricular septal defect. ‡ From associated valve disease in four and from "miscellaneous" causes in three. § From associated valve disease in one.

AMI = acute myocardial infarction; Angio = angiogram; AP = angina pectoris; CA = coronary artery; n = number; Pts. = patients; S = syncope; VF = ventricular fibrillation; ... = not known.

Possibly, the anomalous artery is compressed during its course between the aorta posteriorly and the pulmonary trunk anteriorly in a manner similar to that proposed for the left main coronary artery when it arises from the right sinus of Valsalva and also courses between the two great arteries (Fig. 1). A more likely possibility is diminished flow into the anomalous right coronary artery due to its upright slit-like origin from the aorta and its peculiar orientation to the mid portion of the lumen of the aorta in a manner demonstrated in Figure 5. When both the pulmonary trunk and aorta dilate during exercise, the slit-like ostium surely becomes even more narrowed. The upright nature of the slit-like ostium also prevents blood within the aortic lumen from flowing into the right coronary artery during ventricular diastole without a peculiar direction of flow (Fig. 5).

References

1. **Cheitlin MD, DeCastro CM, McAllister HA.** Sudden death as a complication of anomalous left coronary origin from the anterior sinus of valsalva. A not-so-minor congenital anomaly. Circulation 1974;50:780–7.
2. **Chaitman BR, Lesperance J, Saltiel J, Bourassa MG.** Clinical, angiographic, and hemodynamic findings in patients with anomalous origin of the coronary arteries. Circulation 1976;53:122–31.
3. **Kimbris D, Iskandrian AS, Segal BL, Bemis CE.** Anomalous aortic origin of coronary arteries. Circulation 1978;58:606–15.
4. **Liberthson RR, Dinsmore RE, Fallon JT.** Aberrant coronary artery origin from the aorta. Report of 18 patients, review of literature and delineation of natural history and management. Circulation 1979;59:748–54.
5. **Pedersen DH, Zipes DP, Foster PR, Troup PJ.** Ventricular tachycardia and ventricular fibrillation in a young population. Circulation 1979;60:988–97.
6. **White NK, Edwards JE.** Anomalies of the coronary arteries. Report of four cases. Arch Pathol 1948;45:766–71.
7. **Alexander RW, Griffith GC.** Anomalies of the coronary arteries and their clinical significance. Circulation 1956;14:800–5.
8. **Thompson SI, Vieweg WV, Alport JS, Hagan AD.** Anomalous origin of the right coronary artery from the left sinus of Valsalva with associated chest pain. Report of two cases. Cathet Cardiovasc Diagnosis 1976;2:397–402.
9. **Benge W, Martins JB, Funk DC.** Morbidity associated with anomalous origin of the right coronary artery from the left sinus of Valsalva. Am Heart J 1980;99:96–100.

Separate aortic ostium of the left anterior descending and left circumflex coronary arteries from the left aortic sinus of Valsalva (absent left main coronary artery)

Barry S. Dicicco, M.D.,
Bruce M. McManus, M.D., Ph.D.,
Bruce F. Waller, M.D., and
William C. Roberts, M.D. *Bethesda, Md.*

Ordinarily, of course, only one coronary artery arises from the left sinus of Valsalva and that is the left main (LM) coronary artery. On rare occasion, the LM coronary artery is absent and both left anterior descending (LAD) and left circumflex (LC) coronary arteries arise independently, each from a separate ostium in the left sinus of Valsalva (Figs. 1 to 3). Schlesinger et al.[1] found a separate ostium for both LAD and LC coronary arteries in the left aortic sinus in 2 (0.2%) of 1000 consecutive necropsies, and Zumbo et al.[2] observed coronary arterial anomalies in 33 of 2089 necropsied patients, 21 (1%) of whom had a separate

From the Pathology Branch, National Heart, Lung and Blood Institute, National Institutes of Health.

Received for publication March 11, 1982; accepted March 19, 1982.

Reprint requests: William C. Roberts, M.D., Pathology Branch, NHLBI-NIH, Bldg. 10A, Room 3E-30, Bethesda, MD 20205.

aortic ostium of the LAD and LC coronary arteries. During the past 3 years, we have studied at necropsy four patients (three men) aged 61 to 74 years (mean 67) in whom the LAD and LC arose separately in the left aortic sinus; three died from consequences of coronary atherosclerosis and one from a noncardiac cause.

We call attention to this anomaly because its nonrecognition at angiography or operation could potentially lead to serious consequences. If at coronary angiography contrast material is injected into only one or the other of the two arteries arising from the left aortic sinus, the noninjected artery might mistakenly be interpreted as being totally occluded at its origin from the LM coronary artery. If either the LAD or LC coronary arteries are not visualized by selective injection of contrast material, injection into the sinuses of Valsalva may prevent confusing an anomalously arising coronary artery with a totally occluded coronary artery. If either ostium is not perfused at the time of cardiopulmonary bypass, a portion of left ventricular myocardium might not be adequately oxygenated, as observed in a patient described by Ogden.[3] A theoretical advantage of a separate ostium of both the LAD and LC coronary arteries from the left aortic sinus is the inability to have complications resulting from narrowing of the LM coronary artery. Two of our four patients with separate origin of the LAD and LC coronary arteries, however, had severe (> 75% cross-sectional area) narrowing of both LAD and LC coronary arteries proximal to any major branches and therefore had so-called "LM equiva-

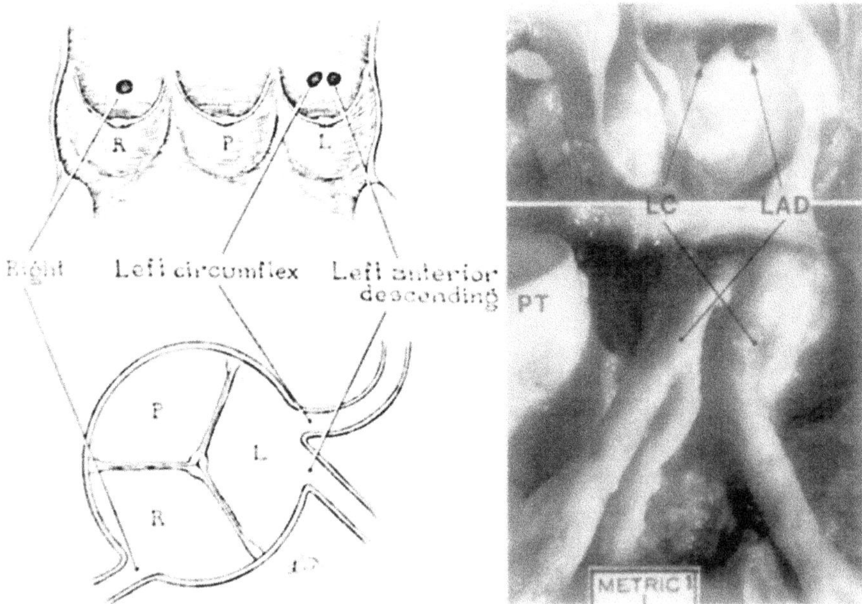

Fig. 1. Drawing *(left)* of aorta showing origin of each of the left circumflex *(LC)* and left anterior descending *(LAD)* coronary arteries from a separate ostium in the left sinus of Valsalva. *Right upper,* Interior of left sinus showing each ostium (SH No. A81-49). *Lower right,* Exterior view showing both LC and LAD coronary arteries arising separately. *PT* = pulmonary trunk. (Photo by M.M.M. Moore.)

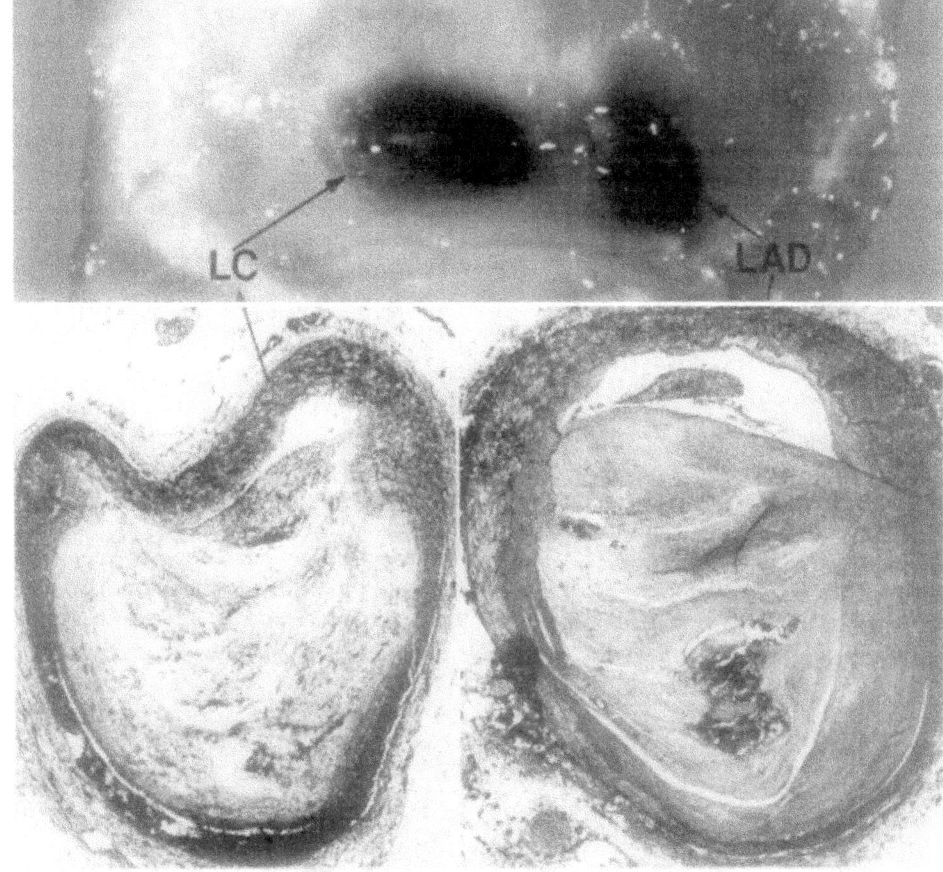

Fig. 2. *Upper,* Portion of aorta behind left sinus showing a separate ostium for each of the left circumflex *(LC)* and left anterior descending (LAD) coronary arteries in 63-year-old woman (GT No. 81A-209). (Photo by M.M.M. Moore.) *Lower left,* Cross-section of LAD coronary artery in its first 5 mm segment. *Lower right,* Cross-section of LC coronary artery in its first 5 mm segment. Both the LAD and LC are considerably narrowed proximally (left main equivalent). (Movat stains; each original magnification ×14.)

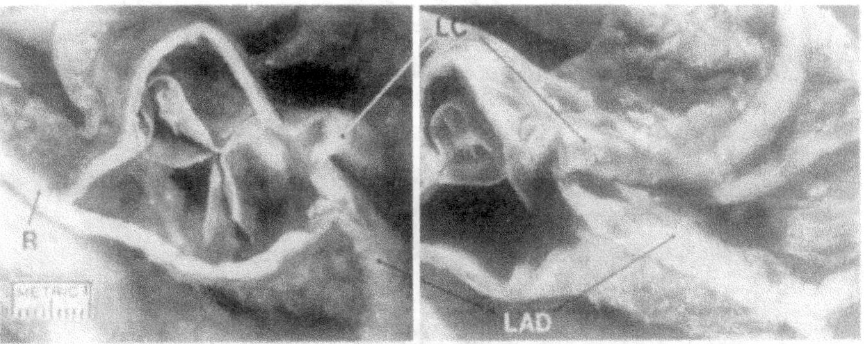

Fig. 3. Aortic valve from above showing separate origins of the right *(R)*, left anterior descending *(LAD)*, and left circumflex *(LC)* coronary arteries from the aorta in a 74-year-old man (GT No. 79A-74). (Photo by M.M.M. Moore.)

lent" narrowing (Fig. 2). This coronary anomaly does not appear to accelerate atherosclerosis in either of the separately arising coronary arteries.[2]

REFERENCES

1. Schlesinger MJ, Zoll PM, Wessler S: The conus artery: A third coronary artery. AM HEART J **38**:823, 1949.
2. Zumbo O, Fani K, Jarmdyeh J, Daoud AS: Coronary atherosclerosis and myocardial infarction in hearts with anomalous coronary arteries. Laboratory Investigation **14**:571, 1965.
3. Ogden JA: Anomalous aortic origin: Circumflex, anterior descending or main left coronary arteries. Arch Pathol **88**:323, 1969.

Origin of the left main from the right coronary artery or from the right aortic sinus with intramyocardial tunneling to the left side of the heart via the ventricular septum: The case against clinical significance of myocardial bridge or coronary tunnel

William C. Roberts, M.D., Barry S. Dicicco, M.D.,
Bruce F. Waller, M.D., Joan C. Kishel, M.D.,
Bruce M. McManus, M.D., Ph.D.,
Stuart L. Dawson, M.D., John C. Hunsaker, III, M.D.,
and James L. Luke, M.D. *Bethesda, Md., and
Washington, D.C.*

From the Pathology Branch, National Heart, Lung and Blood Institute, National Institutes of Health; and the Medical Examiner's Office, Washington, D.C.

Received for publication Apr. 15, 1982; accepted Apr. 19, 1982.

Reprint requests: William C. Roberts, M.D., Pathology Branch, NIH-NHLBI, Bldg. 10A, Room 3E-30, Bethesda, MD 20205.

Recently we studied the hearts of two patients who died from consequences of knife or bullet wounds. Although during life neither ever had clinical evidence of cardiac dysfunction, at necropsy both had origin of the left main (LM) coronary artery from either the right (R) coronary artery or directly from the right anterior sinus of Valsalva with intramyocardial coursing within the ventricular septum to the left side of the heart. The course within the septum was 5.0 cm in the 34-year-old man (Fig. 1) and 4.5 cm in the 48-year-old man (Fig. 2). In each patient, the LM exited from the ventricular septum anteriorly and immediately branched into the left anterior descending (LAD) and left circumflex (LC) coronary arteries which thereafter followed their usual courses. The walls of the tunneled LM in each patient were thinner than that of the R, LAD, or LC coronary arteries. The course of the R coronary artery was normal. The myocardium was normal. The major coronary arteries in both patients were free of atherosclerotic plaques.

Review of previous published reports on patients with origin of the LM from the R coronary artery or from the right anterior aortic sinus disclosed at least 11 necropsy

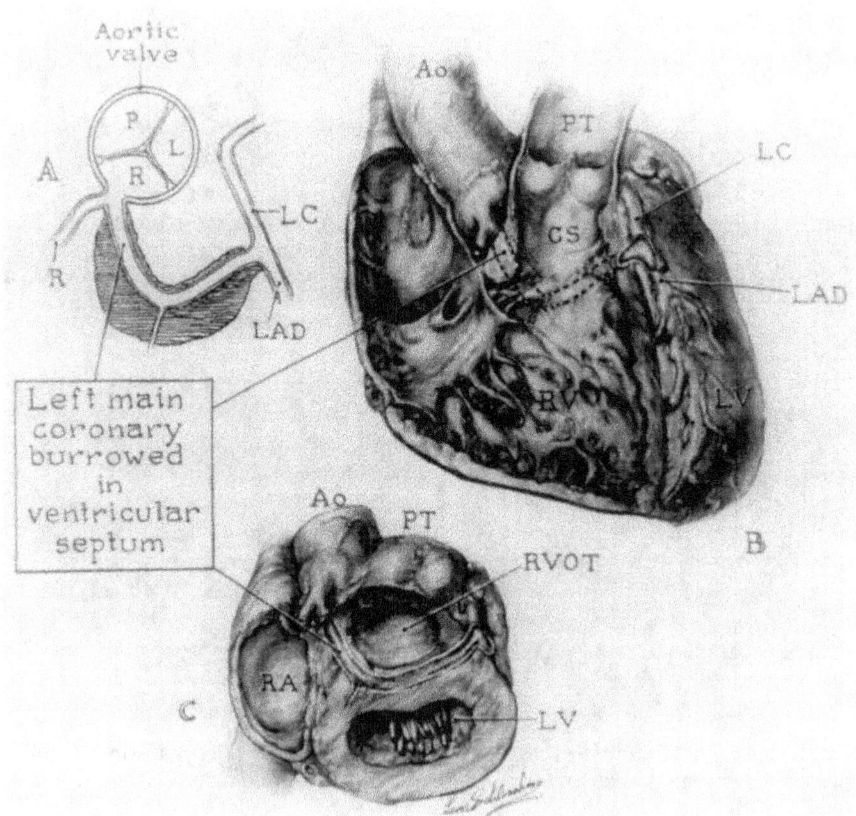

Fig. 1. Drawing of the heart in our 34-year-old man (DCMEO No. 81-09-750). The left main (LM) coronary artery coursed within the ventricular septum beneath the right ventricular outflow tract before branching above the septum into the left anterior descending *(LAD)* and left circumflex *(LC)* coronary arteries. *Ao* = aorta; *CS* = crista supraventricularis; *LV* = left ventricle; *RA* = right atrium; *PT* = pulmonary trunk; *RV* = right ventricle.

"

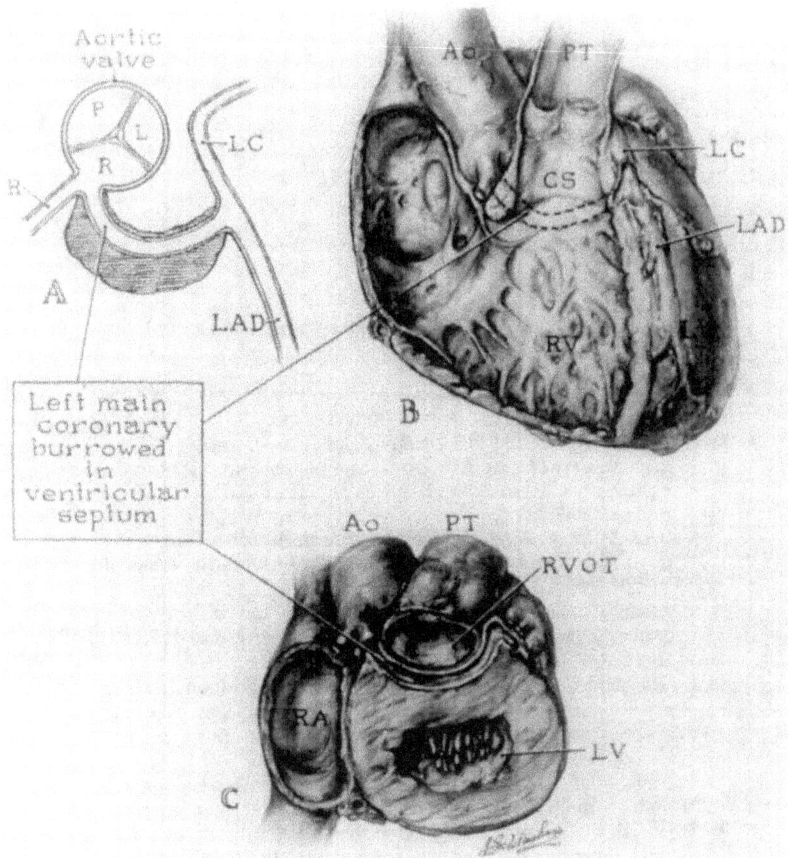

Fig. 2. Drawing of the heart in our 48-year-old man (DCMEO No. 82-03-291). Abbreviations as in Fig. 1.

patients (aged 28 to 87 years [mean = 55]; eight males and three females) in whom the LM arose either from the R coronary artery or directly from the right anterior aortic sinus and thereafter coursed within the ventricular septum to emerge in the epicardium above the anterior portion of septum.[1-7] Of these 11 previously reported necrospy patients, five died from noncardiac conditions and never had evidence of cardiac dysfunction during life; three died from coronary atherosclerotic heart disease[4,6,7]; one died from valvular heart disease[1]; and one died from amyloid heart disease.[5] In the remaining patient (case No. 9 of Cheitlin et al.[7]), a 36-year-old man with repeated episodes of ventricular tachycardia and finally fatal cardiac arrest, it is likely that the coronary anomaly in some way was responsible for the ventricular arrhythmia and sudden death. Although it is of course hazardous to attribute functional importance to a coronary anomaly when only 1 of 11 reported patients appears to have had a fatal or nonfatal cardiac problem not explainable by another cardiac condition, the anomaly in this one patient suggests that this coronary anomaly may occasionally be of clinical importance. We found no reports of this anomaly being diagnosed by coronary angiography during life.[8] In three additional reported necropsy patients (aged 4, 39, and 60 years; two males), the LAD arose from the R coronary artery or right sinus of Valsalva and thereafter

coursed similarly in the ventricular septum; the LC arose from the R coronary artery and coursed behind the aorta before reaching the left atrioventricular sulcus.[9-11] None of these three patients ever had evidence of cardiac dysfunction.

Although angina pectoris[12] and sudden death[13] have been attributed to tunneling of one (LAD) of the four major coronary arteries, the absence of evidences of myocardial ischemia both clinically and at necropsy in our two patients and in 10 of 11 previously reported patients suggests that tunneling is an unlikely cause of myocardial ischemia. In each of our two patients the tunneled LM was over 4 cm in length. When only the LAD is tunneled, the tunneled segment is usually less than 3 cm in length and, of course, only one artery is affected in this circumstance rather than two which is the situation when the LM is tunneled. Tunneling of a major coronary artery within myocardium protects the intramyocardial segment from atherosclerotic plaques.

REFERENCES

1. Gallavardin L, Ravault P: Anomalie d'origine de la coronaire anterieure. Lyon Med **136**:270, 1925.
2. Kintner AR: Anomalous origin and course of the left coronary artery. Arch Pathol **12**:586, 1931.
3. Born E: Uber Missbildungen der Kranzarterien und ihre

Beziehungen zu Zirkulationsstorungen und plotzlichem Tod. Virchows Arch Pathol Anat **290**:688, 1933.

4. Roberts JT, Loube SD: Congenital single coronary artery in man. Report of nine new cases, one having thrombosis with right ventricular and atrial (auricular) infarction. AM HEART J **34**:188, 1947.

5. Snow PJD: A case of single coronary artery with stereographic demonstration of the arterial distribution. Br Heart J **15**:261, 1953.

6. Allen GL, Snider TH: Myocardial infarction with a single coronary artery. Report of a case. Arch Intern Med **117**:261, 1966.

7. Cheitlin MD, De Castro CM, McAllister HA: Sudden death as a complication of anomalous left coronary origin from the anterior sinus of Valsalva. A not-so-minor congenital anomaly. Circulation **50**:780, 1974.

8. Moodie DS, Gill C, Loop FD, Sheldon WC: Anomalous left main coronary artery originating from the right sinus of Valsalva. Pathophysiology, angiographic definition, and surgical approaches. J Thorac Cardiovasc Surg **80**:198, 1980.

9. Bochdalek J: Anomaler Verlauf der Kranzartenen des Herzens. Virchows Arch Pathol Anat **41**:260, 1967.

10. Sanes S: Anomalous origin and course of the left coronary artery in a child. So-called congenital absence of the left coronary artery. AM HEART J **14**:219, 1937.

11. White NK, Edwards JE: Anomalies of the coronary arteries. Report of four cases. Arch Pathol **45**:766, 1948.

12. Rossi L, Dander B, Nidasio GP, Arbustini E, Paris B, Vassanelli C, Buonanno C, Poppi A: Myocardial bridges and ischemic heart disease. Eur Heart J **1**:239, 1980.

13. Morales AR, Romanelli R, Boucek RJ: The mural left anterior descending coronary artery, strenuous exercise and sudden death. Circulation **62**:230, 1980.

Fatal atherosclerotic narrowing of the *right main* coronary artery: Origin of the left anterior descending or left circumflex coronary artery from the right (the true "left-main equivalent")

William C. Roberts, M.D., Bruce F. Waller, M.D., and Charles S. Roberts. *Bethesda, Md.*

Normally the two coronary arteries arise from the aorta: one, the right (R), arises from its right or anterior side and continues as a single artery; and the second, the left main

From the Pathology Branch, National Heart, Lung and Blood Institute, National Institutes of Health.

Received for publication Apr. 16, 1982; accepted May 15, 1982.

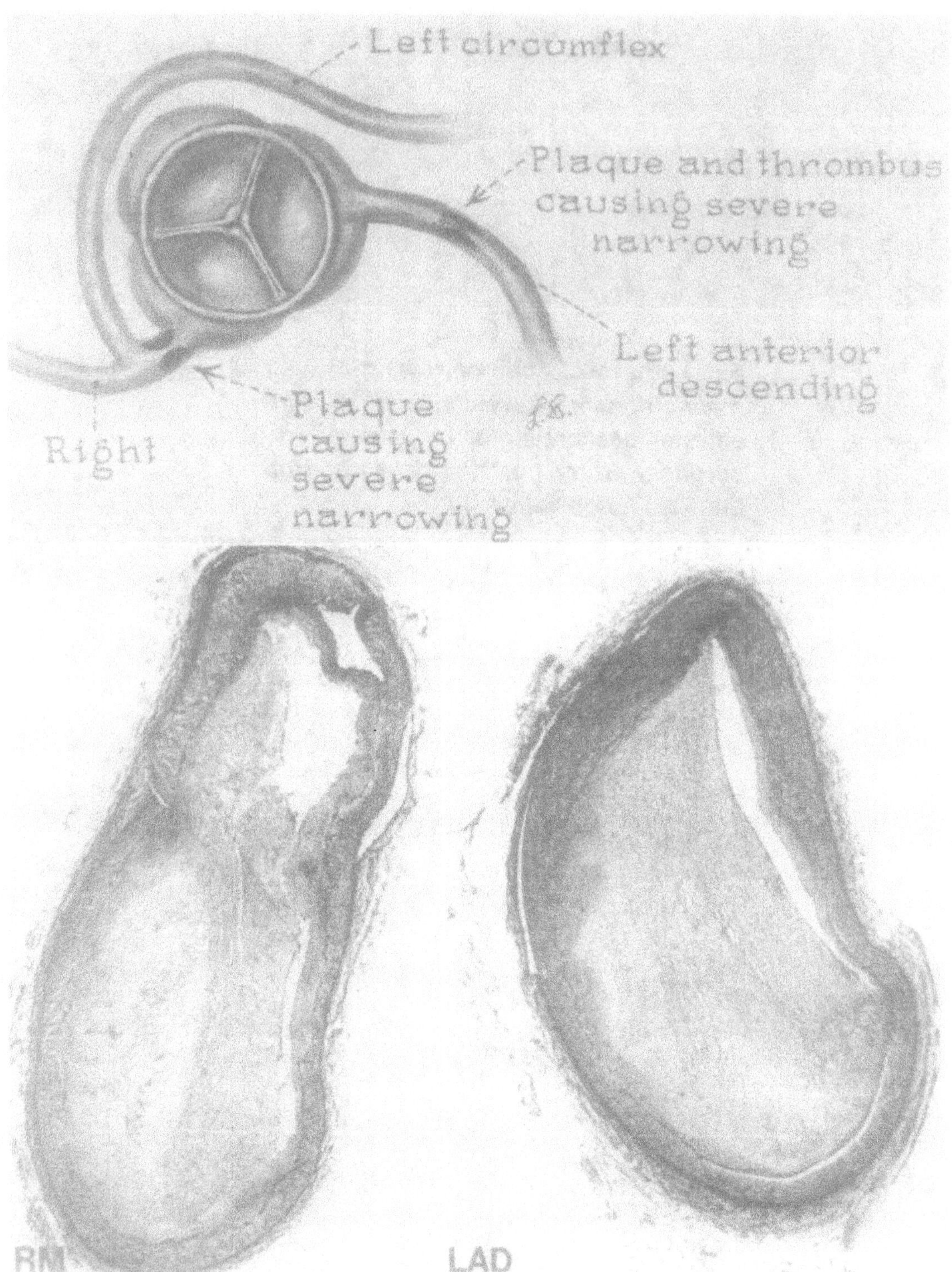

Fig. 1. Drawing *(upper)* of coronary arteries arising from the aorta in the 35-year-old man (WHC No. 79-88). *RM*, Cross section of right main *(RM)* artery before it bifurcates into the left circumflex and right coronary arteries. *LAD*, Cross-section of the left anterior descending *(LAD)* artery in its first 2 cm. Both the RM and LAD are severely narrowed by atherosclerotic plaque. (Movat stains; each original magnification ×25.)

(LM), arises from its left or posterior side and subdivides into two arteries, the left anterior descending (LAD) and the left circumflex (LC) coronary arteries. Severe narrowing of the LM may lead to inadequate oxygenation of left ventricular (LV) myocardium perfused by the LAD and LC. Rarely, the main coronary artery which subdivides into two major branches arises from the right side of the aorta (right main [RM]) rather than from the left side, and when this circumstance exists the main trunk (RM) subdivides either into the R and LC or into the R and

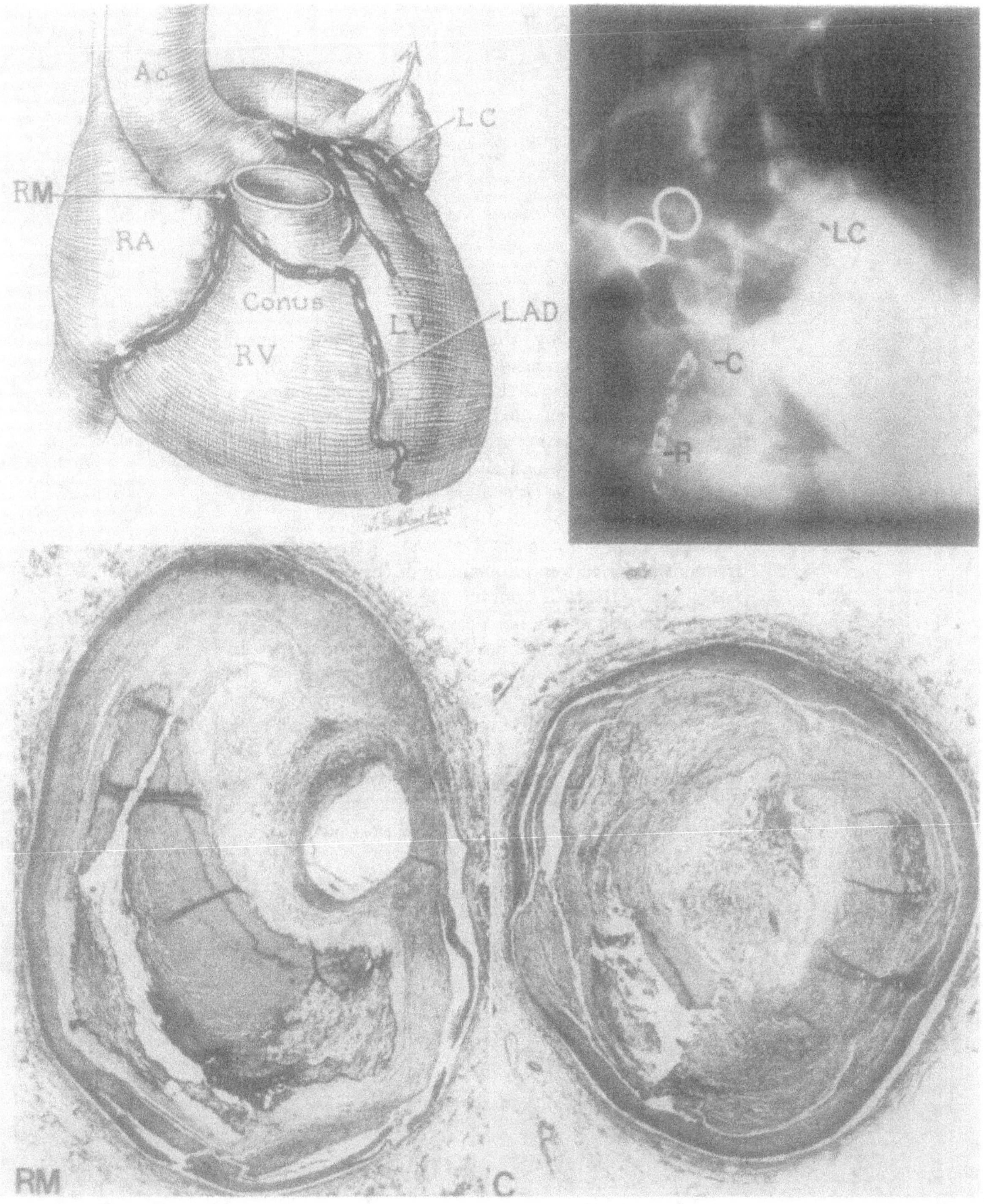

Fig. 2. Coronary arterial pattern in the 60-year-old man (NIH No. A81-63). *RM* = right main; *LAD* = left anterior descending; *LC* = left circumflex coronary arteries. *Upper right*, Radiograph of heart at necropsy showing heavy calcific deposits in the coronary arteries. *RM*, Cross section of RM coronary artery. *C*, Cross section of conus artery in its first 2 cm. Both major coronary arteries are severely narrowed by atherosclerotic plaque. (Movat stains; each original magnification ×23.)

LAD (conus branch). Severe narrowing of the RM in this circumstance is equivalent to severe narrowing of the LM but the LV myocardium deprived or potentially deprived of adequate oxygenation would be that supplied by the R and LC or the R and LAD, not that supplied by the LAD and LC.

Recently, we studied at necropsy the hearts of two patients with fatal atherosclerotic coronary heart disease in whom the main or subdividing coronary artery arose from the right side of the aorta, rather than from the left side, yielding a RM rather than an LM coronary artery. In one patient, a 35-year-old man who died suddenly 42 days after an acute myocardial infarction, the LC and R arose from the RM and the RM was severely narrowed by an atherosclerotic plaque (Fig. 1). In the second patient, a 60-year-old man who died shortly after aortocoronary bypass grafting for severe angina pectoris, the LAD and R arose from the RM which also was severely narrowed by atherosclerotic plaque (Fig. 2), as were all major coronary arteries.

Origin of the LC from the R coronary artery is the most frequent major congenital anomaly of the coronary arteries. Origin of the LAD from the RM, however, is extremely rare. Reports of five necropsy patients with this type anomaly appear only in a thesis[1] and, to our knowledge, in no published reports. Severe narrowing by atherosclerotic plaque of the RM coronary artery—the true equivalent of severe narrowing of the LM coronary artery—has not been reported previously, and indeed the concept of a RM coronary artery, except possibly in the congenital condition, corrected transposition of the great arteries (l-transposition), has not been presented previously.

REFERENCE

1. Ogden JA: Congenital variations of the coronary arteries. A clinicopathologic survey. M.D. Thesis, New Haven, Yale University School of Medicine, 1968, pp 1-384.

Anomalous Origin of the Left Anterior Descending Coronary Artery from the Pulmonary Trunk with Origin of the Right and Left Circumflex Coronary Arteries from the Aorta

WILLIAM C. ROBERTS, MD
MAX ROBINOWITZ, MD

Origin of both right and left main (LM) coronary arteries from the pulmonary trunk (PT) rarely allows survival for more than 2 weeks after birth. Origin of the LM from the PT with origin of the right coronary artery from the aorta allows longer survival, but usually (80%) for no more than 1 year after birth. Origin of the right coronary artery from the PT and the LM from the aorta, in contrast, allows survival into adulthood and maybe a normal life span. Because the LM is equivalent to 2 major coronary arteries, whenever the LM arises from the PT, whether in association with the right artery or when isolated, survival is short. However, when 1 major branch of the LM arises from the PT and both the right and the other major LM branch arises from the aorta, the survival rate should be similar to that in patients in whom the right coronary artery arises from the PT and the LM from the aorta. In this report we describe a man in whom the left anterior descending coronary artery (LAD) arose from the PT and the right and left circumflex (LC) coronary arteries from the aorta.

T.J., a 32-year-old man, died suddenly soon after jogging on December 29, 1981. In November 1979 a continuous murmur "similar to that of a patent ductus arteriosus" had been heard during routine physical examination. He was and always had been asymptomatic. The murmur was grade 3/6 in intensity, and loudest in the third left intercostal space. The systemic blood pressure was 120/50 mm Hg. The electrocardiogram was normal. Chest radiograph showed the cardiac silhouette to be at the upper limits of normal. On the M-mode echocardiogram, the left ventricular cavity in end-diastole was 65 mm and the left atrium was 40 mm. Coronary angiography disclosed the origin of the right artery from the right sinus and the origin of only the LC from the left sinus of Valsalva. Both the right coronary artery and LC communicated through collateral vessels with the LAD, which arose from the PT; it was dilated and tortuous. The ejection fraction on the left ventricular angiogram was 48%. The pulmonary to systemic flow ratio was 1.6:1.

On March 9, 1981, thoracotomy was performed for the purpose of ligating the LAD close to its origin from the PT and insertion of saphenous vein graft from aorta to the more distal portion of the LAD. At operation, rather than ligating the LAD, the proximal LC was ligated instead (Fig. 1). On the second postoperative day, the continuous precordial murmur was still audible and repeat angiography disclosed that both the LAD and the graft were widely patent. Reoperation was performed on March 12, 1981, and this time the LAD near the PT was ligated (Fig. 1).

From the Pathology Branch, National Heart, Lung, and Blood Institute, National Institutes of Health, Bethesda, Maryland, and the Cardiovascular Pathology Department, Armed Forces Institute of Pathology, Washington, DC. Manuscript received and accepted July 24, 1984.

Reevaluation in May 1981 disclosed mild exertional dyspnea postoperatively, but never chest pain. The patient was working full days as a dentist. The blood pressure was 130/85 mm Hg. No precordial murmurs were present. Electrocardiography disclosed Q waves in leads I and aVL and inverted T waves in lead aVL. The Bruce treadmill test to 10 minutes disclosed a heart rate of 175 beats/min, blood pressure 155/75 mm Hg, no symptoms and no ischemic electrocardiographic changes. No symptoms occurred thereafter and he began running 2 miles daily and playing tennis. On December 29, 1981, he complained of dyspnea shortly after a run and died.

Necropsy disclosed the heart weight at 450 g. The proximal LAD was occluded by a thrombus and ligature and the graft was patent (Fig. 1). A transmural scar involved the lateral wall of the left ventricle and ventricular septum at the base and both papillary muscles were focally scarred (Fig. 2).

At least 7 patients (Table I) have been reported in whom the LAD arose from the PT and both right and LC arteries arose from the aorta.[1–6] At the time of the reports 1 patient (patient 1, Table I), a 7-month old girl, had died of an anterior wall acute myocardial infarct; the other 6 (patients 2 to 7, all women) were aged 18 to 55 years (mean 34). Our patient is the only male thus far described. Of the 6 adults, all were symptomatic: 5 with angina pectoris, 1 of whom also had an anterior wall acute myocardial infarct, and 1 with severe fatigue at-

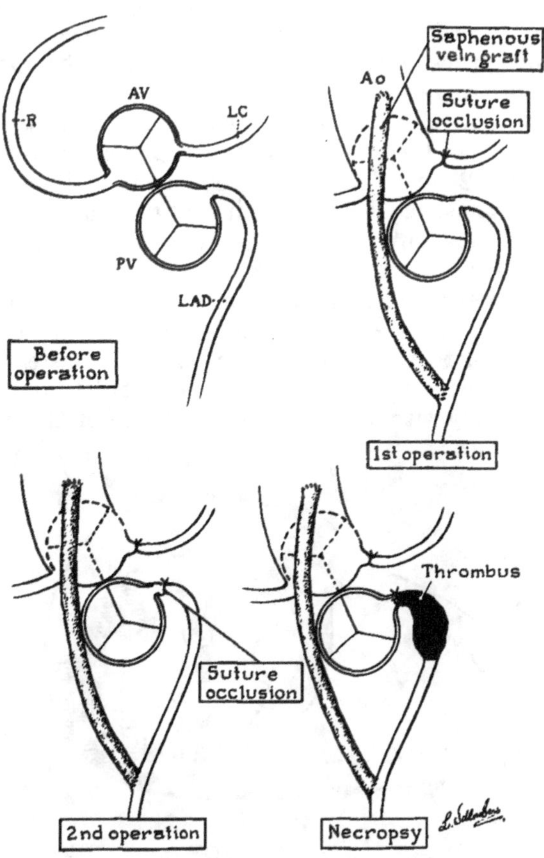

FIGURE 1. Sequence of development before, during and after operation in the patient described. Ao = aorta; AV = aortic valve; PV = pulmonic valve; LAD, LC and R = left anterior descending, left circumflex and right coronary arteries.

TABLE I Certain Observations in 7 Previously Reported Patients (Patients 1 to 7) and in Our Patient (no. 8) in Whom the Left Anterior Descending Coronary Artery Arose from the Pulmonary Trunk

Pt	First Author	Year	Age (yr) & Sex	Age (yr) Onset Symptoms	First Symptom	AMI	Precordial Murmur		Anterior Wall Ischemia (ECG)	CE by X-Ray	CA A	Ligation LAD	Conduit Aorta to LAD	Alive (mo PO)
							Systole	Diastole						
1	Schwartz[1]	1971	7 moF	—	—	0	0	0	+	+	+	0	0	—
2	Probst[2]	1976	35F	18	AP	0	+	+	+	0	+	0	0	+
3	Baltaxe[3]	1977	18F	18	Fatigue	—	+	0	—	+	+	—	—	—
4	Donaldson[4]	1979	24F	24	AP	0	+	0	+	0	+	+	0	+ (12)
5	Donaldson[4]	1979	26F	—	AP	—	—	—	—	—	+	+	0	—
6	Singh[5]	1983	45F	36	AP	0	+	0	+	+	+	+	+	+ (24)
7	Evans[6]	1984	55F	37	AP	+	0	0	+	+	+	+	+	+ (5)
8	Roberts	1984	32M	—	0	0	+	+	0	0	+	+	+	0

A = angiogram; AMI = acute myocardial infarction; AP = angina pectoris; CA = coronary artery; CE = cardiac enlargement; ECG = electrocardiogram; LAD = left anterior descending; PO = postoperatively; + = positive, present or done; 0 = negative or absent; — = no information available or not done or not applicable.

tributed to severe mitral regurgitation from papillary muscle dysfunction. The angina at some time in all 5 patients was stable, but 3 of the 5 (patients 4, 6 and 7) had unstable angina just before cardiac operation. The age at onset of symptoms of myocardial ischemia in the 6 adults ranged from 18 to 37 years (mean 27). Precordial murmurs were described in 4 of 5 previously reported adults. (No information was provided in the "addendum case" of Donaldson et al.[4]): The murmur apparently was present only in systole in 4 patients, and also in diastole in 1. The intensity of the murmurs was mentioned in 2 patients: "soft" in 1 (patient 4) and grade 2/6 in 1 (patient 6). Findings on the electrocardiogram at rest were described in 4 adults: All had poor R-wave progression in leads V_1 to V_3 and at least 2 (patients 6 and 7) had ST–T-wave changes of ischemia in more than 1 lead. Exercise stress tests in 2 patients (patients 2 and 7) disclosed ST-segment ischemic changes in each. Chest x-rays in 5 of the 6 adults disclosed normal-sized cardiac silhouettes in 2 and cardiac enlargement in 3: mild in 2 (patients 4 and 6) and severe in 1 (patient 3). Right-sided cardiac catheterization, performed in at least 5 patients (patients 2 and 4 to 7) disclosed normal pressures in each and oxygen step-up in the pulmonary trunk in only 1 (patient 6). Coronary angiography with injection of contrast material in the right coronary artery and LC in all 6 adults disclosed that each of these 2 arteries in all 6 patients was large, occasionally also tortuous, and that the LAD was filled with extensive collateral vessels from both the right coronary artery and LC. Injection of contrast material into the PT did not cause filling of the LAD; when the LAD, however, was filled by injections into either the right coronary artery or LC, contrast material did enter the PT through the LAD, which was filled by collateral vessels.

Of the 6 previously reported adults, operative treatment was carried out in 4, all of whom preoperatively had angina: In 2 patients (patients 4 and 5) the PT was opened and the ostium of the LAD was obliterated by sutures, and in 2 (patients 6 and 7) the LAD was ligated just proximal to its entrance into the PT and a reversed saphenous vein was inserted from the ascending aorta to the LAD. Of the 4 patients who had operative treatment, angina disappeared in 3 (patients 4 to 6) and persisted in 1 (patient 7). Patients 6 and 7 had repeat coronary and left ventricular angiography 24 and 36 months, respectively, after operation; in each, the right and LC arteries were much smaller than they had been preoperatively and the collateral vessels between the right coronary artery and LC and the LAD had disappeared; patient 7 had persistent angina postoperatively and the distal portions of both the right coronary artery and LC (36 months postoperatively) were quite narrowed; the cause of narrowing was unclear. Left ventricular angiograms, performed in 4 adults, were normal in 2 (patients 2 and 4), and in the other 2 the apical portion of the left ventricle was akinetic in 1 (patient 6) and aneurysmal in 1 (patient 7). Repeat left ventricular angiography in these latter 2 patients disclosed better overall contractions in 1 and no change in 1 (patient 7).

The presence of both subjective and objective evidence of myocardial ischemia in the 6 previously reported adults and the disappearance of angina and of the collateral vessels between the 2 coronary arteries arising from the aorta and the LAD arising from the PT supports the view that operative treatment is proper for patients with this coronary anomaly. Whether LAD ligation alone is enough or whether ligation plus insertion

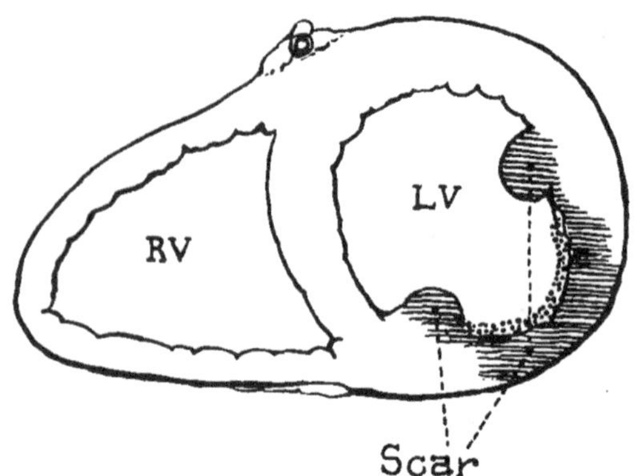

FIGURE 2. Transverse section of cardiac ventricles at level of left ventricular papillary muscles showing transmural left ventricular scar. LV = left ventricle; RV = right ventricle.

of a graft between the aorta and LAD is preferable is unclear. Direct connection of the LAD to aorta in this situation appears technically inadvisable. All 4 patients reported in whom operation was performed had angina pectoris. Our patient was asymptomatic preoperatively. Obviously, no data are available on the advisibility of operation in an asymptomatic person in whom the LAD arises from the PT, but it appears reasonable to believe that the operative therapy in this circumstance is proper. If operation is to be performed, however, clear identification of the anomalous artery before ligation is mandatory.

References

1. **Schwartz RP, Robicsek F.** An unusual anomaly of the coronary system: origin of the anterior (descending) interventricular artery from the pulmonary trunk. J Pediatr 1971;78:123–126.
2. **Probst P, Pachinger O, Koller H, Niederberger M, Kaindl F.** Origin of anterior descending branch of left coronary artery from pulmonary trunk. Br Heart J 1976;38:523–525.
3. **Baltaxe HA, Wixson D.** The incidence of congenital anomalies of the coronary arteries in the adult population. Radiology 1977;122:47–52.
4. **Donaldson RM, Thornton A, Raphael MJ, Sturridge MF, Manuel RW.** Anomalous origin of the left anterior descending coronary artery from the pulmonary artery. Eur J Cardiol 1979;10:295–300.
5. **Singh RN, Taylor PC.** Anomalous origin of the left anterior descending coronary artery from the pulmonary artery: surgical correction in an adult. Cathet Cardiovasc Diagn 1983;9:411–416.
6. **Evans JJ, Phillips JF.** Origin of the left anterior descending coronary artery from the pulmonary artery. Three year angiographic follow-up after saphenous vein bypass graft and proximal ligation. JACC 1984;3:219–224.

Origin of the Right from the Left Main Coronary Artery (Single Coronary Ostium in Aorta)

DEBORAH J. BARBOUR, MD
WILLIAM C. ROBERTS, MD

Origin of both the right and left main (LM) coronary arteries from the aortic wall of the *right* sinus of Valsalva frequently is a lethal anomaly.[1] Origin of both the right and LM coronary arteries from the aortic wall of the *left* sinus of Valsalva, in contrast, usually is a benign anomaly.[2] Although many studies have described origin of both LM and right coronary arteries from the aortic wall of the same sinus of Valsalva, few[1,2] have described origin of the right coronary artery from the LM. Husaini et al[3] described angiographic features of this anomaly in a 52-year-old man who underwent selective coronary angiography after probable acute myocardial infarction. Muus and McManus[4] described this anomaly in a full-term stillborn infant who also had a bicuspid aortic valve. Whether the coronary anomaly played a role in the stillbirth is uncertain. In both of these previously described patients, the anomalously arising right coronary artery coursed between aorta posteriorly and the pulmonary trunk anteriorly.

J.G., a 65-year-old man, never had signs or symptoms of cardiac dysfunction. He did have systemic hypertension and electrocardiographic voltage criteria consistent with left ventricular hypertrophy. He died from carcinoma of the lung. At necropsy, the heart weighed 380 g. The cardiac cavities were of normal size. No foci of myocardial fibrosis or necrosis were present. The origin and courses of the coronary arteries are shown in Figure 1. The anomalous right coronary artery was much smaller than either the left circumflex or left anterior descending branches; it burrowed into the myocardium of the crista supraventricularis for about 2 cm of its length

From The Pathology Branch, National Heart, Lung, and Blood Institute, National Institutes of Health, Bethesda, Maryland 20205. Manuscript received and accepted November 7, 1984.

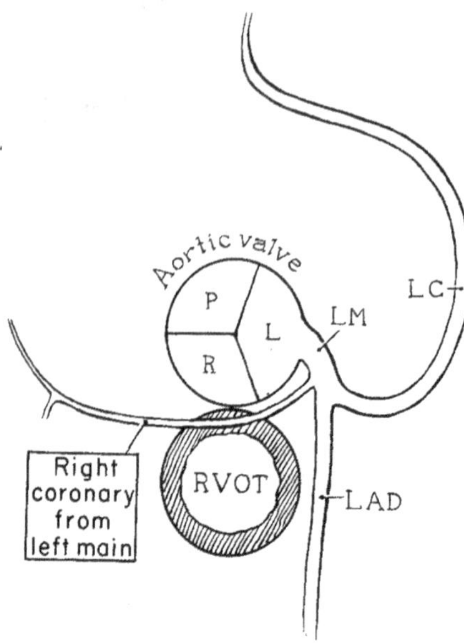

FIGURE 1. Course of the right coronary artery after its anomalous origin from the left main (LM) coronary artery. It burrowed into the myocardium of the crista supraventricularis for 2 cm shortly after its origin. The entire right coronary artery is small and it virtually disappeared after reaching the right margin of the heart. L = left sinus of Valsalva; LAD = left anterior descending coronary artery; LC = left circumflex coronary artery; P = posterior sinus of Valsalva; R = right sinus of Valsalva; RVOT = right ventricular outflow tract.

shortly after its origin from the LM. All epicardial coronary arteries were free of atherosclerotic plaque.

This case demonstrates that origin of the right coronary artery from the LM may be a benign anomaly unassociated with either functional or anatomic evidence of myocardial ischemia.

References

1. **Cheitlin MD, DeCastro CM, McAllister HA.** Sudden death as a complication of anomalous left coronary origin from the anterior sinus of Valsalva. A not-so-minor congenital anomaly. Circulation 1974;50:780–787.
2. **Roberts WC, Siegel RJ, Zipes DP.** Origin of the right coronary artery from the left sinus of Valsalva and its functional consequences: analysis of 10 necropsy patients. Am J Cardiol 1982;49:863–868.
3. **Husaini SN, Beaver WL, Wilson IJ, Lach RD.** Anomalous right coronary artery arising from left mainstem. Cathet Cardiovasc Diagn 1983;9:407–409.
4. **Muus CJ, McManus BM.** Common origin of right and left coronary arteries from the region of left sinus of Valslava: association with unexpected intra-uterine fetal death. Am Heart J 1984;107:1285–1286.

Left Main Coronary Artery Originating From the Right Sinus of Valsalva and Coursing Between the Aorta and Pulmonary Trunk

CHARLES W. BARTH III, MD, WILLIAM C. ROBERTS, MD, FACC

Bethesda, Maryland

Findings are described in five patients who at necropsy were found to have origin of the left main coronary artery from the right sinus of Valsalva and coursing of the anomalously arising artery between aorta and pulmonary trunk to reach the left side of the heart. Three of the five patients were boys and died suddenly at ages 13, 14 and 19 years, respectively: two of them had had one or more episodes of syncope and the third had an abnormal electrocardiogram. The fourth patient, a 64 year old woman, died of chronic congestive heart failure 1 year after an acute myocardial infarction. She had insignificant coronary atherosclerosis. The fifth patient, an 81 year old man, died of chronic alcoholism, having been free of symptoms of cardiac dysfunction during life.

Additionally, clinical and necropsy findings are summarized in 38 previously reported necropsy patients with the coronary anomaly. Of these 38 (34 male [89%]), 23 (61%) died suddenly in the first two decades of life; death in 6 others (16%) appears to have been related to coronary atherosclerosis and 9 patients (24%) died from noncoronary causes. Thus, this anomaly is life-threatening. Why it frequently causes fatal cardiac arrest in some young individuals and allows a normal life span in others remains unclear.

(*J Am Coll Cardiol 1986;7:366–73*)

Although once considered a "minor" coronary anomaly, anomalous origin of the left main coronary artery from the right sinus of Valsalva is now well recognized to cause fatal or nonfatal myocardial ischemia when the left main artery courses between the aorta and pulmonary trunk to reach the left side of the heart (1,2). Symptoms of myocardial ischemia from this anomaly usually develop before the age of 20 years. This report describes findings in 5 patients in whom this anomaly was observed at necropsy and it summarizes observations in 38 previously reported necropsy patients.

Patients Studied

Clinical features. Pertinent findings in the five patients are summarized in Table 1. Three were teenagers and each died suddenly: Patient 1, shortly after running home from school, Patient 2, shortly after mowing the lawn and Patient 3, while jogging. Patients 1 and 2 had one or more episodes of syncope during or shortly after exertion 7 to 12 months before sudden death and Patient 2 had had transient sub-

From the Pathology Branch, National Heart, Lung, and Blood Institute. National Institutes of Health, Bethesda, Maryland.

Manuscript received June 4, 1985; revised manuscript received August 20, 1985, accepted September 4, 1985.

Address for reprints: William C Roberts, MD, Building 10A, Room 3E30, National Institutes of Health, Bethesda, Maryland 20205.

sternal chest pain with exertion on two occasions. Patient 2 had rest and stress electrocardiograms and an echocardiogram after syncope while running 1 month before death. No abnormalities were observed. Patient 3 had ventricular premature complexes and left anterior hemiblock on electrocardiogram 1 year before death. A precordial systolic ejection murmur, grade 2/6, was present in Patient 2.

Patient 4 died at age 64 years. She had been asymptomatic until age 57 when exertional dyspnea and easy fatigability developed. The chest radiograph showed cardiomegaly and the electrocardiogram showed left bundle branch block. She was treated for congestive heart failure with digoxin and diuretic drugs. At age 63 years she had prolonged chest pain and acute myocardial infarction was diagnosed. Three months before death she was hospitalized with chest pain, congestive heart failure and atrial fibrillation. Several days before her death she was again hospitalized with worsening congestive heart failure. She developed ventricular tachycardia followed shortly by fatal ventricular fibrillation. Patient 5 died at age 81 years from chronic alcoholism and was without symptoms of cardiac dysfunction during life.

Necropsy findings. The epicardial coronary arteries in Patients 1 to 4 were free or virtually free of atherosclerotic plaques. Patient 5 had cross-sectional area narrowing by atherosclerotic plaques up to 75% in the right, 50 to 75% in the left circumflex and less than 50% in the left main and

Table 1. Certain Clinical and Necropsy Cardiac Observations in Five Patients in Whom the Left Main Coronary Artery Arose From the Right Sinus of Valsalva and Passed Between the Aorta and Pulmonary Trunk

		Clinical Findings							Time of Death			
Case	Age (yr) & Sex	AP	AMI	S (no.)	D	Duration of Symptoms (mo)	ECG	Mode of Death	During Exertion	Shortly After Exertion	HW (g)	LV Fibrosis
1	13F	0	0	+ (1)	0	12	—	Sudden	0	+	210	0
2	14M	+	0	+ (3)	0	7	Normal	Sudden	0	+	370	+
3	19M	0	0	0	0	0	VPC, LAH	Sudden	+	0	325	0
4	64F	0	+	0	+	84	LBBB	CHF	0	0	500	+
5	81M	0	0	0	0	0	—	Alcoholism	0	0	420	0

AMI = acute myocardial infarction; AP = angina pectoris, CHF = congestive heart failure; D = dyspnea; ECG = electrocardiogram; F = female; HW = heart weight, LAH = left anterior hemiblock; LBBB = left bundle branch block, LV = left ventricular; M = male; S = syncope (no of episodes), VPC = ventricular premature complexes, + = present; 0 = absent; — = no information

left anterior descending coronary arteries. In contrast to normal (Fig. 1). in each of the five patients small wooden sticks placed into the ostium of the left main and right coronary arteries (Fig. 2) were at right angles to each other when viewed from the aorta. The ostium of the right coronary artery was oval in shape with the largest diameter located in a right to left direction with the ostial lumen facing the central portion of aorta. The artery coursed away from the aorta more or less at right angles to it. In contrast, the ostium of the left main coronary artery in Patients 1 to 4 was slit-like with the largest diameter located in a cephalad to caudad direction; the artery coursed parallel to the aortic wall with the ostium pointing directly toward the aortic wall rather than toward the central portion of the aorta. The ostium of the left main coronary artery in Patient 5 was a narrow oval rather than slit-like and the proximal left main

artery had almost circumferential calcified plaque that did not actually cause significant luminal narrowing (Fig. 3). Patient 2 had scarring of one left ventricular papillary muscle (Fig. 4). and Patient 4 had a large healed apical infarct that was aneurysmal and contained a thrombus (Fig. 5). All five patients had a dominant right coronary artery circulation.

Discussion

Classification of the anomaly. Anomalous origin of the left main coronary artery from the right sinus of Valsalva can be classified into four major groups according to the course taken by the left main artery in relation to the aorta and pulmonary trunk en route to the left side of the heart. The left main artery may course anterior to the pulmonary trunk (1,2). posterior to the aorta (3). within the ventricular septum beneath the right ventricular infundibulum (4) or, as in our five patients. between the aorta and pulmonary trunk. When the left main artery passes anterior to the pulmonary trunk over the right ventricular infundibulum, symptoms of myocardial ischemia have not been reported unless significant coronary narrowing due to atherosclerotic plaque was present (1,2). With the exception of the 12 year old girl with this anomaly described by Murphy et al. (3), symptoms of myocardial ischemia have not been reported when the left main artery arises from the right sinus of Valsalva and courses posterior to the aorta.

Review of previous reports. At least 38 necropsy cases have been reported with origin of the left main coronary artery from the right sinus of Valsalva with coursing between the aorta and pulmonary trunk (Tables 2 and 3) (1,5–18). In nine patients, death was unrelated to the anomaly and symptoms of myocardial ischemia were absent during life (Table 2). In the other 29, death was of coronary origin (Table 3). Of these 29 patients. 23 (79%) died before age 20 years (mean 15) and the other 6 (21%) from age 49 to 82 years (mean 61). Of the 23 patients who died young, 22 (96%) died suddenly during or shortly after vigorous exertion and 1 died of acute myocardial infarction, having

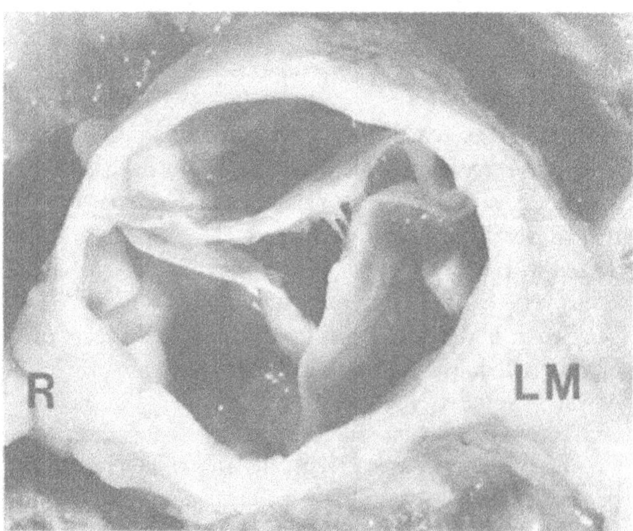

Figure 1. The aortic valve seen from above showing normal origin of the right (R) and left main (LM) coronary arteries. Wooden sticks have been placed in the ostium of each of the normally arising arteries demonstrating the almost perpendicular relation of the proximal portions of these arteries to the center of the aortic lumen.

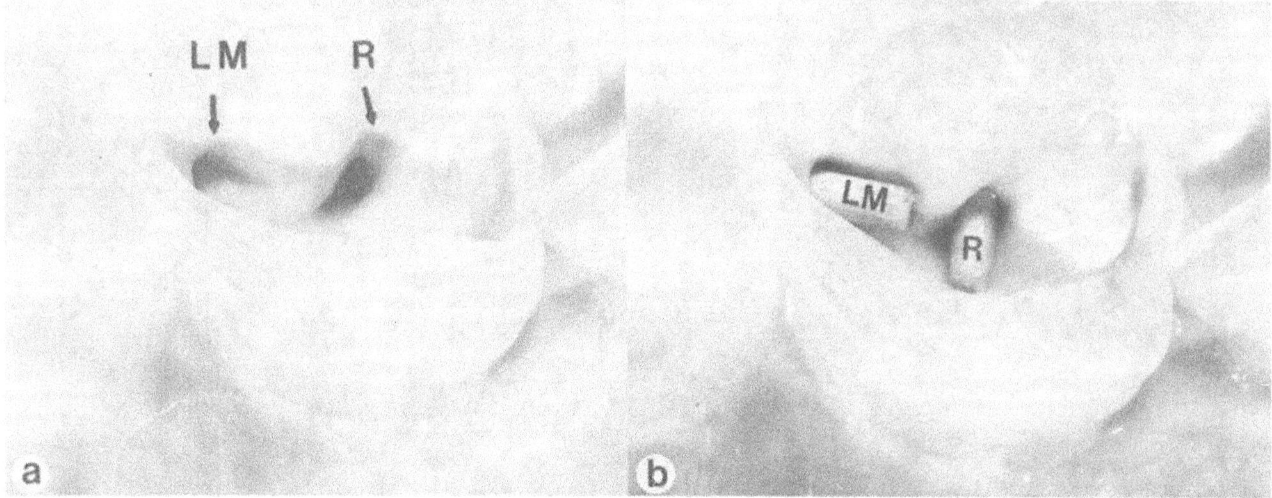

Figure 2. The ostia of the left main (LM) and right (R) coronary arteries in the right sinus of Valsalva viewed from the aortic lumen without (**a**) and with (**b**) wooden sticks in their proximal lumens demonstrating the perpendicular relation of the sticks to each other.

survived for 19 hours after initial collapse, which likewise occurred shortly after exertion. In the 11 cases in which information was provided, 8 patients had had symptoms before the final collapse: exertional syncope in 4, angina in 3 and exertional dyspnea in 1. Of the 23 young patients, 21 were male. At necropsy, 5 of the 23 patients had histologic evidence of myocardial necrosis; 1 patient apparently had atherosclerotic narrowing in the anomalous left main coronary artery.

Mechanism of death in older patients with the anomaly. All six patients who died after age 20 years were men. Three died of acute myocardial infarction and one died suddenly; the mode of death in the other two was not described. Symptoms of cardiac dysfunction were not described in any of the six patients. Histologic evidence of myocardial necrosis was present in four and not discussed in two patients. All six older patients apparently had significant coronary narrowing by atherosclerotic plaque in the abnormal or normal coursing arteries, or both. One patient lacked the circumflex branch of the left main artery.

Although it is clear from current necropsy information that this anomaly can cause sudden death at a young age, the role the anomaly plays in those who have survived past age 20 years is less clear. Our older patient (Case 4) appears to be the only one thus far reported in whom fatal myocardial ischemia could be attributed entirely to the coronary anomaly. Why this patient had fatal myocardial ischemia late in life after decades without symptoms is unclear. Possibly, the excessive cardiac weight (500 g) may have been a factor. Why Patient 5 survived 81 years free of symptoms of cardiac dysfunction is not clear either. Whereas the left main coronary artery arose from the aortic lumen at an acute angle in a manner similar to that in the other four patients, the ostium was not slit-like. This may be due in part to the presence of almost circumferential calcified plaque in the left main artery that caused less than 25% cross-sectional area narrowing but made the artery relatively rigid and less susceptible to dynamic compression. This would, however,

Figure 3. Patient 5. Schematic drawing of the anomalously arising left main coronary artery from the right sinus of Valsalva demonstrating the circumferential calcified atherosclerotic plaque in the proximal left main coronary artery.

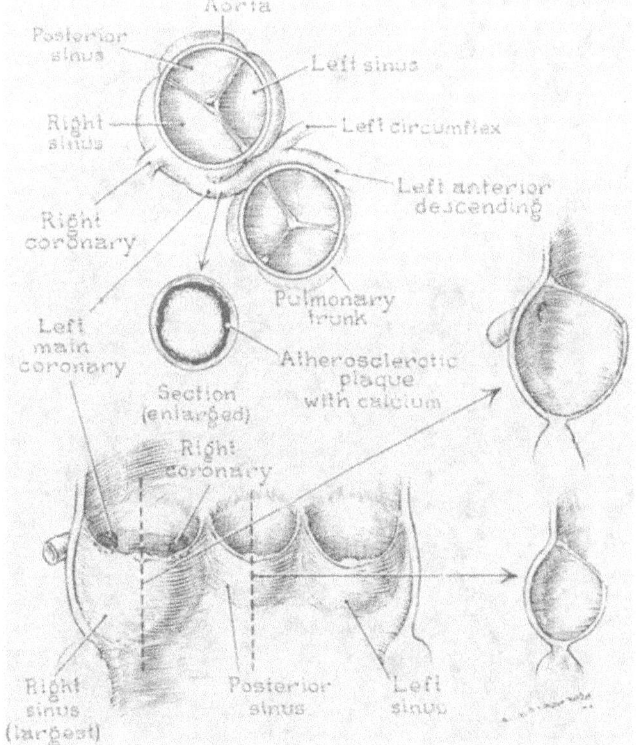

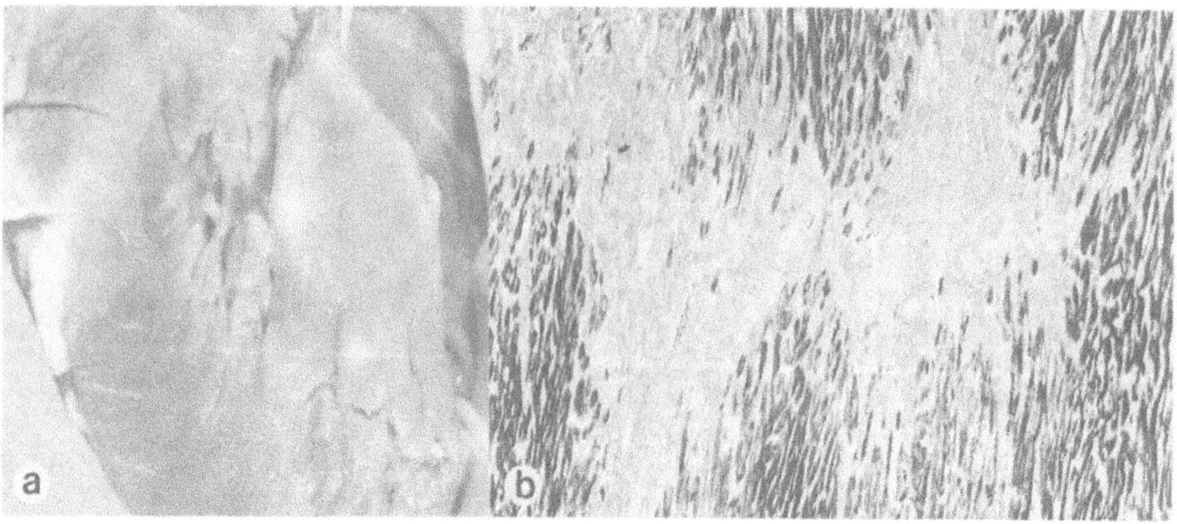

Figure 4. Patient 2. Patchy fibrosis of the anterolateral papillary muscle. **a,** The cut surface of the papillary muscle. **b,** Photomicrograph of the papillary muscle stained with the phosphotungstic acid method demonstrating scar (magnification × 40, reduced by 20%).

not explain why the anomaly did not cause symptoms earlier in life before the plaque would have been present.

Pathogenesis of myocardial ischemia. The precise mechanism by which anomalous origin of the left main

Figure 5. Patient 4. Cut section of the severely dilated left ventricle demonstrating the healed apical infarct with aneurysm containing thrombus (T).

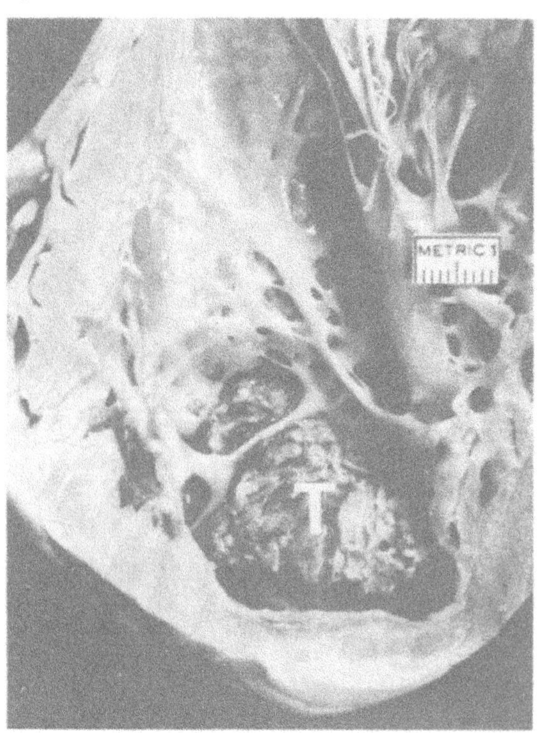

coronary artery from the right sinus of Valsalva with coursing between the pulmonary trunk and aorta causes myocardial ischemia is unclear. In each of our five patients the normal right coronary artery arose at an angle more or less perpendicular to the center of the aortic lumen, and it coursed directly away from the aorta; in contrast, the left main coronary artery arose from the aortic lumen at roughly a 180° angle to the center of the aorta. After takeoff, the anomalously arising left main coronary artery was adherent to the wall of the aorta for roughly 1.5 cm as it coursed to the left side of the heart between pulmonary trunk and aorta. Additionally, the ostium of the anomalously arising left main artery was slit-like in Patients 1 to 4 with the largest diameter in a cephalad-caudal direction; in contrast, the ostium of the normally arising right coronary artery was circular and larger. The firmly anchored root of the pulmonary trunk appears to present a potential barrier against which the left main artery could be compressed by expansion of the aortic root that occurs during increased intraaortic pressure associated with exertion. The left main coronary artery of course is equivalent to two arteries in the sense that it is responsible for supplying coronary blood flow to the major portion of the left ventricle and, therefore, significant reduction of flow through it is particularly perilous. Although it is likely that the narrowed left main coronary orifice has the potential to diminish flow through it, an actual reduction appears to be significant only during or immediately after exertion in those individuals without associated atherosclerosis.

Association of death with exertion. The association of death with exertion can be explained by three factors: 1) myocardial oxygen requirements increase with exertion and therefore any obstruction to coronary flow is more likely to result in myocardial ischemia; 2) it is likely that outward expansion of the roots of both aorta and pulmonary trunk during exertion causes further compression of the ostial lumen of the left main artery (1,13); and 3) the left main artery, as it courses between the aorta and pulmonary trunk,

Table 2. Published Reports of Anomalous Origin of Left Main Coronary Artery From Right Sinus of Valsalva With Coursing of the Left Main Artery Between the Pulmonary Trunk and Aorta: Nine Necropsy Cases With Noncoronary Cause of Death and Without Significant Coronary Atherosclerosis

| | References | | Age (yr) | | LV | |
Case	First Author	Year	& Sex	Cause of Death	Fibrosis	Necrosis
1	Sanes (3)	1937	68F	PE	+	0
2	Nicod (6)	1952	77M	Senility	0	0
3	Alexander (7)	1956	67F	Tuberculosis	0	0
4	Alexander (7)	1956	53M	Hemorrhage	0	0
5	Cheitlin (1)	1974	48M	Cancer	0	0
6	Cheitlin (1)	1974	40M	Endocarditis	0	0
7	Cheitlin (1)	1974	66M	Cirrhosis	—	—
8	Cheitlin (1)	1974	67M	Cancer	0	0
9	Cheitlin (1)	1974	42M	Cardiomyopathy	—	—

PE = pulmonary embolus; other abbreviations as in Table 1.

could be compressed against the root of the pulmonary trunk where it is firmly anchored to the infundibular septum when the aortic root and pulmonary trunk dilate during exertion. The fact that sudden exertional death and nonfatal myocardial ischemia have been seen in persons in whom the left main artery originates from the proximal right coronary artery and then courses between the great arteries (1,6), and who therefore do not have the abnormal oblique takeoff of the left main artery or the slit-like ostium in the right sinus of Valsalva, suggests that hemodynamic compression (hemodynamic vice) of the left main artery between the great arteries cannot be excluded as an additional mechanism of myocardial ischemia. Davia et al. (19) described a 14 year old boy who had two "exertionally related myocardial infarctions" due to this anomaly; he underwent surgical enlargement of the narrowed left main ostium and is asymptomatic during heavy labor 9 years later. This case lends further support to the theory that the primary mechanism causing myocardial ischemia is related to the narrowed left main coronary ostium.

Usefulness of exercise electrocardiography in diagnosis. The usefulness of stress electrocardiography in identifying the ischemic nature of this anomaly in young persons has received little attention. The fact that one of our necropsy patients, the 14 year old boy (Case 2), had a normal stress test 1 month before death prompted us to review previous experience with stress electrocardiography in young patients with isolated anomalous origin of the left main artery from the right sinus of Valsalva with coursing of this artery between the aorta and pulmonary trunk. Results of stress electrocardiography in seven patients are summarized in Table 4 (1,13,20,21). Of these seven, three had an abnormal stress electrocardiogram (evidence of ischemia or ventricular arrhythmia) and four had a normal stress electrocardiogram. In three of the latter four, however, the test was not a maximal effort. Two of the seven, both of whom had a normal submaximal stress electrocardiogram, sub-

sequently died suddenly. The other five patients underwent surgery. It is clear that the stress electrocardiogram, particularly one that is submaximal in effort, is not a reliable screening test for this anomaly in young patients who present with exertional syncope, angina and even acute myocardial infarction.

Differential diagnosis and means of diagnosis. Young patients with this anomaly often present with exertional syncope, dizziness and angina, but other cardiovascular abnormalities, such as hypertrophic cardiomyopathy and aortic valve stenosis, can present in a similar manner and therefore must be distinguished. The diagnostic approach taken with these young patients must take into account the fallibilities of the various noninvasive tests in identifying this potentially fatal coronary anomaly. The rest electrocardiogram is normal in almost all young persons with this anomaly and therefore it is not helpful. Physical examination may provide important clues to the noncoronary causes of these symptoms, that is, murmurs and peripheral pulses characteristic for aortic stenosis or hypertrophic cardiomyopathy. Echocardiography also is helpful in assessing for or confirming aortic stenosis or hypertrophic cardiomyopathy. Liberthson et al. (22) reported a 54 year old woman with angina pectoris in whom cross-sectional echocardiography identified anomalous origin of the left main coronary artery from the proximal right coronary artery with coursing of the left main artery between aorta and pulmonary trunk. Echocardiography, while potentially useful, has not been reported to have successfully identified origin of the left main artery directly from the right sinus of Valsalva. Continuous ambulatory electrocardiography may identify significant arrhythmias, but provides no help in identifying the cause of the arrhythmias. If the noncoronary causes of exertional syncope and angina are not identified, then more extensive evaluation is dictated to exclude the possibility of anomalous origin of the left main coronary artery.

As has been demonstrated, stress electrocardiography does

Table 3. List of Published Reports of Clinical and Necropsy Findings in 29 Patients With Origin of Left Main Coronary Artery From the Right Sinus of Valsalva With Coursing of the Left Main Artery Between the Pulmonary Trunk and Aorta: Death Due to Coronary Disease

| | Reference | | | Clinical Findings | | | | | | | Time of Death | | | LV | | |
Case	First Author	Year	Age (yr) & Sex	AP	AMI	S (no)	D	Duration of Symptoms (mo)	Abnormal ECG	Mode of Death	During Exertion	Shortly After Exertion	HW (g)	Fibrosis	Necrosis	CAD
1	Jokl (8)	1962	14M	0	0	0	0	0	—	Sudden	0	+	350	0	0	0
2	Jokl (9)	1966	16M	0	0	+(1)	+	48	—	Sudden	+	0	—	0	0	0
3	Cohen (10)	1967	11M	0	+	0	0	0	+*	AMI	0	+	280	0	+	0
4	Benson (11)	1968	13M	0	0	0	0	0	—	Sudden	0	+	260	0	0	0
5	Benson (11)	1968	13M	0	0	0	0	0	—	Sudden	0	+	370	0	0	0
6	Benson (12)	1970	54M	+	0	0	0	3	0	Sudden	0	0	460	0	0	+
7	Cheitlin (1)	1974	17M	0	0	+(1)	0	—	—	Sudden	0	+	—	0	0	
8	Cheitlin (1)	1974	14M	—	—	—	—	—	—	Sudden	0	+	—	—	—	0
9	Cheitlin (1)	1974	18M	—	—	—	—	—	—	Sudden	+	0	—	—	—	0
10	Cheitlin (1)	1974	17M	—	—	—	—	—	—	Sudden	+	0	—	—	—	0
11	Cheitlin (1)	1974	18M	—	—	—	—	—	—	Sudden	+	0	—	—	—	0
12	Cheitlin (1)	1974	22M	—	—	—	—	—	—	Sudden	+	0	—	—	—	0
13	Cheitlin (1)	1974	20M	—	—	—	—	—	—	Sudden	+	0	—	—	+	0
14	Cheitlin (1)	1974	22M	—	—	—	—	—	—	Sudden	+	0	—	—	—	0
15	Cheitlin (1)	1974	49M	—	+	—	—	—	—	AMI	—	—	—	—	+	+
16	Cheitlin (1)	1974	49M	—	+	—	—	—	—	AMI	—	—	—	—	+	+
17	Cheitlin (1)	1974	64M	—	—	—	—	—	—	—	—	—	—	—	—	+
18	Cheitlin (1)	1974	69M	—	+	—	—	—	—	AMI	—	—	—	—	+	+
19	Cheitlin (1)	1974	82M	—	—	—	—	—	—	—	—	—	—	—	—	+
20	Pedal (13)	1976	10F	+	0	+(9)	—	26	0	Sudden	0	+	145	+	+	0
21	Liberthson (14)	1979	1M	0	0	0	0	0	—	Sudden	0	+	—	0	0	0
22	Liberthson (14)	1979	11M	+	0	0	0	<1	—	Sudden	+	0	—	0	+	0
23	Liberthson (14)	1979	17M	0	0	0	0	0	—	Sudden	+	0	—	0	+	+
24	Lynch (15)	1980	20M	—	—	—	—	—	—	Sudden	+	0	—	—	—	0
25	Lynch (15)	1980	19M	—	—	—	—	—	—	Sudden	+	0	—	—	—	0
26	Tsung (16)	1982	14M	—	0	—	—	—	—	Sudden	+	0	450	0	0	0
27	Tsung (16)	1982	18M	—	0	—	—	—	—	Sudden	+	0	480	0	0	0
28	Betend (17)	1983	16M	+	0	+(3)	0	32	+†	Sudden	0	+	—	+	0	0
29	Topaz (18)	1985	15F	—	—	—	—	—	—	Sudden	+	0	—	—	—	0

*Supraventricular tachycardia, Q wave in lead V$_1$ and ST segment depression in lead V$_2$; †second degree atrioventricular block. CAD = atherosclerotic coronary artery disease; other abbreviations as in Table 1

Table 4. List of Published Reports of Stress Electrocardiography in Six Young Patients With Isolated Anomalous Origin of the Left Main Coronary Artery From the Right Sinus of Valsalva With Coursing of the Left Main Between the Pulmonary Trunk and the Aorta, Who Died Suddenly or Had Symptoms of Myocardial Ischemia

First Author	Year	Age (yr) & Sex	S	AP	AMI	SD	Normal Rest ECG	Time Before Death (mo)	Type of Stress Test	Response	Follow-up
Cheitlin (1)	1974	14M	+	0	0	0	+	0	Treadmill†	Normal	Surgery
Pedal (13)	1976	10F	+	+	+	+	+	<36	15 Knee bends	Normal	SD
Mustafa (20)	1981	12M	0	+	0	0	+	0	Treadmill	Normal	Surgery
Donaldson (21)	1983	*M	+	0	0	0	+	0	Treadmill	VT	Surgery
Donaldson (21)	1983	*M	0	+	0	0	+	0	Treadmill	Ischemia	Surgery
Donaldson (21)	1983	*M	0	+	0	0	+	0	Treadmill	Ischemia	Surgery

*Ages of 15, 21 and 32 years in this series could not be identified to individual patients; †submaximal SD = sudden death; VT = ventricular tachycardia, other abbreviations as in Table 1

not always identify myocardial ischemia in young patients with this coronary anomaly who are at risk for sudden death, but it should be done and it should be carried to maximal effort if evidence of myocardial ischemia is not identified at lower levels of exercise. If stress electrocardiography is abnormal, then angiographic assessment of coronary anatomy is dictated. If maximal stress electrocardiography is normal, then coronary angiography must still be considered in boys with clear-cut exercise-induced symptoms. The usefulness of thallium stress electrocardiography for diagnosis of this anomaly is uncertain. Patient 3 (Table 4) had a normal thallium stress test (20). Finally, in the specific case of frank exertional syncope at a young age, particularly in a male patient, coronary angiography should be performed after a second episode of syncope. Angiography should be considered after a single episode if no other clear cause of exertional syncope is evident by noninvasive testing.

Contrast to origin of both coronary arteries from left sinus. In contrast to origin of both coronary arteries from the right sinus of Valsalva with coursing of the left main artery between the great arteries, origin of both left main and right coronary arteries from the left sinus of Valsalva with coursing of the right coronary artery between the great arteries is usually, but not always, a benign congenital anomaly (23). Among 10 necropsy patients with the latter anomaly reported by Roberts et al. (23), the anomaly was an incidental necropsy finding in 7 patients and had nothing to do with their death, but in the other 3, it appeared to have caused fatal cardiac arrest with exertion.

Management of patients with the anomaly. Once the origin of both left main and right coronary arteries from the right aortic sinus with coursing of the left main artery between the great arteries has been diagnosed, at least in younger individuals, operative therapy appears warranted for the prevention of sudden death and for relief of exercise-induced symptoms of myocardial ischemia. Various operative approaches for revascularization have been described. Aortocoronary conduits, either saphenous vein or mammary artery, or both, to the left anterior descending and left circumflex coronary systems have resulted in relief of symptoms and in relief of objective evidence of myocardial ischemia in several patients (22,24,25). Other surgical approaches also have been successful. Davia et al. (19) described a 14 year old boy who had two myocardial infarcts and underwent surgical enlargement of the narrowed left main coronary ostium by extending an incision from the ostium through the common wall of the aorta and the anomalous artery over the intercoronary commissure. He was free of symptoms and active 9 years later, despite the presence of mild aortic regurgitation due to the procedure. Four patients, aged 12 to 36 years, have undergone an operation of a similar nature to reestablish the normal anatomic location of the left main artery origin to the left sinus of Valsalva by incising along the course of the common wall between the aorta and anomalous artery to the region of the left sinus of Valsalva and joining the intima of the vessel to the aorta, resulting in a new ostium (20,21). No evidence of ischemia was present in a follow-up period of 10 to 36 months.

References

1. Cheitlin MD, DeCastro CM, McCallister HA. Sudden death as a complication of anomalous left coronary origin from the anterior sinus of Valsalva. A not so minor congenital anomaly. Circulation 1974, 50:780–7.

2 Liberthson RR, Dinsmore RE, Bharati S, et al. Aberrant coronary artery origin from the aorta. Diagnosis and clinical significance. Circulation 1974;50:774–9.

3. Murphy DA, Roy DL, Sohal M, Chandler BM. Anomalous origin of left main coronary artery from anterior sinus of Valsalva with myocardial infarction. J Thorac Cardiovasc Surg 1978;75:282–5.

4 Roberts WC, Waller BF, McManus BM, Dawson SL, Hunsaker JC, Luke JL. Origin of the left main from the right coronary artery or from the right aortic sinus with intramyocardial tunneling to the left side of the heart via ventricular septum: the case against clinical significance of myocardial bridge or tunnels. Am Heart J 1982;104:303–5.

5 Sanes S Anomalous origin and course of the left coronary artery in a child. Am Heart J 1937;14:219–29

6. Nicod JL. Anomalie coronaire et mort subite Cardiologia 1952; 20.172–9.

7. Alexander RW, Griffith GC. Anomalies of the coronary arteries and their clinical significance. Circulation 1956,14:800–5

8. Jokl E, McClellan JT, Ross GD. Congenital anomaly of left coronary artery in young athlete. JAMA 1962;182:174–5.

9. Jokl E, McClellan JT, Williams WC, Gouze FJ, Bartholomew RD. Congenital anomaly of left coronary artery in young athletes. Cardiologia 1966;49:253–8.

10. Cohen LS, Shaw LD. Fatal myocardial infarction in an 11 year old boy associated with a unique coronary artery anomaly. Am J Cardiol 1967;19:420–3.

11. Benson PA, Lack AR. Anomalous aortic origin of the left coronary artery. Arch Pathol 1968;86:214–6.

12. Benson PA. Anomalous aortic origin of coronary artery with sudden death: case report and review. Am Heart J 1970;70:254–7

13. Pedal I. Aortale Ursprungsanomalie einer Koronararterie Dtsch Med Wochenschr 1976;101:1601–4

14. Liberthson RR, Dinsmore RE, Fallon JT. Aberrant coronary artery origin from the aorta. Report of 18 patients, review of the literature and delineation of natural history and management Circulation 1979;59:748–54.

15. Lynch P. Soldiers, sport and sudden death Lancet 1980;1.1235–7.

16. Tsung SH, Huang TY, Chang HH Sudden death in young athletes. Arch Pathol Lab Med 1982;106.168–70.

17. Betend B, Gillet P, Moreau P, David L. Origine aortique anormale de l'artère coronaire gauche. A propos de la mort subite d'un adolescent. Arch Fr Pediatr 1983;40:479–81.

18. Topaz O. Edwards JE. Pathologic features of sudden death in children, adolescents, and young adults. Chest 1985;87:476–82.

19 Davia JE. Green DC. Cheitlin MD, DeCastro C. Brott WH. Anomalous left coronary artery origin from the right coronary sinus. Am Heart J 1984;108:165–6.

20. Mustafa I, Gula G, Radley-Smith R. Durrer S, Yacoub M Anomalous origin of the left coronary artery from the anterior aortic sinus: a potential cause of sudden death. J Thorac Cardiovasc Surg 1981:82:297–300

21 Donaldson RM. Raphael M, Radley-Smith R. Yacoub MH. Ross DN. Angiographic identification of primary coronary anomalies causing impaired myocardial perfusion. Cathet Cardiovasc Diagn 1983;9:237–49.

22. Liberthson RR. Zaman L. Weyman A, et al Aberrant origin of the left coronary artery from the proximal right coronary artery: diagnostic features and pre- and postoperative course. Clin Cardiol 1982;5:377–81.

23 Roberts WC, Siegel RJ, Zipes DP. Origin of the right coronary artery from the left sinus of Valsalva and its functional consequences: analysis of 10 necropsy patients Am J Cardiol 1982;49:863–8.

24 Moodie DS. Gill C, Loop FD, Sheldon WC. Anomalous left main coronary artery originating from the right sinus of Valsalva. Pathophysiology, angiographic definition and surgical approaches J Thorac Cardiovasc Surg 1980;80:198–205.

25 Sacks JH, Londe SP, Rosenbluth A. Zalis EG. Left main coronary artery bypass for aberrant (aortic) intramural left coronary artery. J Thorac Cardiovasc Surg 1977;73:733–7

Major anomalies of coronary arterial origin seen in adulthood

William C. Roberts, M.D. *Bethesda, Md.*

Both coronary arteries normally arise, of course, from ostia located in the sinus of Valsalva portions of the aorta. The right coronary artery (RCA) arises from the right aortic sinus, usually but not always in its central portion, and the left main (LM) coronary artery arises from the left aortic sinus, nearly always from its central portion. If the aorta contains only two cusps or one cusp rather than its usual three, the location of the coronary ostia are usually as they would be were the valve tricuspid rather than bicuspid or unicuspid. A deviation of origin of a coronary artery from the normal falls under the category of "anomaly of coronary arterial origin," and these anomalies will be reviewed in this article. Anomalies of origin are particularly common in hearts in which other major congenital cardiovascular malformations are present. This review, however, will be limited to those anomalies of origin observed in hearts without other major malformations of the heart or great vessels (Table I).

ORIGIN OF 1 OR MORE CORONARY ARTERIES FROM THE PULMONARY TRUNK *AND* ORIGIN OF 1 OR MORE CORONARY ARTERIES FROM THE AORTA

When both right and LM coronary arteries arise from the pulmonary trunk (PT) or when only one coronary artery is present and it arises from the PT, survival past 1 year of life is impossible unless an associated anomaly is present which allows persistence of pulmonary hypertension after birth (Fig. 1). In these two circumstances, no coronary artery arises directly from the aorta.

When one coronary artery, however, arises from the PT and one or more coronary arteries arise from the aorta, survival past 15 years of age may occur. The most common anomaly in this category is origin of the LM coronary artery from the PT and origin of

the RCA from the aorta (Fig. 1). Far less common is origin of the right or left anterior descending coronary artery (LAD) from the PT, and these anomalies are usually associated with survival into adulthood (Fig. 1).

Left main from the pulmonary trunk

Historic background. This anomaly was described first by Maude Abbott in 1908.[1] Her patient was a woman who lived for 60 years, and this is the longest survival reported with this anomaly. Abriskossoff[2] in 1911 first described findings in an infant with this anomaly. In 1933, Bland et al.[3] described clinical and necropsy findings in a 3-month-old boy with this anomaly, and subsequently this anomaly in infants has often been referred to as the "Bland-White-Garland Syndrome." The infant described by Bland et al. was the son of a physician who observed " . . . the paroxysmal attacks of acute discomfort precipitated by the exertion of nursing." These attacks, which also included inspiratory and expiratory grunts followed by marked pallor and cold sweats, were interpreted by Bland et al. as evidence of angina pectoris. The ECG (three limb leads only) disclosed marked T wave inversions and the chest radiograph showed marked enlargement of the cardiac silhouette. The clinical diagnosis in the infant was "congenital idiopathic hypertrophy of the heart." The coronary anomaly was discovered at necropsy.

Frequency. This anomaly was observed only once among 357 patients with congenital heart disease studied at necropsy by Fontana and Edwards[4] from January, 1920, through June 30, 1954, dates which precede cardiopulmonary bypass operations. Fontana and Edwards[4] also found published reports describing 58 necropsy patients with origin of the LM from the PT. More than half of the 58 patients died between ages 3 and 6 months; 46 patients (79%) were dead by 13 months of age; the remaining 12 patients (21%) lived longer than 15 years. The major cause of death during the first year of life was congestive heart failure; 8 of the 12 adults died suddenly and unexpectedly. Fontana and Edwards[4]

From the Pathology Branch, National Heart, Lung, and Blood Institute, National Institutes of Health.

Received for publication Oct. 7, 1985; accepted Nov. 8, 1985.

Reprint requests: William C. Roberts, M.D., Bldg. 10A, Room 3E-30, NIH, Bethesda, MD 20892.

Table I. Anomalies of coronary arterial origin

I. *Origin of 1 or more coronary arteries from the pulmonary trunk (PT) and 1 or more coronary arteries from the aorta*
    A. Left main (LM) from PT
    B. Right (R) from PT
    C. Left anterior descending (LAD) from PT
    D. Left circumflex (LC) from PT
    E. Accessory coronary artery from PT

II. Origin of 1 or 2 coronary arteries from the pulmonary trunk without origin of a coronary artery from the aorta
    A. R and LM from PT
    B. "Single coronary artery" from PT

III. *Anomalous origin of 1 or more coronary arteries from the aorta*
    A. LM and R from right aortic sinus
    B. LM and R from left aortic sinus
    C. LM and R from the posterior aortic sinus
    D. R and LC from right aortic sinus (or LC from R) and LAD from left sinus
    E. R and LAD from right aortic sinus (or LAD from R) and LC from left sinus
    F. R from posterior aortic sinus and LM from left sinus
    G. LM from posterior aortic sinus and R from right sinus
    H. LAD and LC from a separate ostium in the left aortic sinus and R from right aortic sinus

IV. *Origin of only 1 coronary artery from the aorta without origin of a coronary artery from the PT (single coronary ostium)*
    A. From the right aortic sinus
        1. R crosses crux and continues as the LC which continues as the LAD
        2. LM from R
            a. Coursing of LM posterior to aorta before dividing into LAD and LC
            b. Coursing of LM between aorta and PT before branching into LAD and LC
            c. Coursing of LM anterior to PT
            d. Coursing of LM in ventricular septum beneath right ventricular infundibulum

        3. LAD and LC from R with coursing of LC posterior to aorta and LAD anterior to right ventricle (RV)
        4. LAD from R with coursing anterior to RV with R crossing crux to form LC
        5. LAD from R with coursing between aorta and PT with R crossing crux to continue as LC
        6. LAD from R with coursing between aorta and PT and LC from R with retroaortic course
        7. LAD from R coursing anterior to RV, LC from R coursing between aorta and PT
        8. LAD from R coursing retroaortic with R crossing crux to continue as LC
        9. LAD from R with coursing to left side in ventricular septum beneath right ventricular outflow tract and LC from R with retroaortic course to left atrioventricular sulcus
    B. From left aortic sinus
        1. LAD and LC from single coronary artery with LC crossing crux to continue as R
        2. R, LAD, and LC from single coronary artery
            a. R posterior to aorta
            b. R between aorta and PT
            c. R anterior to RV
        3. R and LC from single coronary artery and LAD from R
            a. R between aorta and PT
            b. R posterior to aorta
        4. R and LAD from single coronary artery and of LC from LAD
            a. R between aorta and PT
            b. R posterior to PT
    C. From posterior aortic sinus
        1. Single coronary artery between aorta and PT with trifurcation into R, LAD, and LC
        2. Single coronary artery to left of PT with trifurcation into R, LAD, and LC
        3. Single coronary artery to right and when anterior to aorta giving rise to R and LM which subdivides into LAD and LC

---

found no reports of death in patients with this anomaly from age 13 months to 16 years. Thus, if a patient with this anomaly is able to survive the first year of life, the chances are good that the child will survive until adulthood. Origin of the LM from the PT occurs about equally often in both sexes. I have studied at necropsy 11 patients (seven females) in whom the LM arose from the PT: nine were aged 1 to 18 months (means seven); 1 was 3.5 years old, and one died suddenly at age 41 years. The latter patient was known to have a continuous precordial murmur but never had symptoms of cardiac dysfunction. Her sudden death was clearly the result of the coronary anomaly.

The frequency of this anomaly among adults having coronary arterial angiograms for suspected ischemic heart disease is of course quite low. Among 1750 adults having coronary angiograms reported by Thomas et al.[5] two had origin of the LM from the PT: one was a 45-year-old woman and the other was a 40-year-old woman. Among 9152 patients having coronary angiograms reported by Donaldson et al.,[6] six had origin of the LM from the PT.

Flow in the anomalous artery. Why some patients with anomalous origin of the LM coronary artery from the PT die during the first year of life or soon thereafter and why others survive into adulthood (without operative intervention) is related to the development of collaterals between the coronary artery attached to the ascending aorta (the right

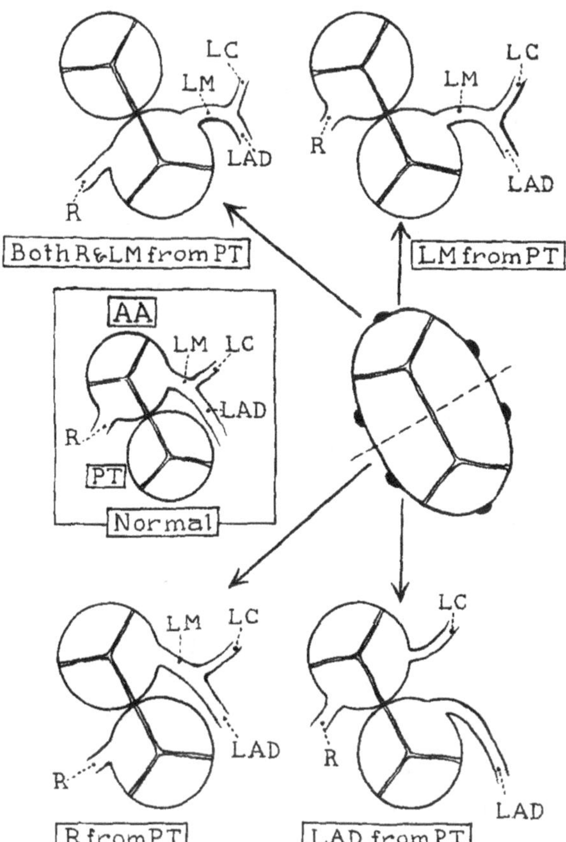

Fig. 1. Diagram illustrating the common arterial trunk arising from the heart in its early development with six potential coronary arterial ostia and the possible coronary anomalies resulting when inappropriate ostia do not regress. *AA* = ascending aorta; *LAD* = left anterior descending coronary artery; *LC* = left circumflex coronary artery; *LM* = left main coronary artery; *PT* = pulmonary trunk; *R* = right coronary artery.

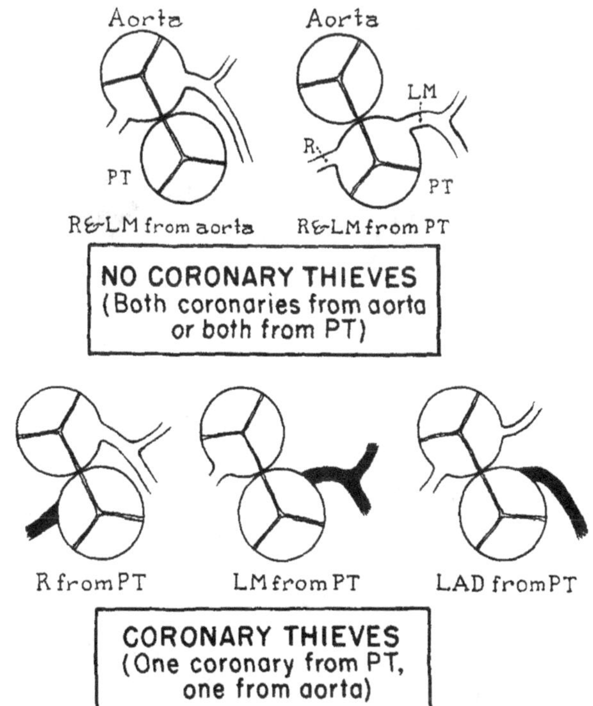

Fig. 2. Diagram showing the coronary anomalies not associated with the "coronary steal" phenomenon and those associated with this phenomenon. Abbreviations as in Fig. 1.

one) and the coronary artery attached to the PT (the LM).[7,8] At birth and during roughly the first 2 months of life, the systolic and diastolic pressures in the ascending aorta and PT are similar and consequently the LM coronary artery is perfused by blood within the PT. At about 2 months of life, the pressure in the PT falls so that by about 12 months of life the systolic pressure in the PT is about one fourth of that in the aorta. Survival is dependent on the development of collateral channels between the normally and abnormally arising coronary arteries, so that flow in the anomalous LM coronary artery is retrograde, it being entirely supplied by blood from the normally arising RCA. The anomalous artery "steals" blood from the normally arising artery (Fig. 2), placing considerable myocardium at risk of ischemia or necrosis (Fig. 3). It would appear that an extensive collateral system must develop for survival to occur. During the period of transition from ante-grade to retrograde flow in the anomalously arising LM coronary artery, death is common.

Morphologic features. The heart is quite different in the infant dying with this anomaly compared to that of the patient surviving to adulthood. In the infant, the cardiac mass is increased (this anomaly provides the best evidence available that chronic myocardial ischemia causes an increase in cardiac mass) and the ventricular cavities are dilated. The area occupied by the mitral valve appears small in comparison to the entire left ventricular cavity. The left ventricular papillary muscles appear to arise in the left ventricle at about the junction of the cephalad and middle thirds of the wall. Normally, the papillary muscles tend to arise about the level of the middle and caudal thirds of the left ventricle. The arterolateral papillary muscle is much smaller than the posteromedial papillary muscle. Additionally, the anterolateral papillary muscle is scarred, often calcified, and in contrast, the myocardium of the posteromedial muscle is preserved. The endocardium of the left ventricle may be thickened so that it has the appearance of diffuse endocardial fibroelastosis. The margin of the anterior mitral leaflet is often thickened. The left atrium is dilated.

In contrast to the appearance in the infant heart,

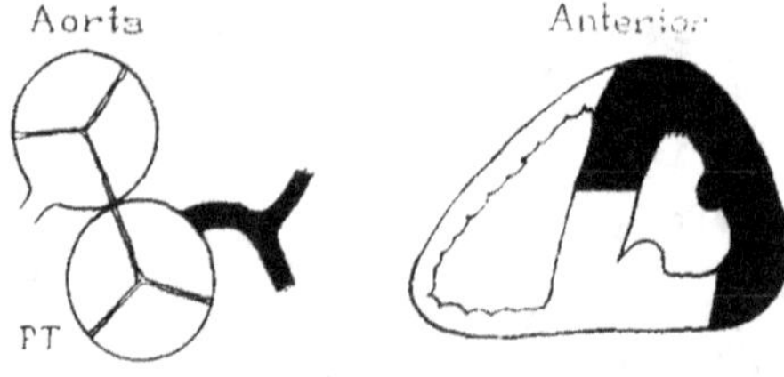

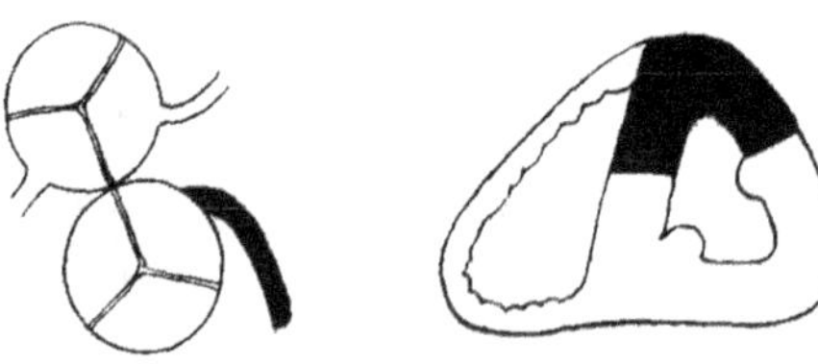

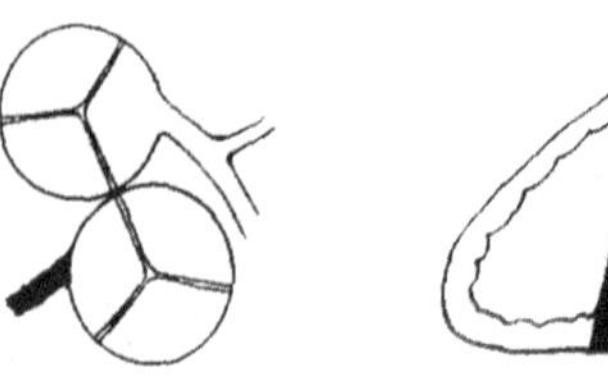

Fig. 3. Diagram showing the portion of left ventricular myocardium at risk of ischemia or necrosis when the left main, left anterior descending, or right coronary artery arises from the pulmonary trunk *(PT)*.

the survivors of this anomaly into adulthood have hearts which are distinguished primarily by the appearances of the epicardial coronary arteries. The right one is dilated and tortuous. The branches of the LM, in contrast, are straighter, not as dilated, but have a thinner wall (like a vein). Vascular channels connecting the RCA to the branches of the LM are visible on the surface of the heart. The mass of the heart is usually increased and the ventricular cavities are usually dilated. The anterolateral papillary muscle is usually scarred and it also contains calcific deposits. One of 10 adults (aged 15 to 54 years [mean 31]) reported by Moodie et al.[9] had extensive left ventricular calcific deposits. Left ventricular endocardial fibroelastosis, which is commonly observed in the infants at necropsy, is usually absent in the adults with this anomaly.

Symptoms of cardiac dysfunction. Symptoms of cardiac dysfunction occur in about 80% of infants in whom the LM arises from the PT, and the symptom complex was reported by Bland et al.[3] and has been substantiated by others.[10-19] In adults or in children

surviving the first year of life, the symptoms complex is far more varied. Many patients with the adult form of anomalous LM arising from the PT are asymptomatic despite extremely active lives. A 29-year-old woman reported by Sabiston et al.[20] had had five full-term normal deliveries without difficulty. The 18-year-old boy reported by Harthorne et al.[16] was a star basketball player who eventually developed excessive dyspnea, chest pain, and finally syncope, only in association with the strenuous exertion of athletic endeavors. The 18-year-old boy reported by Jurishica[10] was a star football player.

The asymptomatic older patients with this anomaly were usually brought to medical attention by the detection of a precordial murmur (often a continuous one) on precordial examination, by the finding of an abnormal ECG showing ischemic changes, or by the occurrence of sudden unexpected death. The latter, unfortunately, is common. Of 14 adults aged 16 to 60 years (mean 36) with this anomaly reviewed by George and Knowlan,[11] 10 died suddenly and unexpectedly and of the 10, sudden death was the initial clinical manifestation of the coronary anomaly in eight. The sudden death was usually associated with sudden physical exertion.

Other reported symptoms in adults with this anomaly have included angina pectoris, exertional dyspnea, and syncope. Clinical features consistent with acute myocardial infarction have not been described, to my knowledge, in adults with this anomaly. Likewise, overt evidence of congestive heart failure is rare in adults, except possibly in those with clinical evidence of mitral regurgitation.[21,22]

Means of diagnosis. The definitive diagnosis of this anomaly is by angiography by injection of contrast material into the lumen of the right coronary artery (or aortic root) with drainage via collaterals into the LM branches and visualization of the connection of the LM to the PT. Although angiography is the only definitive test, other procedures provide important clues to the diagnosis. The presence of a precordial continuous murmur is very helpful. In infants the ECG showing ischemic myocardial changes (anterior wall) is most helpful.[19] In adults with this anomaly, unfortunately, the ECG is not as helpful. The ischemic changes in adults may or may not be present, and even if they are present they could be attributed to coronary narrowing from atherosclerosis. ECG evidence of left ventricular hypertrophy is common in adults with the anomaly.

The echocardiogram may provide clues to diagnosis. In each of three infants, Fisher et al.[23] demonstrated by cross-sectional echocardiography attachment of the LM coronary artery to the PT and markedly dilated poorly contracting left ventricles. Terai et al.,[24] also in an infant, demonstrated by cross-sectional echocardiography origin of the LM from the PT as well as a very large right coronary artery arising from the ascending aorta. Robinson et al.[26] cautioned that the only reliable echocardiographic finding in the anomaly was the actual demonstration of the LM arising from the PT, not the absence of identification of the origin of the LM from the aorta. King et al.,[27] by pulsed Doppler echocardiography, demonstrated in a 2-month-old infant bidirectional Doppler flow in the proximal portion of the PT. The late systolic flow pattern on the Doppler flow tracing indicated a left-to-right shunt through the LM arising from the PT. Whether echocardiography will be as useful in adults with this anomaly as in infants remains to be determined.

The presence of mitral regurgitation in a young person with ischemic changes on the ECG might suggest the presence of the coronary anomaly. Mitral regurgitation may be the dominant clinical feature of this coronary anomaly. Both Usman et al.[21] and Burchell and Brown[22] described a patient whose dominant clinical problem was mitral regurgitation.

Radionuclide angiography may be useful in distinguishing patients with origin of the LM from the PT from those with idiopathic dilated cardiomyopathy.[28] Origin of the LM from the PT cannot usually be seen by injecting contrast material into the PT. However, the LM can be seen arising from the PT if a balloon is inflated in the PT just distal to the site of contrast material injection.[29]

Operative treatment and results. A number of operative procedures have been utilized for treatment of this anomaly[5, 9, 14, 16, 19, 20, 23, 30-46]: (1) ligation of the LM coronary artery at its attachment to the PT; (2) obliteration of the LM ostium by covering it within the lumen of the PT with artificial or biologic material; (3) ligation of the LM artery or closure of its ostium plus insertion of a conduit, usually a reversed saphenous vein, from ascending aorta to left anterior descending coronary artery; (4) anastomosis of the LM to the ascending aorta either directly or via an artificial (polytetrafluoroethylene) or biologic graft, with closure of the site of origin of the LM from the PT; (5) division of the LM artery close to its ostium in the PT and direct anastomosis of a subclavian or common carotid artery to the LM in an end-to-end fashion. In the procedures in which a conduit has been interposed between the aorta and the LM coronary artery, the conduit has been located posterior to the PT, within the PT as a tunnel, and anterior to the PT. Despite the multiple different procedures utilized for treatment, the best one is unclear. Good results have been obtained with most of them.

An early operative procedure to correct this anomaly was a simple ligation of the LM coronary artery. This procedure has produced good long-term results in infants, children, and adults. Shrivastava et al.[41] followed two infants and two children (aged 6 and 7 years) for >10 years after simple LM ligation and all were asymptomatic postoperatively, although the ECG remained abnormal in two. Wilson et al.,[42] by polling many cardiovascular surgeons, collected 13 patients who had LM ligation only when they were aged 13 years or older. The mean age at last follow-up was 37 ± 9 years and the mean follow-up period was 9 years. Although there had been no deaths at operation or in the early postoperative period, three patients died later (2, 6, and 7 years after operation). These same authors also described results in 16 patients who had had LM ligation plus insertion of a saphenous vein between the ascending aorta and the LAD coronary artery at age 13 years or older. At a mean age of last follow-up of 38 ± 11 years and a mean of 5 ± 3 years after operation, there was only one death and that was in the early postoperative period. Wilson et al.[42] concluded that the probability of survival was similar following either LM ligation alone or LM ligation plus aorto-LAD grafting. About half the patients in both their two operative groups were improved symptomatically by the operation.

Moodie et al.[9] described operative results in 10 patients aged 15 to 54 years (mean 31) at the time of closure of the LM ostium from within the PT plus aorto-LAD grafting (six patients), isolated closure of the LM ostium from inside the PT (three patients), and transfer of the LM ostium with a cuff of PT directly to the ascending aorta (one patient). The 10 patients were followed 4 months to 16 years (mean 6 years): six were asymptomatic postoperatively, three were functional class II (each was class III preoperatively [New York Heart Association classification]), and one died late. Postoperative stress ECGs showed no evidence of myocardial ischemia in six of six patients and normal stress thallium tests in eight of eight patients.

The present commonly employed operative procedures for this anomaly—namely, LM ligation with aorto-LAD grafting or connection of the LM to the aorta either directly or via a graft—appear to have similar effects on the sizes of the collaterals between the branches of the RCA and the branches of the LAD and LC coronary arteries and the size of the RCA postoperatively. Early after operation and as long as 3 years postoperatively, the sizes of the collaterals and RCA postoperatively may be similar to their sizes preoperatively. By 3 years after operation, however, the collaterals are usually much smaller or have disappeared and the lumen of and the tortuosity of the RCA is much less than preoperatively. In a patient reported by Chaitman et al.,[37] however, who was evaluated at age 36 (over 8 years after LM ligation and aorto-LAD grafting via a saphenous vein), large collaterals were still present between the LM branches and the RCA.

These operations have variable effects on the degree of mitral regurgitation postoperatively if mitral regurgitation was present preoperatively. The valvular lesion may disappear or be unchanged or it may lessen postoperatively. If there is ECG evidence of left ventricular hypertrophy preoperatively, that condition usually persists after operation. Left ventricular function, however, is usually improved by operation. Bagger et al.[46] described a 19-year-old woman who had LM ligation and saphenous vein grafting between the aorta and LAD; evaluation 6 months postoperatively disclosed disappearance of the collaterals, normal left ventricular contractions compared to preoperative studies, a 100% increase in coronary sinus blood flow and a 128% increase during pacing, whereas preoperatively pacing did not increase the coronary sinus blood flow.

Right coronary artery from pulmonary trunk

Historic background. The first report of origin of the RCA from the PT was by Sir John Brooks, an anatomist, who studied two cadavers and postulated in 1885 that blood flow in the anomalously arising RCA was reversed: blood from the aorta entered the LM coronary artery, passed through collaterals to the RCA, and then drained into the PT.[47] Monckelberg[48] in 1914 studied at necropsy a 30-year-old man who had died shortly following an epileptic seizure and found the RCA anomaly. Schley[49] in 1925 described the anomaly in a 61-year-old man who died of syphilis. Jordan et al.[50] also found the anomaly in a patient at necropsy, as did Cronk et al.[51] The latter patient had lived 90 years before he died, shortly following seizures. These latter authors described severe atherosclerosis in the branches of the LM coronary artery and no atherosclerosis in the RCA, a finding which proves that the pressure in the RCA was venous and that in the left coronary arteries was arterial. Cronk et al.[51] also noted that the intramural coronary arteries in the right ventricular wall were numerous and in the left ventricular free wall they were relatively sparse. The left coronary artery (probably the LAD) had a maximal diameter of 20 mm and the RCA had a maximal diameter of 6 mm. The first patient with this anomaly who was treated operatively was reported by Tingelstad et al.[52] in 1972.

Frequency. This anomaly is far less common than is origin of the LM from the PT. In their 1962 book, Fontana and Edwards[4] found reports of only four necropsy cases of origin of the RCA from the PT, while at the same time finding reports of 58 necropsy cases of origin of the LM from the PT. From review of the necropsy reports at Yale–New Haven Hospital from 1952 to 1968, Ogden[53] found four cases of origin of the RCA from the PT and 39 cases of origin of the LM from the PT. By 1979, Lerberg et al.[54] found reports describing 14 patients with origin of the RCA from the PT and reports describing 140 patients with origin of the LM from the PT.

Flow in the anomalous artery. Flow in the anomalous artery, be it right, LM, LAD, or LC from the PT, should be similar and variable, depending on the patient's age. Although flow through the anomalously arising LM has been demonstrated to be antegrade early in life and retrograde after approximately a year (sometimes earlier) of life, antegrade flow has not been demonstrated in infancy when the RCA has arisen from the PT and the LM has arisen from the aorta. The reason of course is that diagnosis of origin of the RCA from the PT has not been made during infancy; indeed, the youngest child in whom this diagnosis has been established was 6 years old and that patient was described by Lerberg et al.[54] Retrograde flow through the anomalous RCA has been established both by angiogram and by visualization at operation.

Morphologic features. Whereas increase in ventricular mass, left ventricular scarring, anterolateral papillary muscle fibrosis and calcification, right ventricular and left ventricular dilatation, and diffuse left ventricular endocardial fibroelastosis (of variable degree) might be expected in cases of origin of the LM from the PT, none of these morphologic findings appear to be the consequence of origin of the RCA from the PT. Indeed, the only predictable morphologic finding is an increase in the size of the LM coronary artery and its branches and an increase (but less so) in the size of the RCA with thinning of its wall (compared to normal).

Clinical manifestations. This anomaly usually produces no symptoms of cardiac dysfunction and no evidence of myocardial ischemia. Of nine necropsy cases reported up to 1979 and summarized by

Lerberg et al.[54] one patient, a 2-year-old boy, was found dead in his crib without preceding evidence of any illnes. Another, an 11-year-old girl, had cardiac arrest, and another, a 72-year-old man, had evidence of chronic congestive cardiac failure. None of the three patients had another condition that could be responsible for their deaths. All six remaining necropsy patients were either free of clinical evidence of cardiac dysfunction or they had another cardiac disorder (aortic regurgitation or systemic hypertension or mitral stenosis) which could readily explain any cardiac dysfunction. These six patients were aged 30 to 90 years (mean 62). Five other patients up to 1979 had the anomaly diagnosed by angiography and each of them had operative therapy.[54] Their ages at operation were 11, 12, 25, 42, and 64 years, and three were female.[54-58] Three of them were asymptomatic and were found to have a continuous precordial murmur (left sternal border), one (age 64 years) presented with evidence of congestive cardiac failure,[56] and one (age 25 years) had cardiac arrest with successful resuscitation.[58] A year earlier, however, the latter patient had had one syncopal episode. Thus, anomalous origin of the RCA from the PT is a cause of cardiac arrest, and this fact by itself justifies operative intervention if this coronary anomaly is known to be present, even though the individual may be asymptomatic.

Recently, Mintz et al.[59] reported a 47-year old man who had angina pectoris for 2 months. The resting ECG and the chest radiogram were normal. Thallium-201 myocardial perfusion scanning disclosed a decrease in perfusion in the 4-hour-study. Total anterograde LM coronary flow was 1440 to 1680 ml/min, but only 240 to 280 ml/min supplied the myocardium and the remainder passed to the PT via the RCA. Thus there was a 5:1 intercoronary shunt. This study was the first to quantitate the degree of the "coronary steal" in this anomaly (Fig. 2).

In contrast to its usefulness when the LM coronary artery arises from the PT, the ECG in origin of the RCA from the PT is usually of no benefit. Ischemic changes are usually absent and signs of ventricular hypertrophy are usually absent or only borderline. The chest radiogram usually shows mild enlargement of the cardiac silhouette, but the cardiac size may be entirely normal. Cross-sectional echocardiography may be useful for diagnosis. Origin of the RCA from the PT must be demonstrated—not absence of origin of the RCA from the aorta.[60] The finding of a large LM coronary artery or a large RCA by echocardiography might provide the initial suspicion of the pressure of this anomaly.

Certain diagnosis is established by angiography, with injection of contrast material in the LM coronary artery arising from the aorta, and visualization of the RCA via collaterals from the LM branches and finally the appearance of contrast material in the PT.

Operative treatment and results. The operation of choice for this anomaly appears to be transsection of the RCA from the PT and direct anastomosis of the RCA to the aorta (end-to-side). Tingelstad et al.[52] were the first to report this technique. Their patient was a 12-year-old asymptomatic boy who was found to have a continuous precordial murmur. The left-to-right shunt from the LM to the RCA was calculated to have been 1.7 to 1. Others[53, 54, 56-61] have also successfully utilized this transsection technique. The patient operated on by Bregman et al.[58] had presented with cardiac arrest and was successfully resuscitated. The patient was asymptomatic 2 years postoperatively.

Left anterior descending coronary artery from pulmonary trunk.

At least eight patients have been reported in whom the LAD arose from the PT and both right and LC arteries arose from the aorta, and the findings in these patients were summarized by Roberts and Robinowitz.[62] At the time of their 1984 report, one patient (a 7-month-old girl) had died of an anterior wall acute myocardial infarct; the other seven (six women) were aged 18 to 55 years (mean 34). The patient reported by Roberts and Robinowitz[62] is the only male thus far described. Of the seven adults, six were asymptomatic, five with angina pectoris, one of whom also had an anterior wall acute myocardial infarct, and one with severe fatigue attributed to severe mitral regurgitation from papillary muscle dysfunction. The angina at some time in all five patients was stable, but three of the five had unstable angina just before cardiac operation. The age at onset of symptoms of myocardial ischemia in the six adults ranged from 18 to 37 years (mean 27). Precordial murmurs were described in five or six adults. (No information was provided in the "addendum case" of Donaldson et al.[63]) The murmur apparently was present only in systole in four patients, and also in diastole in two. The intensity of the murmurs was mentioned in three patients; it was "soft" in one, grade 2/6 in one, and grade 3/6 in one. Findings on the ECG at rest were described in five adults: four had poor R wave progression in leads V_1 to V_3 and at least two had ST-T-wave changes of ischemia in more than one lead. In one patient the ECG was normal. Exercise stress tests in two patients disclosed ST segment

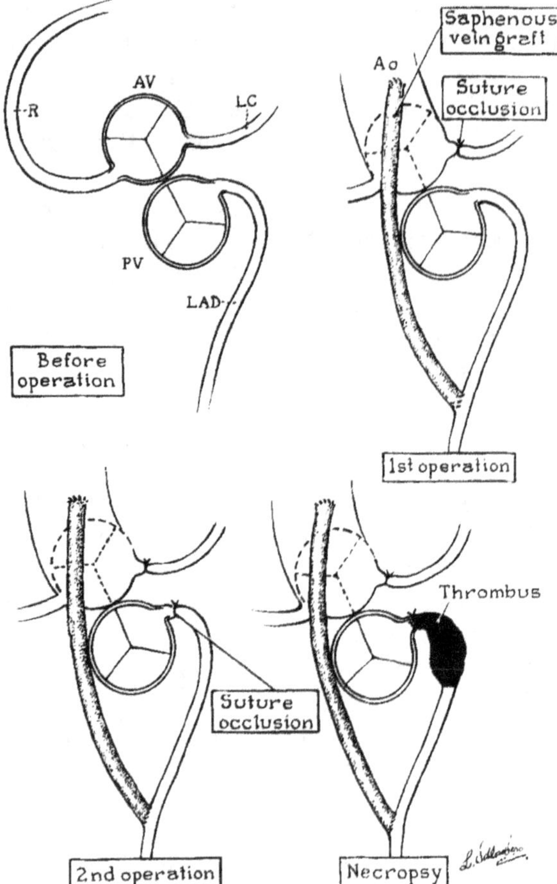

Fig. 4. Diagram showing sequence of events in a 32-year-old man in whom the left anterior descending *(LAD)* coronary artery arose from the pulmonary trunk. Before operation he was asymptomatic but had a precordial continuous murmur. At the first operation, the left circumflex *(LC)* coronary artery was inadvertently ligated rather than the LAD. At the second operation, performed 3 days after the first, a conduit was inserted between ascending aorta and LAD. The patient died suddenly soon after jogging 9 months after the cardiac operations. Obviously, if operation is to be performed for this anomaly, the anomalously arising artery must be clearly identified before ligation. *Ao* = aorta; *AV* = aortic valve; *LC* = left circumflex coronary artery; *PV* = pulmonic valve; *R* = right coronary artery. (From Roberts WC, and Robinowitz M: Am J Cardiol **54**:1381, 1984. Reproduced by permission.)

ischemic changes in each. Chest x-ray films in six of the seven adults disclosed normal-sized cardiac silhouettes in three and cardiac enlargement in three; the latter was mild in two and severe in one. Right-sided cardiac catheterization, performed in at least six patients, disclosed normal pressures in each and oxygen step-up in the PT in two. Coronary angiograpy with injection of contrast material in the right and LC coronary arteries in all seven adults disclosed that each of these two arteries in all seven patients was large, occasionally also tortuous, and

that the LAD was filled by extensive collateral vessels from both the right and LC coronary arteries. Injection of contrast material into the PT did not cause filling of the LAD; when the LAD, however, was filled by injections into either the right or LC coronary artery, contrast material did enter the PT through the LAD, which was filled by collateral vessels.

Of the eight reported adults, operative treatment was carried out in six, four of whom preoperatively had angina; in two patients, the PT was opened and the ostium of the LAD was obliterated by sutures, and in two the LAD was ligated just proximal to its entrance into the PT and a reversed saphenous vein was inserted from the ascending aorta to the LAD. One patient, a 32-year-old asymptomatic man reported by Roberts and Robinowitz,[62] inadvertently had suture occlusion of the LC rather than of the LAD, with insertion of a saphenous vein from the aorta to the LAD at the first operation (Fig. 4). At the second operation 3 days later, the LAD was ligated proximally (Fig. 4). This patient died suddenly while jogging 9 months postoperatively. Of the five symptomatic patients who had operative treatment, angina disappeared in three and persisted in one. Two patients had repeat coronary and left ventricular angiography 24 and 36 months, respectively, after operation; in each, the right and LC coronary arteries were much smaller than they had been preoperatively, and the collateral vessels between the right and LC coronary arteries and the LAD coronary artery had disappeared. One patient had persistent angina postoperatively and the distal portions of both the right and LC coronary arteries (36 months postoperatively) were quite narrowed; the cause of narrowing was unclear. Left ventricular angiograms, performed in five adults, were normal in three, and in the other two the apical portion of the left ventricle was akinetic in one and aneurysmal in one. Repeat left ventricular angiography in these latter two patients disclosed better overall contractions in one and no change in one.

The presence of both subjective and objective evidence of myocardial ischemia in six of the eight reported adults and the disappearance of angina and of the collateral vessels between the two coronary arteries arising from the aorta and the LAD arising from the PT supports the view that operative treatment is proper for patients with this coronary anomaly. Whether LAD ligation alone is enough, or whether ligation plus insertion of a conduit between the aorta and LAD is preferable, is unclear. Direct connection of the LAD to aorta in this situation appears technically inadvisable. Four of the six patients in whom operation was performed had angina pectoris. Two patients were asymptomatic preoperatively. Obviously, no data are available on the advisability of operation in an asymptomatic person in whom the LAD arises from the PT, but it appears reasonable to believe that the operative therapy in this circumstance is proper. If an operation is to be performed, however, clear identification of the anomalous artery before ligation is mandatory.

Left circumflex coronary artery from the pulmonary trunk.

Effler et al.[64] mentioned an 8-year-old boy (their case No. 7) who by angiogram had a LC coronary artery attached to a pulmonary artery (which one was not mentioned); the correct diagnosis was not confirmed anatomically. Honey et al.[65] described a 13-year-old boy who had aortic isthmic coarctation, right aortic arch, bicuspid aortic valve, and origin of the LC coronary artery from the right main pulmonary artery. Chaitman et al.[66] described a 14-year-old asymptomatic girl in whom the LC apparently arose from the PT. Ott et al.[67] described an 8-year-old girl, also with a bicuspid aortic valve, in whom the LC coronary artery arose from the right main coronary artery. No adults have been reported with origin of the LC coronary artery from any pulmonary artery.

Accessory coronary artery from pulmonary trunk.

The most common accessory coronary artery arising from the PT is a conus artery. Origin of this small coronary artery from the PT is of no functional significance.

ORIGIN OF 1 OR 2 CORONARY ARTERIES FROM THE PULMONARY TRUNK WITHOUT ORIGIN OF A CORONARY ARTERY FROM THE AORTA

At least 12 patients with origin of both LM and right coronary arteries from the PT have been reported, and all died during the first month of life, usually in the first 1 or 2 days.[68-77] Thus, nearly all of these infants had patent ductus arteriosus. Most had other major anomalies of the heart or great arteries. At least two patients have been described in whom a single coronary artery arose from PT and no coronary artery arose from the aorta.[78, 79] Feldt et al.[78] described a 7-year-old girl who had a ductus closed at age 6 and a ventricular septal defect (VSD) closed just before death. At necropsy, a single coronary arose for the PT and the mitral valve was stenotic. Monselise et al.[79] described a 1-year-old boy with a VSD and a single coronary artery arising from the PT. Survival in these two patients was made possible by the presence of the associated congenital anomalies which allowed systemic pressure in the PT.

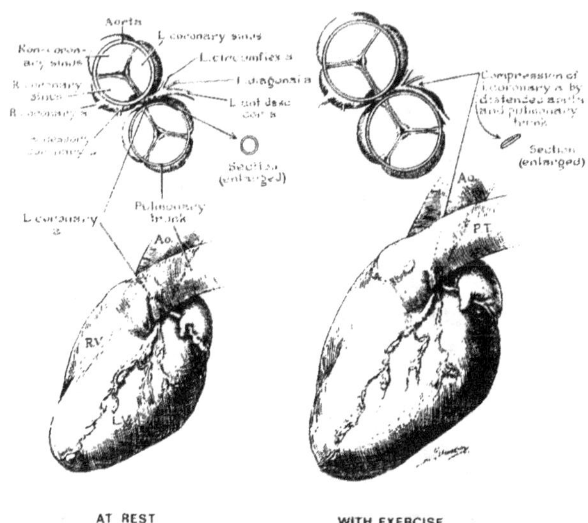

Fig. 5. Diagram showing a proposed mechanism by which origin of the left *(L)* main coronary artery *(a)* from the right sinus of Valsalva causes nonfatal or fatal cardiac dysfunction.

ANOMALOUS ORIGIN OF 1 OR MORE CORONARY ARTERIES FROM THE AORTA

Both *left main* and right coronary arteries from the *right* aortic sinus

Classification of the anomaly. This condition has been reviewed recently by Barth and Roberts.[80] Anomalous origin of the LM coronary artery from the right sinus of Valsalva can be classified into four major groups, according to the course taken by the LM in relation to the aorta and PT en route to the left side of the heart. The LM may course anterior to the PT, posterior to the aorta,[81] within the ventricular septum beneath the right ventricular infundibulum,[82] or between the aorta and PT (Fig. 5). When the LM passes anterior to the PT over the right ventricular infundibulum, symptoms of myocardial ischemia have not been reported unless significant coronary arterial narrowing due to atherosclerotic plaque was present. With the exception of the 12-year-old girl with this anomaly described by Murphy et al,[83] symptoms of myocardial ischemia have not been reported when the LM arises from the right sinus of Valsalva and courses posterior to the aorta.

Review of published reports. At least 43 necropsy patients have been reported with origin of the LM coronary artery from the right sinus of Valsalva, with coursing between the aorta and PT.[80, 81, 84-96] In nine, death was unrelated to the anomaly and symptoms of myocardial ischemia were absent during life. In the other 34 patients, death was of coronary origin. Of the 34 patients, 26 (76%) died

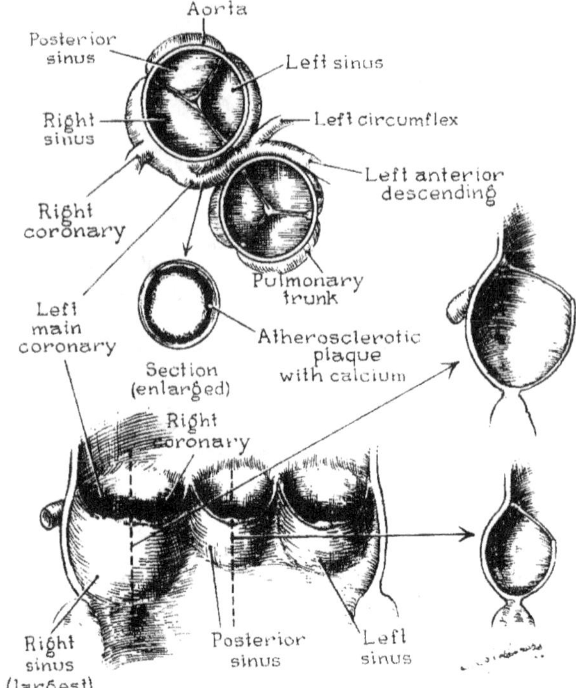

Fig. 6. Drawing of an anomalously arising left main coronary artery from the right sinus of Valsalva in an 81-year-old man (DCMEO No. 80-04-332) who never had evidence of cardiac dysfunction and who died of a noncardiac condition. The wall of the anomalously arising left main coronary artery is heavily calcified. (From Barth CW III, and Roberts WC: J Am Coll Cardiol **7**:366, 1986. Reproduced by permission.)

before age 20 years and the other eight (24%) died at ages ranging from 49 to 82 years (mean 64). Of the 26 patients who died young, 25 (96%) died suddenly during or shortly after vigorous exertion and one died of acute myocardial infarction, having survived for 19 hours after initial collapse, which likewise occurred shortly after exertion. Of the 14 patients where information was provided, 10 had had symptoms before the final collapse; there was exertional syncope in six, angina in four, and exertional dyspnea in one. Of the 26 young patients, 24 (92%) were male. At necropsy, 5 of the 26 patients had histologic evidence of myocardial necrosis; one patient apparently had atherosclerotic narrowing in the anomalous LM coronary artery.

Mechanism of death in older patients with the anomaly. Of the eight patients who died after age 20 years, seven were men. Four died of consequences of acute myocardial infarction: one died suddenly; one died of a noncardiac cause (alcoholism) (Fig. 6); the mode of death in the other two was not described. Symptoms of cardiac dysfunction were described in only one of the eight patients. Histologic evidence of myocardial necrosis or fibrosis was present in five, absent in one, and not discussed in two patients. Of the eight older patients, six apparently had significant coronary narrowing by atherosclerotic plaque in the abnormal and/or normally coursing arteries. One patient lacked the circumflex branch of the LM artery.

While it is clear from current necropsy information that this anomaly can cause sudden death at a young age, the role the anomaly plays in those who have survived past age 20 years is less clear. One of the two older patients reported by Barth and Roberts[80] appears to be the only one thus far reported in whom fatal myocardial ischemia could be attributed entirely to the coronary anomaly. Why this patient had fatal myocardial ischemia late in life after decades without symptoms is unclear. Possibly, the excessive cardiac weight (500 gm) was a factor. Why other older patients survive into the ninth decade free of symptoms of cardiac dysfunction is not clear either.

Pathogenesis of myocardial ischemia. The precise mechanism by which anomalous origin of the LM coronary artery from the right sinus of Valsalva with coursing between the PT and aorta causes myocardial ischemia is unclear. In each of the five patients reported by Barth and Roberts,[80] the normal RCA arose at an angle more or less perpendicular to the center of the aortic lumen, and it coursed directly away from the aorta; in contrast, the LM coronary artery arose from the aortic lumen at roughly a 180-degree angle to the center of the aorta. After takeoff, the anomalously arising LM was adherent to the wall of the aorta for roughly 1.5 cm as it coursed to the left side of the heart between the PT and aorta. Additionally, the ostium of the anomalously arising LM was slit-like, with the largest diameter in a cephalad-caudal direction; in contrast, the ostium of the normally arising RCA was circular and larger. The firmly anchored root of the PT appears to present a potential barrier against which the LM could be compressed by expansion of the aortic root that occurs during increased intra-aortic pressure associated with exertion. The LM coronary artery, of course, is equivalent to two arteries in the sense that it is responsible for supplying coronary blood flow to the major portion of the left ventricle; therefore significant reduction of flow through it is particularly perilous. While it is likely that the narrowed LM orifice has the potential to diminish flow through it, an actual reduction appears to be significant only during or immediately following exertion in those individuals without associated atherosclerosis.

Association of death with exertion. The association of death with exertion can be explained by three factors. (1) Myocardial oxygen requirements increase with exertion; therefore, any obstruction to coronary flow is more likely to result in myocardial ischemia. (2) It is likely that outward expansion of the roots of both the aorta and PT during exertion causes further compression of the ostial lumen of the LM. (3) The LM, as it courses between the aorta and PT, could be compressed against the root of the PT where it is firmly anchored to the infundibular septum when the aortic root and PT dilate during exertion. The fact that sudden exertional death and nonfatal myocardial ischemia have been seen in persons in whom the LM originates from the proximal RCA and then courses between the great arteries[81, 85]—and who therefore do not have the abnormal oblique take-off of the LM nor the slit-like ostium in the right sinus of Valsalva—suggests that hemodynamic compression (hemodynamic vise) of the LM between the great arteries cannot be excluded as an additional mechanism of myocardial ischemia. Davia et al.[97] described a 14-year-old boy who had two "exertionally related myocardial infarctions" due to this anomaly, underwent surgical enlargement of the narrowed LM ostium, and is asymptomatic during heavy labor 9 years later. This case lends further support to the theory that the primary mechanism causing myocardial ischemia is related to the narrowed LM ostium.

Usefulness of exercise electrocardiography in diagnosis. The usefulness of stress electrocardiography in identifying the ischemic nature of this anomaly in young persons has received little attention. The fact that one patient reported by Barth and Roberts,[80] a 14-year-old boy, had a normal stress test 1 month before death prompted them to review previous experience with stress electrocardiography in young patients with isolated anomalous origin of the LM from the right sinus of Valsalva with coursing of the LM between the aorta and PT. Results of stress electrocardiography[6, 81, 91, 98] in seven patients disclosed that three had abnormal stress ECGs (ECG evidence of ischemia or ventricular arrythmia) and four had normal stress ECGs. In three of the latter four, however, the test was not at maximal effort. Two of the seven, both of whom had normal submaximal stress electrocardiography, subsequently died suddenly. The other five patients had surgery. It is clear that the stress ECG, particularly that which is submaximal in effort, is not a reliable screening test for this anomaly in young patients who present with exertional syncope, angina, and even acute myocardial infarction.

Differential diagnosis and means of diagnosis. Young patients with this anomaly often present with exertional syncope, dizziness, and angina, but other cardiovascular abnormalities, such as hypertrophic cardiomyopathy and aortic valve stenosis, can present in a similar manner and therefore must be distinguished. The diagnostic approach taken with these young patients must take into account the fallibilities of the various noninvasive tests in identifying this potentially fatal coronary anomaly. The resting ECG is normal in almost all young persons with this anomaly and therefore it is not helpful. Physical examination may provide important clues to the noncoronary causes of these symptoms, i.e., murmurs and peripheral pulses characteristic for aortic stenosis or hypertrophic cardiomyopathy. Echocardiography also is helpful in assessing for or confirming aortic stenosis or hypertrophic cardiomyopathy. Liberthson et al.[99] reported a 54-year-old woman with angina pectoris in whom cross-sectional echocardiography identified anomalous origin of the LM coronary artery from the proximal RCA with coursing of the LM between the aorta and PT. Echocardiography, while potentially useful, has not been reported to have successfully identified origin of the LM directly from the right sinus of Valsalva. Continuous ambulatory electrocardiography may identify significant arrhythmias, but it provides no help in identifying the cause of the arrhythmias. If the noncoronary causes of exertional syncope and angina are not identified, then more extensive evaluation is dictated to exclude the possibility of anomalous origin of the LM. As has been demonstrated, stress electrocardiography does not always identify myocardial ischemia in young patients with this coronary anomaly who are at risk for sudden death, but it should be done and it should be carried to maximal effort if evidence of myocardial ischemia is not identified at lower levels of exercise. If stress electrocardiography is abnormal, then angiographic assessment of coronary anatomy is dictated.[100, 101] If maximal stress electrocardiography is normal, then coronary angiography must still be considered in boys with clear cut exercise-induced symptoms. The usefulness of thallium stress electrocardiography for diagnosis of this anomaly is uncertain. The patient reported by Mustafa et al.[98] had normal thallium stress electrocardiography. Finally, in the specific case of exertional syncope at a young age, particularly in males, coronary angiography should be done after a second episode of syncope. Angiography should be considered, however, after a single episode if no other clear cause of exertional syncope is evident by noninvasive testing.

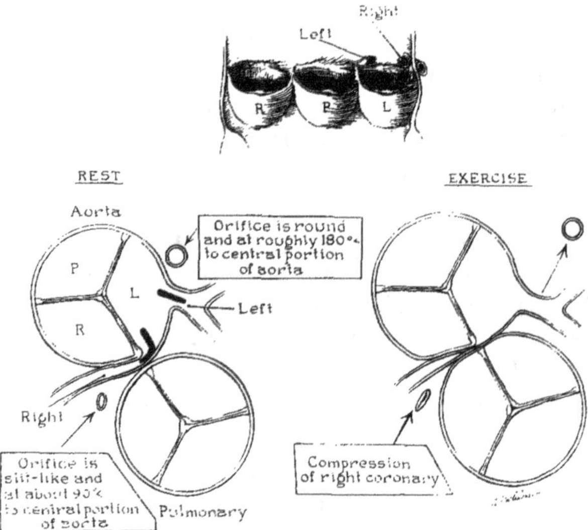

Fig. 7. Diagram showing mechanism by which origin of the right coronary artery arising from the left sinus of Valsalva might cause fatal or nonfatal cardiac dysfunction. (From Roberts WC, et al: Am J Cardiol **49**:863, 1982. Reproduced by permission.)

Management of patients with the anomaly. Once the origin of both LM and right coronary arteries from the right sinus with coursing of the LM between the great arteries has been diagnosed, at least in younger individuals, operative therapy appears warranted for the prevention of sudden death and for relief of exercise-induced symptoms of myocardial ischemia. Various operative approaches for revascularization have been described. Aortocoronary conduits, either saphenous vein or mammary artery, or both, to the LAD and LC coronary systems have resulted in relief of symptoms and in relief of objective evidence of myocardial ischemia in several patients.[99, 102, 103] Other surgical approaches have also been successful. Davia et al.[97] described a 14-year-old boy who had had two myocardial infarcts and subsequently underwent surgical enlargement of the narrowed LM coronary ostium by the extension of an incision from the ostium through the common wall of the aorta and the anomalous artery over the intercoronary commissure. He was free of symptoms and active 9 years later, despite the presence of mild aortic regurgitation due to the procedure. Four patients, aged 12 to 36 years, have undergone an operation of a similar nature to reestablish the normal anatomic location of the LM origin to the left sinus of Valsalva by incising along the course of the left sinus of Valsalva and joining the intima of the vessel to the aorta, resulting in a new ostium.[6, 98] No evidence of ischemia was present in a follow-up period of 10 to 36 months.

BOTH LEFT MAIN AND *RIGHT* CORONARY ARTERIES FROM THE *LEFT* AORTIC SINUS.

Origin of the RCA from the left sinus of Valsalva has until recently been considered a minor congenital anomaly of no clinical significance.

Frequency. This anomaly is missed probably as frequently at necropsy as it is observed. Its true occurrence at necropsy therefore is really not known. It appears, however, that this anomaly is more frequent than origin of both right and LM coronary arteries from the right sinus with subsequent coursing of the LM between the aorta and PT. At necropsy, I have seen five cases of origin of both LM arteries and RCAs from the right sinus and 16 cases of origin of both coronary arteries from the left sinus of Valsalva, with coursing of either the LM or RCA between the aorta and PT.

Angiographically, origin of both coronary arteries from the left sinus is more frequent than origin of both from the right sinus, because patients with the former are more likely to have evidence of myocardial ischemia. Liberthson et al.,[92] during the same time period, observed at coronary angiography nine patients in whom both LM and RCA arose from the right sinus and nine in whom both arose from the left sinus of Valsalva, with either the LM or the RCA passing between the aorta and PT.

Evidence of myocardial ischemia. With patients in whom both coronary arteries arise from the left aortic sinus with the RCA passing between the aorta and PT, it is unclear how many during life have evidence of myocardial ischemia and how many do not. Roberts et al.[104] collected reports describing at necropsy 26 patients with origin of both coronary arteries from the left sinus, and not a single patient had had symptoms of cardiac dysfunction and in none could death be attributed to the anomaly. In contrast, analysis of published data on 34 other patients in whom this congenital anomaly was detected by coronary angiography disclosed that at least 12 had had symptoms of cardiac dysfunction unassociated with significant coronary atherosclerosis or a noncoronary cardiac condition.[81, 92, 105-111] Of the 12, three had had acute myocardial infarcts, seven had angina pectoris, one had syncope, and one had nonfatal ventricular fibrillation. Of the 12 necropsy patients with this coronary anomaly reported by Roberts et al.[104] three died suddenly, two clearly during exertion, and two of them previously had had either angina or syncope. One of the three patients, a 23-year-old woman, became symptomatic only after she became a long-distance runner; she had frequent episodes of ventricular tachycardia. At necropsy, two of these three symptomatic patients had grossly visible left ventricular scars. Subsequently, Hanzlick and Stivers[112-114] reported a 26-year-old marathon runner who was training for the Iron-man Triathlon. He collapsed and died just past the finish line of a 13.5-mile race. This patient previously had had two episodes of abnormally severe dyspnea after long runs. Brandt et al.[111] reported a 35-year-old man who had at that age developed periodic substernal chest pain, one episode being acute myocardial infarction. He underwent operation with placement of a cephalic vein between the ascending aorta and the RCA. Doppler probe studies of this patient objectively confirmed that the coronary anomaly caused left ventricular functional impairment and that it impaired coronary artery reserve. Coronary reserve was returned to normal by the operation and the patient had been asymptomatic during the entire 9-month period after operation. Isner et al.[115] reported a 23-year-old man who developed severe chest pain after ingestion of a heavy meal, went to bed, and later was found dead in bed. This patient had had occasional episodes of chest pain before his sudden death.

Mechanism of myocardial ischemia. The mechanism of ischemia appears to be the same as in patients in whom both coronary arteries arise from the right sinus of Valsalva, just as long as one of the major coronary arteries courses between the aorta and PT. There are three possibilities: (1) the slit-like orifice of the anomalously arising coronary artery is compressed closed or nearly so as the aorta dilates with exertion; (2) the anomalous artery itself is compressed by the aorta and PT as it courses between these two arteries, which dilate with exertion; or (3) both factors 1 and 2 (Fig. 7). The upright nature of the slit-like orifice of the anomalous artery prevents blood within the aortic lumen from flowing into the RCA during ventricular diastole without a peculiar direction of flow. In a 60-year-old man with this coronary anomaly, Keren et al.[110] demonstrated angiographically significant narrowing of the RCA as it coursed between the two great arteries during ventricular *systole.*

Treatment. In contrast to the situation in which both coronary arteries arise from the right aortic sinus, therapy in the situation in which both coronary arteries arise from the left aortic sinus is not as clear-cut. In the former group of patients, operative intervention is indicated, even in the asymptomatic patient, to prevent fatal or nonfatal myocardial ischemia. In that situation, however, it is the LM coronary artery which has a slit-like orifice and which courses between the aorta and PT. The LM, of course, is not one but really two major coronary

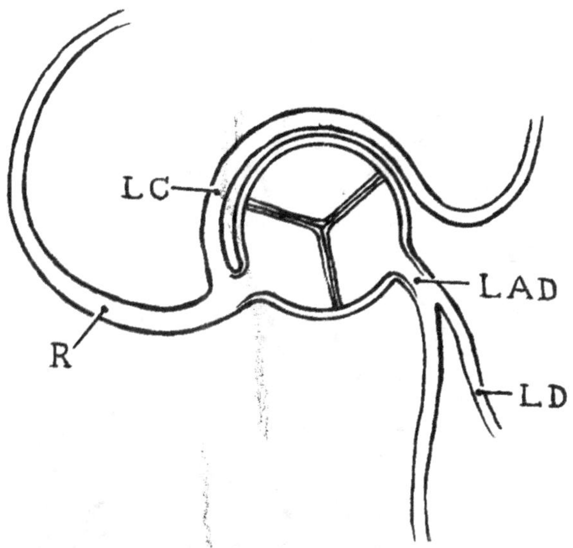

Fig. 8. Diagram showing origin of left circumflex *(LC)* coronary artery arising as the first branch of the right *(R)* coronary artery and then coursing posterior to the aorta before reaching the left atrioventricular sulcus. The left anterior descending *(LAD)* coronary artery arises from the left sinus of Valsalva. *LD* = left diagonal.

arteries. When both coronary arteries arise from the left aortic sinus, only one major coronary artery, the RCA, arises from a slit-like orifice and courses between the aorta and PT. In the latter situation, there appears no justification for operative intervention unless the patient has developed clinical signs of symptoms of myocardial ischemia. Sudden death as the initial manifestation of this coronary anomaly is extremely rare. Sudden death in almost all reported patients has been preceded by other symptoms of myocardial ischemia. If symptoms or signs of myocardial ischemia, however, have occurred, operative therapy is clearly warranted.

BOTH LEFT MAIN AND RIGHT CORONARY ARTERIES FROM THE POSTERIOR AORTIC SINUS.

To my knowledge, origin of both LM arteries and RCAs from the posterior sinus of Valsalva has never been reported.

BOTH RIGHT AND LEFT CIRCUMFLEX CORONARY ARTERIES FROM THE RIGHT AORTIC SINUS (OR ORIGIN OF THE LEFT CIRCUMFLEX FROM THE RIGHT CORONARY ARTERY) AND THE LEFT ANTERIOR DESCENDING CORONARY ARTERY FROM THE LEFT AORTIC SINUS

Initial description. The first description of this anomaly was by Antopol and Kugel[116] in 1933. These authors described four cases in adults (one a man; sex in other three not stated) at necropsy. In three the LC arose from the right sinus of Valsalva and in

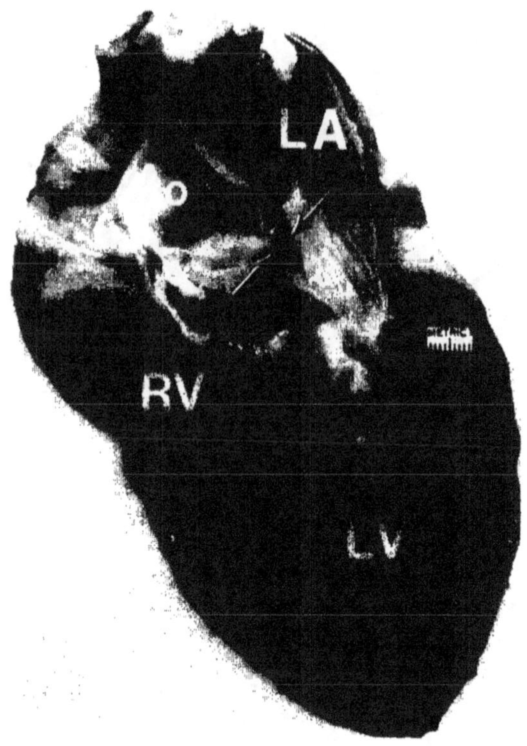

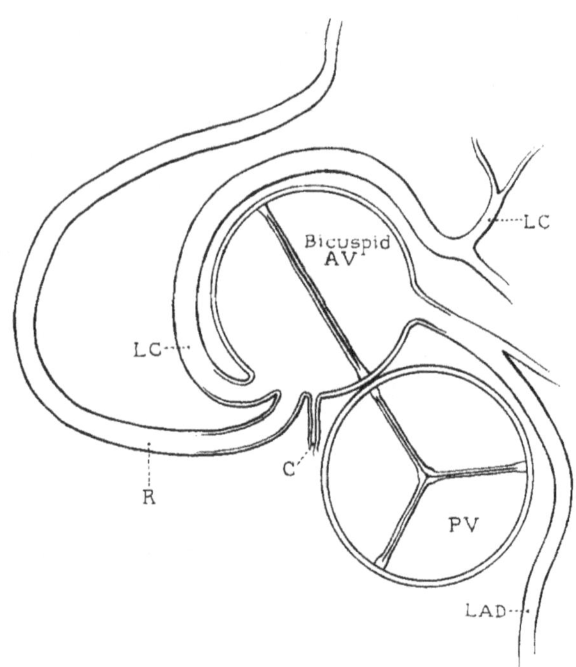

Fig. 9. Anteroposterior longitudinal view of the heart (SH No. A81-20) showing the course of an anomalously arising left circumflex coronary artery *(arrows)* between the aorta *(Ao)* and the left atrium *(LA)* before reaching the left atrioventricular sulcus. The left circumflex arose as the first branch of the right coronary artery. RV = right ventricle; LV = left ventricle.

Fig. 10. Origin of left circumflex *(LC)* coronary artery directly from the right anterior aspect of the aorta with retroaortic coursing to the left atrioventricular sulcus in a 43-year-old man (No. A81-5757) who died of complications of severe coronary atherosclerosis. Although congenitally biscuspid, the aortic valve *(AV)* appeared to have functioned normally. C = conus coronary artery; LAD = left anterior descending coronary artery; PV = pulmonic valve; R = right coronary artery.

one, from the RCA. In all four, the RCA coursed retrograde to the aorta before reaching the left atrioventricular sulcus. The LAD arose from the left sinus of Valsalva, and it coursed directly to this usual location. The LM was absent. When, however, the LC arises as the first branch of the RCA, the initial portion of the RCA then is equivalent to the normal "LM" coronary artery[117] (Fig. 8). When the LC arises directly from the right sinus of Valsalva or as the first branch of the RCA, the LC always follows a retroaortic course to the left atrioventricular sulcus (Fig. 9).

Frequency. Origin of the LC from the right aortic sinus or from the RCA is the most common anomaly of coronary arterial origin. Among 600 hearts of patients aged 30 to 89 years (100 hearts in each of the six decades), White and Edwards[118] found two cases of this anomaly—both were men, one aged 76 and one aged 81 years. Thus there is a frequency of 1 per 300 adults at necropsy. Ogden[53] found this anomaly in 14 necropsy patients studied in a 16-year period at the Yale–New Haven Hospital. I have seen this anomaly at necropsy in 15 patients aged 22 to 71 years (mean 50) (11 men); 12 had no associated

anomalies and three had valvular heart disease (rheumatic heart disease in two and a normally functioning bicuspid aortic valve in 1 [Fig. 10]). In 14 patients the coronary anomaly clearly was of no clinical significance; in one, a 22-year-old man who died suddenly while playing basketball, the anomaly may have been important. In eight patients the LC arose directly from the right aortic sinus and in seven patients it arose as the first branch of the RCA.

Of 2996 patients having selective coronary angiography, Page et al.[119] found that 20 (16 men) had origin of the LC from the right sinus of Valsalva or as the first branch of the RCA. In none of the 20 patients could cardiac dysfunction be attributed to the presence of this coronary anomaly (1 of the 20 also had origin of the LAD from the PT). Among 3750 coronary arteriograms reviewed by Chaitman et al.[105] 31 adults had anomalies of coronary origin, the most common (17 patients) being origin of the LC from the right sinus of Valsalva or as the first branch of the RCA. The sex of the 17 patients was not stated. Of 200 coronary angiograms reviewed by Ray et al.,[120] two—men aged 60 and 62 years—had

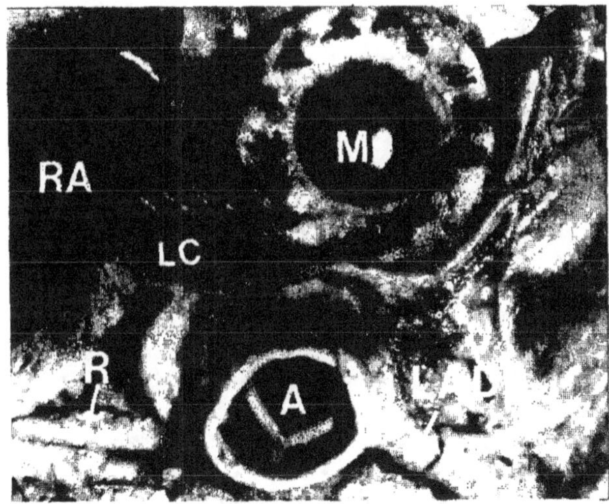

Fig. 11. Compression *(arrows)* of an anomalously arising left circumflex *(LC)* coronary artery from the right *(R)* coronary artery by the rings of prosthetic valves in both the aortic *(A)* and mitral *(M)* valve positions. *LAD* = left anterior descending coronary artery; *RA* = right atrium. (From Roberts WC, and Morrow AG: J Thorac Cardiovasc Surg **57**:834, 1969. Reproduced by permission.)

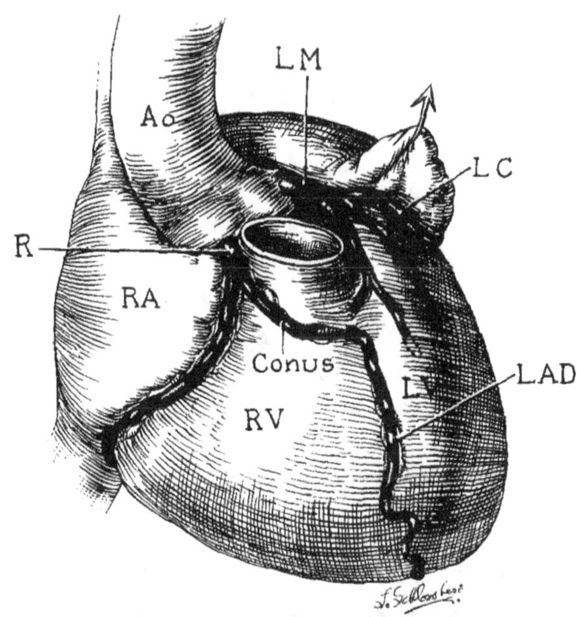

Fig. 12. Origin of the left anterior descending *(LAD)* from the right *(R)* coronary artery with coursing anterior to the right ventricular *(RV)* outflow tract in a 60-year-old man (No. A81-63) who died of consequences of severe coronary atherosclerosis. *Ao* = aorta; *LM* = left main; *LC* = left circumflex; *LV* = left ventricle; *RA* = right atrium. (From Robers WC, et al: AM HEART J **104**:638, 1982.)

origin of the LC from the RCA. Baltaxe and Wixson[121] reviewed 1000 consecutive coronary arteriograms performed mainly because of angina pectoris, and various coronary anomalies were found in nine; two of these, a 51-year-old woman and a 56-year-old man, had origin of the LC as the first branch of the RCA. Of 7000 patients having coronary angiograms, Kimbiris et al.[106] found anomalous aortic origin of one or more coronary arteries in 45; origin of the LC from the right sinus of Valsalva or as the first branch of the RCA was the most common of the five anomalies found, occurring in 26 patients (58%). The sex of the 26 patients was not stated. Of 21 cases of anomalous coronary origin reported by Liberthson et al.[122] (9 obtained at necropsy in a cardiovascular registry and 11 by selective coronary angiography), 11 had origin of the LC from the right sinus of Valsalva or as the first branch of the RCA. The mean age of the 11 patients was 54 years and eight were men.

Clinical significance. None, unless cardiac surgery is performed. If coronary perfusion during coronary bypass is limited to the artery arising from the left sinus of Valsalva, then the myocardium in the distribution of the LC coronary artery is not perfused. If perfusion is to the artery arising from the right sinus of Valsalva and if the LC arises as the first branch of the RCA, the tip of the perfusing cannula might be past the origin of the LC and again the myocardium dependent on the LC is deprived. If

both right and LC coronary arteries arise from the right sinus of Valsalva, one artery would be deprived by cannulation of only one of the coronary ostia in this sinus. If this anomaly is present in the patient who has replacement of both mitral and aortic valves, the fixation rings of the prostheses may compress the lumen of the LC coronary artery which courses in a path between the prosthetic anuli[123] (Fig. 11).

BOTH RIGHT AND LEFT ANTERIOR DESCENDING FROM THE RIGHT AORTIC SINUS (OR LAD FROM THE RIGHT CORONARY ARTERY) AND LEFT CIRCUMFLEX CORONARY ARTERY FROM THE LEFT AORTIC SINUS.

This is a rare anomaly in hearts without other congenital anomalies of the heart or great anterior vessels. Several varieties have been recognized or are possible: (1) origin of the LAD from the right sinus or from the RCA with coursing to the left side of the heart anterior to the right ventricular infundibulum (Fig. 12); (2) origin of the LAD from the right sinus of Valsalva or directly from the RCA with coursing to the left side of the heart between the aorta and PT (to my knowledge, this pattern has not been observed but is theoretically possible); (3) origin of the LAD from the right aortic sinus or directly from the aorta with coursing to the left side of the heart in

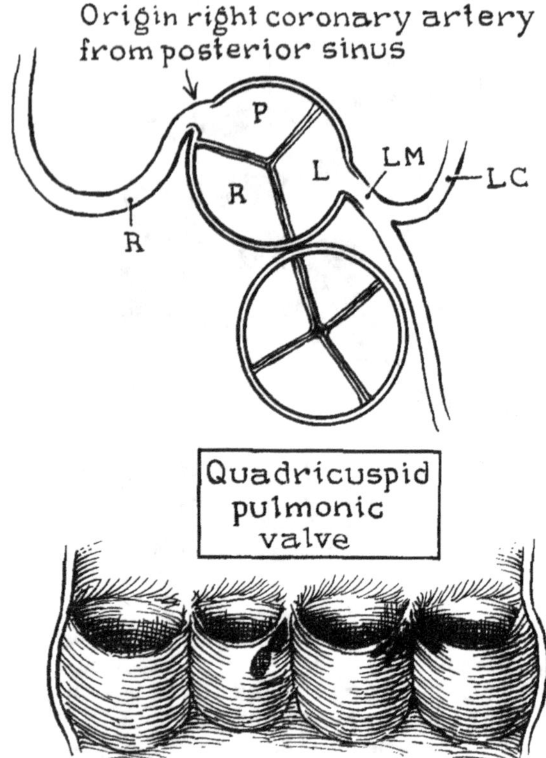

Fig. 13. Origin of the right *(R)* coronary artery from the posterior *(P)* aortic sinus in a 19-year-old man (DCMEO No. 83-09-602) who died suddenly while playing basketball. The pulmonic valve was quadricuspid. The cause of sudden death was not determined. Whether the coronary anomaly played a role in the sudden death is unclear.

the ventricular septum beneath the right ventricular infundibulum.

RIGHT CORONARY ARTERY FROM THE POSTERIOR AORTIC SINUS AND THE LEFT MAIN CORONARY ARTERY FROM THE LEFT AORTIC SINUS.

This is an extremely rare anomaly in hearts without other congenital anomalies. Vlodaver et al.[124] found this anomaly in only one heart among their huge collection. That patient was a 72-year-old man who died from atherosclerotic coronary artery disease. I have seen this anomaly once (Fig. 13). The patient was a 19-year-old boy who died suddenly while playing basketball (DCMEO No. 83-09-602). It seemed unlikely that the anomaly was associated with the boy's sudden death because the heart weighed 450 gm, a weight which is clearly abnormal. The cause of the cardiomegaly, however, is unknown. I have observed one heart in which the ostium of the RCA was located just cephalad to the most cephalad extension of the commissures between the right and posterior aortic valve cusps (GT No. 85A-143). This patient was a 79-year-old man who died of consequences of atherosclerosis.

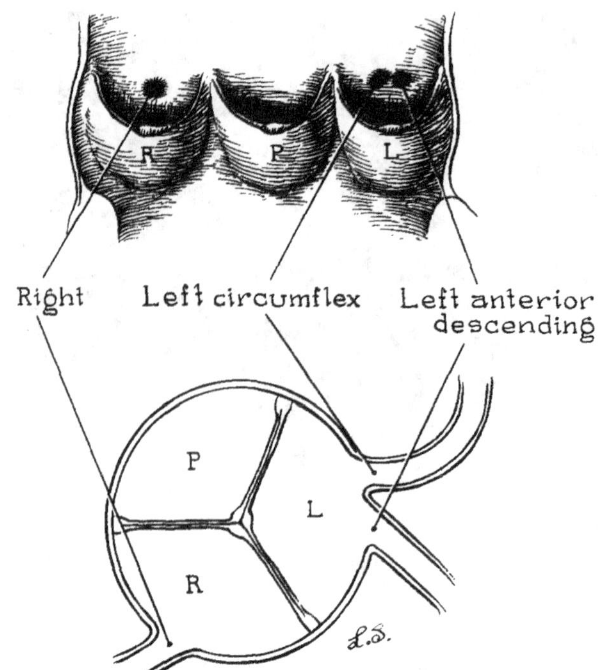

Fig. 14. Drawing of aorta showing origin of each of the left circumflex and left anterior descending coronary arteries from a separate ostium in the left *(L)* sinus of Valsalva. *R* = right and *P* = posterior sinus of Valsalva or cusp. (From Dicicco BS, et al: AM HEART J **104:**153, 1982.)

LEFT MAIN CORONARY ARTERY FROM THE POSTERIOR AORTIC SINUS AND RIGHT CORONARY ARTERY FROM THE RIGHT AORTIC SINUS.

To my knowledge this anomaly has not been reported in a patient without other anomalies of the heart or great vessels. I have examined a heart, however, in which the ostium of the LM coronary artery arose just above the commissure between the left and posterior aortic valve cusps (SGAH No. A82-1). The patient was a 54-year-old man who died from atherosclerotic coronary artery disease. The anomaly did not appear to have clinical significance.

BOTH LEFT ANTERIOR DESCENDING AND LEFT CIRCUMFLEX CORONARY ARTERIES FROM A SEPARATE OSTIUM IN THE LEFT AORTIC SINUS WITH THE RIGHT CORONARY ARTERY FROM THE RIGHT AORTIC SINUS.

This anomaly is fairly common. Ogden[53] found this anomaly in six necropsy patients in a 16-year period. I have observed it at necropsy in nine patients aged 35 to 82 years (mean 60) (seven men), all seen in a 7-year period. Two of the nine patients were reported previously[125] (Fig. 14). In none of the 9 patients was the anomaly of clinical significance. One of the nine patients was a 60-year-old man (A82-79) who also had congenitally bicuspid pulomonic and aortic valves; both LAD and LC arose from a separate ostium to the left of the raphe or in the location of the normal left aortic sinus of Valsalva (Fig. 15). Zumbo et al.[126] found this anomaly in 21 of 2089 hearts at necropsy.

ORIGIN OF ONLY 1 CORONARY ARTERY FROM THE AORTA WITHOUT ORIGIN OF A CORONARY ARTERY FROM THE PULMONARY TRUNK (SINGLE CORONARY OSTIUM IN AORTA)

History. According to Smith,[127] "single coronary artery" (a misnomer in my view—"single aortic coronary ostium without a pulmonary artery coronary ostium" is better) was first described in Banchi[128] in 1903.

Classification. Several authors have suggested classifications for single coronary ostium. Smith[127] in 1950 suggested three groups. (1) A single coronary artery that follows the course of the RCA with continuation into the LC which continues as the LAD, *or* a single LM which branches into the LAD and LC, the latter of which extends across the crux to form the RCA. (2) After its origin from a single aortic ostium, the main trunk branches quickly into a right and LM coronary artery or into a right, LAD, and LC coronary artery which reach their usual location a relatively short distance from the aortic ostium. (3) The single coronary artery branches so atypically that there is little similarity to the normal coursing of the three major (right, LAD, and LC) coronary arteries. In Smith's review of previously reported necropsy cases, there were nine in group one unassociated with other major cardiovascular anomalies (aged 33 to 66 years; six men), 15 in group 2 (aged 35 to 65; 10 men), and only two in group 3 (aged 22 and 38; one man). Smith actually found 15 patients in group 3 but 13 of them had various other congenital anomalies of the heart and great arteries.

Ogden and Goodyear[129] in 1970 suggested a classification employing five types subdivided by the letters "R" and "L" to indicate whether the single coronary ostium was in the right or left aortic sinus of Valsalva. These authors followed this letter by numbers 1 to 5 to indicate the pattern of anatomic distribution of the branches according to their initial divisions. In cases of single right coronary ostium, types 1 to 5, the letters "a," "b," and "c" were added to indicate the course of the branches. This classification has logic, but it is incomplete.

Lipton et al.[130] proposed a classification based on their angiographic studies, and it employed features

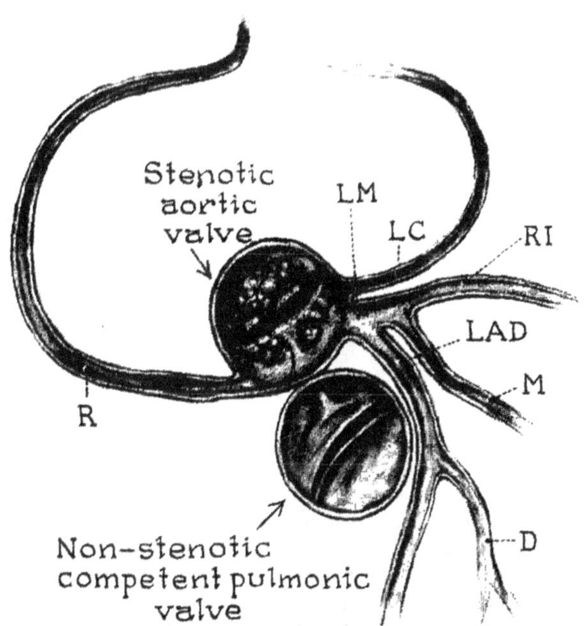

Fig. 15. Drawing showing origin of both left-sided coronary arteries directly from the left anterior side of the aorta in a 60-year-old man (No. A82-79) in whom both semilunar valves were congenitally bicuspid and the aortic valve was also stenotic. *D* = diagonal; *LAD* = left anterior descending; *LC* = left circumflex; *LM* = "left main"; *M* = marginal; *R* = right; *RI* = ramus intermedius.

of the classifications of both Smith[127] and Ogden and Goodyear.[129] These authors used the latter authors' "R" and "L" and "a" and "b" systems, but incorporated these letters into the three groups proposed by Smith. Thus, group 1 was designated R1 and L1; group 2 was designated R2-a and L2-a, R2-b and L2-b, and R2-p and L2-p; and group 3 included cases in which the LC and LAD arose separately from a single trunk arising from the right aortic sinus. The letter "a" indicated that the "transverse" branch from the single coronary artery passed "anterior" to the right ventricular infundibulum; "b" that it passed "between" the aorta and PT, and "p" that it passed retroaortic. This classification provides more easily memorable numbers and letters than that proposed by Ogden and Goodyear. I like this newer classification, but their group 3 is incomplete.

A purely descriptive classification of "single coronary artery" is presented in Table I.

Frequency. "Single coronary anomaly" is rare, particularly in the absence of other anomalies of the heart and great vessels. In 1968, Ogden (quoted by Ogden and Goodyear[129]) compiled 142 cases including 10 of his own. The male-to-female ratio was 1.4 to 1. The single coronary artery arose from the right aortic sinus in 70 cases (49%) and from the left aortic sinus in 64 cases (45%). Unfortunately, Ogden

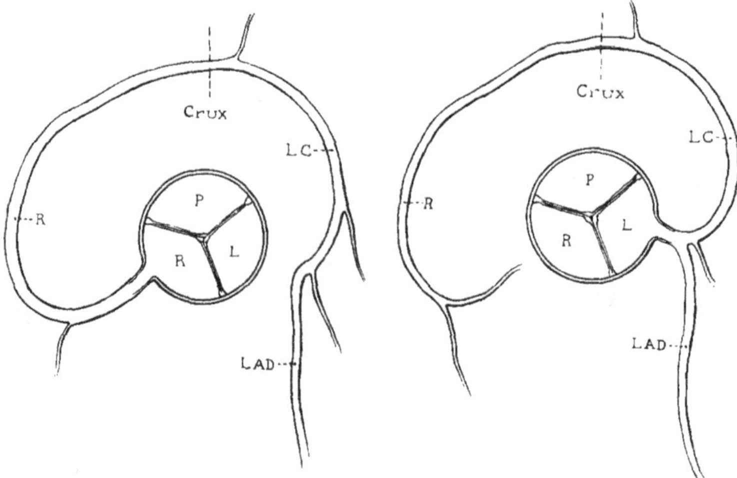

Fig. 16. Drawings of the two most common varieties of single coronary ostium. In one (*left*), the single ostium arises in the right aortic sinus and in the other (*right*), the single ostium arises in the left (*L*) aortic sinus. When the single coronary artery arises from the right aortic ostium, the right (*R*) coronary artery crosses the crux to continue as the left circumflex (*LC*), which in turn continues as the left anterior descending (*LAD*). When the single ostium is located in the left aortic sinus, the left main gives rise to the LAD and the LC, and LC crosses the crux to continue as the right coronary artery.

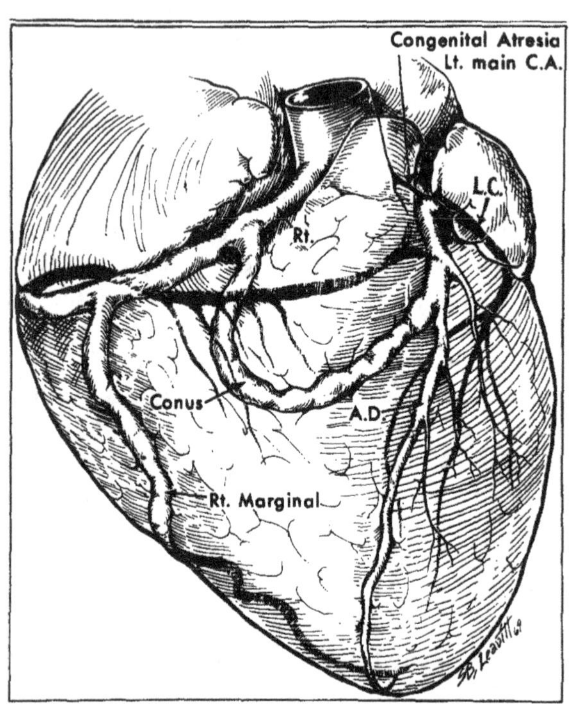

Fig. 17. Diagram of epicardial coronary arteries in a 60-year-old man (No. A69-61) who died suddenly as a consequence of severe coronary narrowing by atherosclerotic plaques but in whom the left (*Lt*) main coronary artery (*CA*) was congenitally atretic. This anomaly is equivalent to single coronary ostium with the single ostium in the right sinus of Valsalva. (From Fortuin NJ, and Roberts WC: Am J Med **50**:385, 1971. Reproduced by permission.)

included four cases in which a single LM coronary artery arose from the PT. The ages of the 142 patients ranged from 7 months to 20 years, and 41 (68%) of them had associated anomalies of the heart or great vessels; of the 82 patients aged 20 years or older, only five (6%) had associated anomalies of the heart or great arteries. Of the 46 cases with associated anomalies of the heart or great vessels, 17 (37%) had transposition of the great arteries, 10 (22%) had coronary artery fistula, and seven (15%) had bicuspid aortic valves; the remaining 12 patients (26%) had a variety of anomalies.

I have studied five adults at necropsy with single coronary ostium unassociated with other congenital cardiovascular defects. In two cases, both men, aged 39 and 73 years, a single LM pattern was present (Fig. 16). In one case, a 60-year-old man, the LM was congenitally atretic and the coronary pattern was of the single RCA type (Fig. 17). In one case, a 65-year-old man, the single artery arose in the left aortic sinus but the RCA coursed to the right between the aorta and PT after taking origin from the LM (Fig. 18). In the final case, a 69-year-old man with cardiovascular features of the Marfan syndrome but without the skeletal features of this syndrome, the single ostium was in the right aortic sinus with immediate origin of the LC with retroaortic course from the RCA and immediate origin of the LAD from the RCA, with coursing anterior to the right ventricular outflow tract.

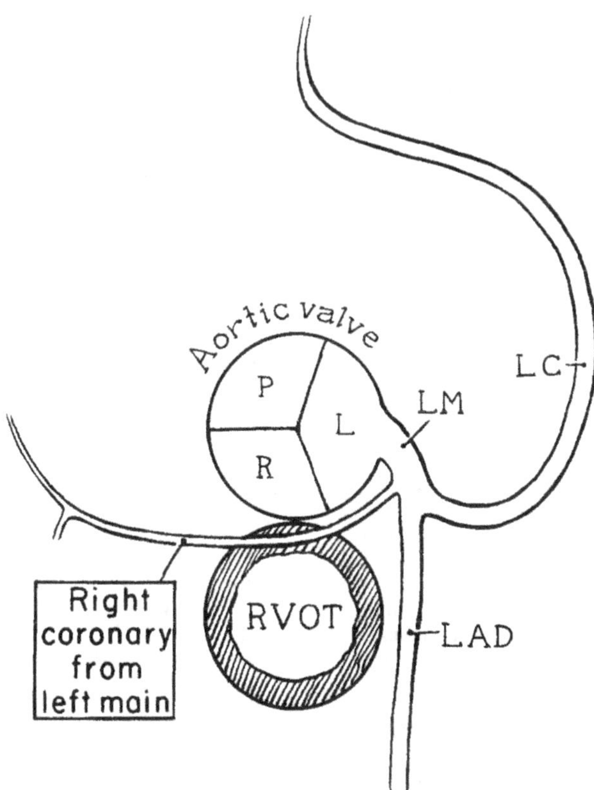

Fig. 18. Single coronary ostium with origin of the right coronary artery from the left main *(LM)* and coursing of the right coronary artery between aortic valve and right ventricular outflow tract *(RVOT)* on its way to the right atrioventricular sulcus in a 65-year-old man (DCVAH No. 84A-112) who never had signs or symptoms of cardiac dysfunction. *L* = left aortic sinus; *LAD* = left anterior descending; *LC* = left circumflex; *P* = posterior aortic sinus; *R* = right aortic sinus. (From Barbour DJ, and Roberts WC: Am J Cardiol **55**:609, 1985. Reproduced by permission.)

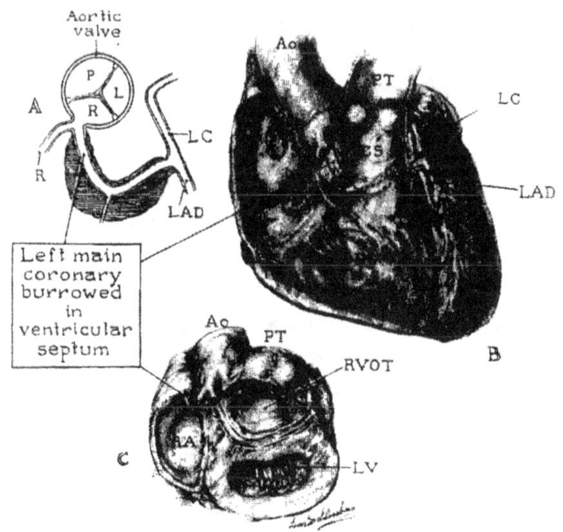

Fig. 19. Drawing of the heart in which the left main coronary artery arose from the right *(R)* aortic sinus and then the left main coursed behind the right ventricular outflow tract and within the crista supraventricular *(CS)* myocardium before entering the epicardium just anterior to the ventricular septum. The left main then divided into the left anterior descending *(LAD)* and left circumflex *(LC)* coronary arteries. This anomaly caused no cardiac dysfunction. *Ao* = ascending aorta; *L* = left aortic sinus; *LV* = left ventricle; *P* = posterior aortic sinus; *PT* = pulmonary trunk; *LV* = left ventricle; *R* = either right aortic sinus or right coronary artery; *RA* = right atrium; *RV* = right ventricle. (From Roberts WC, et al: Am Heart J **104**:303, 1982.)

Of the 142 cases analyzed by Ogden and Goodyear,[129] 31 (23%) had a single artery which did not branch (their type 1); 21 (15%) had two major branches with one coursing posterior to the aorta (type 2); 15 (11%) had two major branches with one branch coursing between the aorta and PT (type 3); 18 (13%) had two major branches with one branch coursing anterior to the PT (type 4); and seven patients (5%) had three major branches, all with origin of the single coronary artery in the right aortic sinus (type 5).

Of the 10 cases of single coronary artery diagnosed angiographically by Lipton et al.,[130] five had group 2R (a in one, b in two, and p in one), one had group 1L, and four had group 2L (b in three, and p in one). None of these 10 patients had other associated congenital cardiovascular anomalies; they ranged in aged from 39 to 64 years and eight were men.

Clinical significance. Although some patients have been described in whom symptoms of myocardial ischemia have occurred, the symptomatic patients nearly always have had associated atherosclerotic coronary disease, or valvular heart disease, or other major congenital anomalies of the heart or great arteries. Of course, severe atherosclerotic narrowing of the single coronary artery before it divides or narrowing of its ostium in the aorta may have particularly devastating consequences.

ORIGIN OF THE LM OR BOTH LAD AND LC CORONARY ARTERY FROM THE RCA WITH INTRAMYOCARDIAL COURSING TO THE LEFT SIDE OF THE HEART OF THE LM OR LAD IN THE VENTRICULAR SEPTUM BENEATH THE RIGHT VENTRICULAR INFUNDIBULUM.

At least 13 necropsy patients (10 men) have been described in whom a single aortic coronary ostium, located in the right aortic sinus, gave rise to the RCA. This in turn gave rise to the LM coronary artery, which coursed in the ventricular septum beneath the right ventricular infundibulum for about 5 cm before emerging in the epicardium just anterior to the ventricular septum where it gave off the LAD and LC branches (Fig. 19). These cases have been summarized by Roberts et al.[82] In none of the 13 patients was death, or myocardial dysfunction (if present) related to the coronary anomaly. These cases in which the LM coronary artery was in an intramyocardial location for about 5 cm indicate that tunneling of a major coronary artery—indeed, an artery equivalent to two major coronary arteries—has no functional significance in myocardium. Saner et al.[131] and Schulte et al.[132] reported single cases (a 73-year-old man and a 71-year-old woman) in whom the LAD arose either from the right aortic sinus or from the RCA and coursed in the ventricular septum beneath the right ventricular infundibulum before emerging just anterior to the ventricular septum. In neither patient had there been clinical evidence of myocardial ischemia.

REFERENCES

1. Abbott ME: Anomalous origin from the pulmonary arteries. *In* Osler W, editor: Osler's modern medicine, Its theories and practice. Philadelphia, 1908, Lea & Febiger, p. 420.
2. Abrikossoff A: Aneurysm des Linken Herzventrikels mit Abnromer Abganstelle der Linken Koronararterie von der Pulmonalis Bei Einem Funfmonatlichen Kinde. Virchows Arch Pathol Anat **203**:413, 1911.
3. Bland EF, White PD, Garland J: Congenital anomalies of the coronary arteries: Report of an unusual case associated with cardiac hypertrophy. Am Heart J **8**:787, 1933.
4. Fontana RS, Edwards JE: Congenital cardiac disease: A review of 357 cases studied pathologically. Philadelphia, 1962, W.B. Saunders Co., p. 291.
5. Thomas CS, Campbell WB, Alford WC Jr, Burrus GR, Stoney WS: Complete repair of anomalous origin of the left coronary artery in the adult. J Thorac Cardiovasc Surg **66**:439, 1973.
6. Donaldson RM, Raphael M, Radley-Smith R, Yacoub MH, Ross DN: Angiographic identification of primary coronary anomalies causing impaired myocardial perfusion. Cathet Cardiovasc Diagn **9**:237, 1983.
7. Edwards JE: Anomalous coronary arteries with special reference to arteriovenous-like communications. Circulation **17**:1001, 1958.
8. Edwards JE: The direction of blood flow in coronary arteries arising from the pulmonary trunk. Circulation **29**:163, 1964.
9. Moodie DS, Fyfe D, Gill CC, Cook SA, Lytle BW, Taylor PC, Fitzgerald R, Sheldon WC: Anomalous origin of the left coronary artery from the pulmonary artery (Bland-White-Garland syndrome) in adult patients: Long-term follow-up after surgery. Am Heart J **106**:381, 1983.
10. Jurishica AJ: Anomalous left coronary artery. Adult type. Am Heart J **54**:429, 1957.
11. George JM, Knowlan DM: Anomalous origin of the left coronary artery from the pulmonary artery in an adult. N Engl J Med **261**:993, 1959.
12. Lampe CFJ, Verheught APM: Anomalous left coronary artery. Adult type. Am Heart J **59**:769, 1960.
13. Liebman J, Hellerstein HK, Ankeney JL, Tucker A: The problem of the anomalous left coronary artery arising from the pulmonary artery in older children. Report of three cases. N Engl J Med **269**:486, 1963.
14. Talner NS, Halloran KH, Mahdavy M, Gardner TH, Hipona F: Anomalous origin of the left coronary artery from the pulmonary artery. A clinical spectrum. Am J Cardiol **15**:689, 1965.
15. Likar I, Criley JM, Lewis KB: Anomalous left coronary artery arising from the pulmonary artery in an adult. A review of the therapeutic problem. Circulation **33**:727, 1966.
16. Harthorne JW, Scannell JG, Dinsmore RE: Anomalous origin of the left coronary artery. Remediable cause of sudden death in adults. N Engl J Med **275**:660, 1966.
17. Wesselhoeft H, Fawcett JS, Johnson AL: Anomalous origin of the left coronary artery from the pulmonary trunk. Its clinical spectrum, pathology, and pathophysiology, based on a review of 140 cases with seven further cases. Circulation **38**:403, 1968.
18. Perry LW, Scott LP: Anomalous left coronary artery from pulmonary artery. Report of 11 cases; review of indications for and results of surgery. Circulation **41**:1043, 1970.
19. Askenazi J, Nadas AS: Anomalous left coronary artery originating from the pulmonary artery. Report of 15 cases. Circulation **51**:976, 1975.
20. Sabiston DC Jr, Floyd WL, McIntosh HD: Anomalous origin of the left coronary artery from the pulmonary artery in adults. Surgical management. Arch Surg **97**:963, 1968.
21. Usman A, Fernandez B, Uricchio JF, Nichols HT: Aberrant origin of left coronary artery combined with mitral regurgitation in an adult. Am J Cardiol **8**:130, 1961.
22. Burchell HB, Brown AL Jr: Anomalous origin or coronary artery from pulmonary artery masquerading as mitral insufficiency. Am Heart J **63**:388, 1962.
23. Fisher EA, Sepehri B, Lendrum B, Luken J, Levitsky S: Two-dimensional echocardiographic visualization of the left coronary artery in anomalous origin of the left coronary artery from the pulmonary artery. Pre- and postoperative studies. Circulation **63**:698, 1981.
24. Terai M, Nagai Y, Toba T: Cross-sectional echocardiographic findings of anomalous origin of left coronary artery from pulmonary artery. Br Heart J **50**:104, 1983.
25. Caldwell RL, Hurwitz RA, Girod DA, Weyman AE, Feigenbaum H: Two-dimensional echocardiographic differentiation of anomalous left coronary artery from congestive cardiomyopathy. Am Heart J **106**:710, 1983.
26. Robinson PJ, Sullivan ID, Kumpeng V, Anderson RH, MaCartney FJ: Anomalous origin of the left coronary artery from the pulmonary trunk. Potential for false negative diagnosis with cross sectional exhocardiography. Br Heart J **52**:272, 1984.
27. King DH, Danford DA, Huhta JC, Gutgesell HP: Noninvasive detection of anomalous origin of the left main coronary artery from the pulmonary trunk by pulsed Doppler echocardiography. Am J Cardiol **55**:608, 1985.
28. Gutgesell HP, Pinksy WW, DePuey EG: Thallium-201 myocardial perfusion imaging in infants and children; value in distinguishing anomalous left coronary artery from congestive cardiomyopathy. Circulation **61**:596, 1980.
29. Shem-Tov AA, Hegesh J, Schneeweiss A, Neufeld HN: Visualization of left coronary artery in anomalous origin of left coronary artery from pulmonary artery. Am Heart J **108**:621, 1984.
30. Sabiston DC Jr, Neill CA, Taussig HB: The direction of blood flow in anomalous left coronary artery arising from the pulmonary artery. Circulation **22**:591, 1960.
31. Rowe GG, Young WP: Anomalous origin of the coronary arteries with special reference to surgical treatment. J Thorac Cardiovasc Surg **39**:777, 1960.
32. Roche AHG: Anomalous origin of the left coronary artery from the pulmonary artery in the adult. Report of uneventful ligation in two cases. Am J Cardiol **20**:561, 1967.
33. Baue AE, Baum S, Blakemore WS, Zinsser HF: A later stage of anomalous coronary circulation with origin of the left coronary artery from the pulmonary artery. Coronary artery steal. Circulation **36**:878, 1967.

34. Reis RL, Cohen LS, Mason DT: Direct measurement of instantaneous coronary blood flow after total correction of anomalous left coronary artery. Circulation **39** and **40** (suppl I):229, 1969.

35. Somerville J, Ross DN: Left coronary artery from the pulmonary artery. Physiological considerations of surgical correction. Thorax **25**:207, 1970.

36. Neches WH, Mathews RA, Park SC, Lenox CC, Zuberbuhler JR, Siewers RD, Bahnson HT: Anomalous origin of the left coronary artery from the pulmonary artery. A new method of surgical repair. Circulation **50**:582, 1974.

37. Chaitman BR, Bourassa MG, Lesperance J, Grondin P: Anomalous left coronary artery from the pulmonary artery. An eight year angiographic follow-up after saphenous vein bypass graft. Circulation **51**:552, 1975.

38. Pinsky WW, Fagan LR, Mudd JGH, Willman VL: Subclavian–coronary artery anastomosis in infancy for the Blank-White-Garland syndrome. A three-year and five-year follow-up. J Thorac Cardiovasc Surg **72**:15, 1976.

39. Grace RR, Angelini P, Cooley DA: Aortic implantation of anomalous left coronary artery arising from pulmonary artery. Am J Cardiol **39**:608, 1977.

40. Wilson CL, Dlabal, PW, Holeyfield RW, Akins CW, Knauf DG: Anomalous origin of left coronary artery from pulmonary artery. Case report and review of literature concerning teenagers and adults. J Thorac Cardiovasc Surg **73**:887, 1977.

41. Shrivastava S, Castaneda AR, Moller JH: Anomalous left coronary artery from pulmonary trunk. Long-term follow-up after ligation. J Thorac Cardiovasc Surg **76**:130, 1978.

42. Wilson CL, Dlabal PW, McGuire SA: Surgical treatment of anomalous left coronary artery from pulmonary artery: Follow-up in teenagers and adults. AM HEART J **98**:440, 1979.

43. Donaldson RM, Raphael MJ, Yacoub MH, Ross DN: Hemodynamically significant anomalies of the coronary arteries. Surgical aspects. Thorac Cardiovasc Surg **30**:7, 1982.

44. Fisher J, McDonald G, Brinker J, Neill CA, Donahoo JS, Baughman KL: Transpulmonary artery correction of anomalous origin of the left coronary artery by saphenous vein graft. Cathet Cardiovasc Diagn **9**:373, 1983.

45. Savage RW, Glover MU, Utley JR: Reoperation for correction of anomalous origin of left coronary artery from the pulmonary artery with return of left ventricular function. Cathet Cardiovasc Diagn **10**:37, 1984.

46. Bagger JP, Vesterlund T, Nielsen TT: Cardiac metabolism and coronary hemodynamics before and after bypass surgery for anomalous origin of the left main coronary artery from the pulmonary trunk. Am J Cardiol **55**:864, 1985.

47. Brooks H St J: Two cases of an abnormal coronary artery of the heart arising from the pulmonary artery: with some remarks upon the effect of this anomaly in producing cirsoid dilation of the vessels. J Anat Physiol **20**:26, 1885 and 1886.

48. Monchelberg JG: Uber eine seltene Anomalie des Koronarterienabgangs. Zentralbl Herz Krankheiten **6**:441, 1914.

49. Schley J: Abnormer Ursprung der rechten Kranzarterie aus der Pulmonalis bei einem 61-jahringer Mann. Frankfurt Z Pathol **32**:1, 1925.

50. Jordan RA, DRy TJ, Edwards JE: Anomalous origin of the right coronary artery from the pulmonary trunk. Mayo Clin Proc **25**:673, 1950.

51. Cronk ES, Sinclair JG, Rigdon RH: An anomalous coronary artery arising from the pulmonary artery. AM HEART J **42**:906, 1951.

52. Tingelstad, JB, Lower RR, Eldredge WJ: Anomalous origin of the right coronary artery from the main pulmonary artery. Am J Cardiol **30**:670, 1972.

53. Ogden JA: Congenital anomalies of the coronary arteries. Am J Cardiol **25**:474, 1970.

54. Lerberg DB, Ogden JA, Zuberbuhler JR, Bahnson HT: Anomalous origin of the right coronary artery from the pulmonary artery. Ann Thorac Surg **27**:87, 1979.

55. Wald S, Stonecipher K, Baldwin BJ, Hutter DO: Anomalous origin of the right coronary artery from the pulmonary artery. Am J Cardiol **27**:677, 1971.

56. Eugstes GS, Oliva PB: Anomalous origin of the right coronary artery from the pulmonary artery. Chest **63**:294, 1973.

57. Achtel RA, Zaret BL, Iben AB, Hurley EJ: Surgical correction of congenital left coronary artery–main pulmonary artery fistula in association with anomalous right coronary artery. J Thorac Cardiovasc Surg **70**:46, 1975.

58. Bregman D, Brennan FJ, Singer A, Vinci J, Parodi EN, Cassarella WJ, Edie RN: Anomalous origin of right coronary artery from the pulmonary artery. J Thorac Cardiovasc Surg **72**:626, 1976.

59. Mintz GS, Iskandrian AS, Bemis CE, Mundth ED, Owens JS: Myocardial ischemia in anomalous origin of the right coronary artery from the pulmonary trunk. Proof of a coronary steal. Am J Cardiol **51**:610, 1983.

60. Worsham C, Sanders SP, Bulger BM: Origin of the right coronary artery from the pulmonary trunk: Diagnosis by two-dimensional echocardiography. Am J Cardiol **55**:232, 1985.

61. van Meurs-van Woezik H, Serruys PW, Reiber JH, Bos E, deVilleneuve VH: Coronary artery changes 3 years after reimplantation of an anomalous right coronary artery. Eur Heart J **5**:175, 1984.

62. Roberts WC, Robinowitz M: Anomalous origin of the left anterior descending coronary artery from the pulmonary trunk with origin of the right and left circumflex coronary arteries from the aorta. Am J Cardiol **54**:1381, 1984.

63. Donaldson RM, Thornton A, Raphael MJ, Sturridge MF, Emanuel RW: Anomalous origin of the left anterior descending coronary artery from the pulmonary trunk. Eur J Cardiol **10**:295, 1979.

64. Effler DB, Sheldon WC, Turner JJ, Groves LK: Coronary arteriovenous fistulae: Diagnosis and surgical management. Report of fifteen cases. Surgery **61**:41, 1967.

65. Honey M, Lincoln JCR, Osborne MP, de Bono DP: Coarctation of the aorta with right aortic arch. Report of surgical correction in 2 cases: One with associated anomalous origin of left circumflex coronary artery from the right pulmonary artery. Br Heart J **37**:937, 1975.

66. Chaitman BR, Bourassa MG, Lesperance J, Dominquez JLD, Saltiel J: Aberrant course of the left anterior descending coronary artery associated with anomalous left circumflex origin from the pulmonary artery. Circulation **52**:955, 1975.

67. Ott DA, Cooley DA, Pinsky WW, Mullins CE: Anomalous origin of circumflex coronary artery from right pulmonary artery. Report of a rare amonaly. J Thorac Cardiovasc Surg **76**:190, 1978.

68. Grayzel DM, Tennant R: Congenital atresia of the tricuspid orifice and anomalous origins of the coronary arteries from the pulmonary artery. Am J Pathol **10**:791, 1934.

69. Limbourg M: Uber den Ursprung der Kranzarterien des Herzens aus der Arteria pulmonalis. Beitr Pathol Anat **100**:191, 1937.

70. Williams JW, Johnson WS, Boulware JR Jr: Case of tetralogy of Fallot with both coronary arteries arising from pulmonary artery. J Fla Med Assoc **37**:561, 1951.

71. Swan WC, Werthammer S: Aberrant coronary arteries: Experiences in diagnosis with report of three cases. Ann Intern Med **42**:873, 1955.

72. Alexander RW, Griffith GC: Anomalies of the coronary arteries and their clinical significance. Circulation **14**:800, 1956.

73. Schulze WB, Rodin AE: Anomalous origin of both coronary arteries. Report of a case with discussion of teratogenic theories. Arch Pathol **72**:36, 1961.

74. Roberts WC: Anomalous origin of both coronary arteries from the pulmonary artery. Am J Cardiol **10**:595, 1962.

75. Blake HA, Manion WC, Mattingly TW, Baroldi G: Coronary artery anomalies. Circulation **390**:927, 1964.

76. Gonzales-Angulo A, Reyes HA, Wallace SA: Anomalies of the origin of coronary arteries (special reference to single coronary artery). Angiology 17:96, 1966.

77. Kecton BR, Keenan DJM, Monro JL: Anomalous origin of both coronary arteries from the pulmonary trunk. Br Heart J 49:397, 1983.

78. Feldt RH, Ongley PA, Titus JL: Total coronary arterial circulation from pulmonary artery with survival to age seven: Report of case. Mayo Clin Proc 40:539, 1965.

79. Monselise MB, Vlodaver Z, Neufeld HN: Single coronary artery; origin from the pulmonary trunk in association with ventricular septal defect. Chest 58:613, 1970.

80. Barth CW III, Roberts WC: Left main coronary artery originating from the right sinus of Valsalva and coursing between aorta and pulmonary trunk. J Am Col Cardiol 7:366, 1986.

81. Cheitlin MD, DeCastro CM, McCallister HA: Sudden death as a complication of anomalous left coronary origin from the anterior sinus of Valsalva. A not so minor congenital anomaly. Circulation 50:780, 1974.

82. Roberts WC, Dicicco BS, Waller BF, Kishel JC, McManus BM, Dawson SL, Hunsaker JC III, Luke JL: Origin of the left main from the right coronary artery or from the right aortic sinus with intramyocardial tunneling to the left side of the heart via the ventricular septum: The case against clinical significance of myocardial bridge or coronary tunnel. Am Heart J 104:303, 1982.

83. Murphy DA, Roy DL, Sohal M, Chandler BM: Anomalous origin of left main coronary artery from anterior sinus of Valsalva with myocardial infarction. J Thorac Cardiovasc Surg 75:282, 1978.

84. Sanes S: Anomalous origin and course of the left coronary artery in a child. Am Heart J 14:219, 1978.

85. Nicod JL: Anomalie coronaire et mort subite. Cardiologia 20:172, 1952.

86. Alexander RW, Griffith GC: Anomalies of the coronary arteries and their clinical significance. Circulation 14:800, 1956.

87. Jokl E, McClellan JT, Ross GD: Congential anomaly of the left coronary artery in young athlete. JAMA 182:174, 1962.

88. Jokl E, McClellan JT, Williams WC, Gouze FJ, Bartholomew RD: Congenital anomaly of left coronary artery in young athletes. Cardiologia 49:253, 1966.

89. Benson PA, Lack AR: Anomalous aortic origin of the left coronary artery. Arch Pathol 86:214, 1968.

90. Benson PR: Anomalous aortic origin of coronary artery with sudden death: Case report and review. Am Heart J 79:254, 1970.

91. Pedal I: Aortale ursprungsanomalie einer koronararterie. Dtsch Med Wochenschr 101:1601, 1976.

92. Liberthson RR, Dinsmore RE, Fallon JT: Abberant coronary artery origin from the aorta. Report of 18 patients, review of the literature and delineation of natural history and management. Circulation 59:748, 1979.

93. Lynch P: Soldiers, sport and sudden death. Lancet 1:1235, 1980.

94. Tsung SH, Huant TY, Change HH: Sudden death in young athletes. Arch Pathol Lab Med 106:168, 1982.

95. Betend B, Gillet P, Moreau P, David L: Origine aortique anormale de l'artere coronaire gauche. A propos del la mort subite d'un adolescent. Arch Fr Pediatr 40:479, 1983.

96. Topaz O, Edwards JE: Pathologic features of sudden death in children, adolescent, and young adults. Chest 87:476, 1985.

97. Davia JE, Green DC, Cheitlin MD, DeCastro C, Brott WH: Anomalous left coronary artery origin from the right coronary sinus. Am Heart J 108:165, 1984.

98. Mustafa I, Gula G, Radley-Smith R, Durrer S, Yacoub M: Anomalous origin of the left coronary artery from the anterior aortic sinus: A potential cause of sudden death. J Thorac Cardiovasc Surg 82:297, 1981.

99. Liberthson RR, Zaman L, Weyman A, et al: Aberrant origin of the left coronary artery from the proximal right coronary artery: Diagnostic features and pre- and postoperative course. Clin Cardiol 5:377, 1982.

100. Ishikawa T, Brandt PW: Anomalous origin of the left main coronary artery from the right anterior aortic sinus: Angiographic definition of anomalous course. Am J Cardiol 55:770, 1985.

101. Kimbiris D: Anomalous origin of the left main coronary artery from the right sinus of Valsalva. Am J Cardiol 55:765, 1985.

102. Moodie DS, Gill C, Loop FD, Sheldon WC: Anomalous left main coronary artery originating from the right sinus of Valsalva. Pathophysiology, angiographic definition and surgical approaches. J Thorac Cardiovasc Surg 80:198, 1980.

103. Sacks JH, Londe SP, Rosenbluth A, Zalis EG: Left main coronary artery bypass for aberrant (aortic) intramural left coronary artery. J Thorac Cardiovasc Surg 73:733, 1977.

104. Roberts WC, Siegel RJ, Zipes DP: Origin of the right coronary artery from the left sinus of Valsalva and its functional consequences: Analysis of 10 necropsy patients. Am J Cardiol 49:863, 1982.

105. Chaitman BR, Lesperance J, Saltiel J, Bourassa MG: Clinical, angiographic, and hemodynamic findings in patients with anomalous origin of the coronary arteries. Circulation 53:122, 1975.

106. Kimbiris D, Iskandrian AS, Segal BL, Bemis CE: Anomalous aortic origin of coronary arteries. Circulation 58:606, 1978.

107. Thompson SI, Vieweg WVR, Alpert JS, Hagan AD: Anomalous origin of the right coronary artery from the left sinus of Valsalva with associated chest pain. Report of 2 cases. Cathet Cardiovasc Diagn 2:397, 1976.

108. Benge W, Martins JB, Funk DC: Morbidity associated with anomalous origin of the right coronary artery from the left sinus of Valsalva. Am Heart J 99:96, 1980.

109. Bloomfield P, Erhlich C, Folland ED, Bianco JA, Tow DE, Parisi AF: Anomalous right coronary artery: A surgically correctable cause of angina pectoris. Am J Cardiol 51:1235, 1983.

110. Keren A, Tzivoni D, Stern S: Functional consequences of right coronary artery originating from left sinus of Valsalva (Letter). Am J Cardiol 51:1241, 1983.

111. Brandt B III, Martins JB, Marcus ML: Anomalous origin of the right coronary artery from the left sinus of Valsalva. N Engl J Med 309:596, 1983.

112. Hanzlick R, Stivers RR: Sudden death in a marathon runner with origin of the right coronary artery from the left sinus of Valsalva (Letter). Am J Cardiol 51:1467, 1983.

113. Hanzlick RL, Stivers RR: Sudden death due to anomalous right coronary artery in a 26-year-old marathon runner. Am J Forensic Med Pathol 4:265, 1983.

114. Hanzlick R, Stivers RR: Anomalous right coronary artery (Letter). Am J Forensic Med Pathol 5:285, 1984.

115. Isner JM, Shen EM, Martin ET, Fortin RV: Sudden unexpected death as a result of anomalous origin of the right coronary artery from the left sinus of Valsalva. Am J Med 76:155, 1984.

116. Antopol W, Kugel MA: Anomalous origin of the left circumflex coronary artery. Am Heart J 8:802, 1933.

117. Roberts WC, Waller BF, Roberts CS: Fatal atherosclerotic narrowing of the right main coronary artery: Origin of the left arterior descending or left circumflex coronary artery from the right (the true "left main equivalent"). Am Heart J 104:638, 1982.

118. White NK, Edwards JE: Anomalies of the coronary arteries: Report of four cases. Arch Pathol 45:766, 1948.

119. Page HL Jr, Engel JH, Campbell WB, Thomas CS: Anomalous origin of the left circumflex coronary artery. Recognition, angiographic demonstration and clinical significance. Circulation 50:768, 1974.

120. Ray PR, Saunders A, Sowton GE: Review of variations in origin of left circumflex coronary artery. Br Heart J 37:287, 1975.

121. Baltaxe HA, Wixson D: The incidence of congenital anomalies of the coronary arteries in the adult population. Radiology **122**:47, 1977.
122. Liberthson RR, Dinsmore RE, Bharati S, Rubenstein JJ, Caulfeld J, Wheeler EO, Harthorne JW, Lev M: Aberrant coronary origin from the aorta. Diagnosis and clinical significance. Circulation **50**:774, 1974.
123. Roberts WC, Morrow AG: Compression of anomalous left circumflex coronary arteries by prosthetic valve fixation rings. J Thorac Cardiovasc Surg **57**:834, 1969.
124. Vlodaver Z, Neufeld HN, Edwards JE: Coronary arterial variations in the normal heart and in congenital heart disease. New York, 1975, Academic Press, Inc., p. 171.
125. DiCicco BS, McManus BM, Waller BF, Roberts WC: Separate aortic ostium of the left anterior descending and left circumflex coronary arteries from the left aortic sinus of Valsalva (absent left main coronary artery). Am Heart J **104**:153, 1982.
126. Zumbo O, Fani K, Jarmolych J, Daoud AS: Coronary atherosclerosis and myocardial infarction in hearts with anomalous coronary arteries. Lab Invest **14**:571, 1965.
127. Smith JC: Review of single coronary artery with report of 2 cases. Circulation **1**:1168, 1950.
128. Banchi A: Morfologia della arteriae coronariae cordis. Arch Ital Anat Embriol **3**:89, 1903.
129. Ogden JA, Goodyear AVN: Patterns of distribution of the single coronary artery. Yale J Biol Med **43**:11, 1970.
130. Lipton MJ, Barry WH, Obrez I, Silverman J, Wexler L: Isolated single coronary artery: Diagnosis, angiographic classification, and clinical significance. Radiology **130**:39, 1979.
131. Saner HE, Saner BD, Dykoski RK, Edwards JE: Origin of anterior descending coronary artery from right aortic sinus. Intramyocardial tunneling to the left side of the heart. Arch Pathol Lab Med **108**:642, 1984.
132. Schulte MA, Waller BF, Hull MT, Pless JE: Origin of the left anterior descending coronary artery from the right aortic sinus with intramyocardial tunneling to the left side of the heart via the ventricular septum: A case against clinical and morphologic significance of myocardial bridging. Am Heart J **110**:499, 1985.

CONGENITAL CORONARY ARTERIAL ANOMALIES UNASSOCIATED WITH MAJOR ANOMALIES OF THE HEART OR GREAT VESSELS

William C. Roberts, M.D.

ORIGIN OF 1 OR MORE CORONARY ARTERIES FROM THE PULMONARY TRUNK *AND* ORIGIN OF 1 OR MORE CORONARY ARTERIES FROM THE AORTA

When both right and left main coronary arteries arise from the pulmonary trunk or when only 1 coronary artery is present and it arises from the pulmonary trunk, survival past 1 year of life is impossible unless an associated anomaly is present that allows persistence of pulmonary hypertension after birth (Fig. 1). In these 2 circumstances, no coronary artery arises directly from the aorta.

When 1 coronary artery, however, arises from the pulmonary trunk and 1 or more coronary arteries arise from the aorta, survival past 15 years of age may occur. The most common anomaly in the category is origin of the left main coronary artery from the pulmonary trunk and origin of the right coronary artery from the aorta (see Fig. 1). Far less common is origin of the right or left anterior descending from the pulmonary trunk, and these anomalies are usually associated with survival into adulthood (see Fig. 1).

LEFT MAIN FROM THE PULMONARY TRUNK

Historic Background

This anomaly was described first by Maude Abbott in 1908.[1] Her patient was a woman who lived for 60 years, and this is the longest survival reported with this anomaly. Abriskossoff[2] in 1911 first described findings in an infant with this anomaly. In 1933, Bland and associates[3] described clinical and necropsy findings in a 3-month-old boy with this anomaly, and subsequently this anomaly in infants often has been referred to as the "Bland-White-Garland syndrome." The infant described by Bland and associates was the son of a physician who observed " . . . the paroxysmal attacks of acute discomfort precipitated by the exertion of nursing." These attacks, which also included inspiratory and expiratory grunts followed by marked pallor and cold sweats, were interpreted by Bland and associates as evidence of

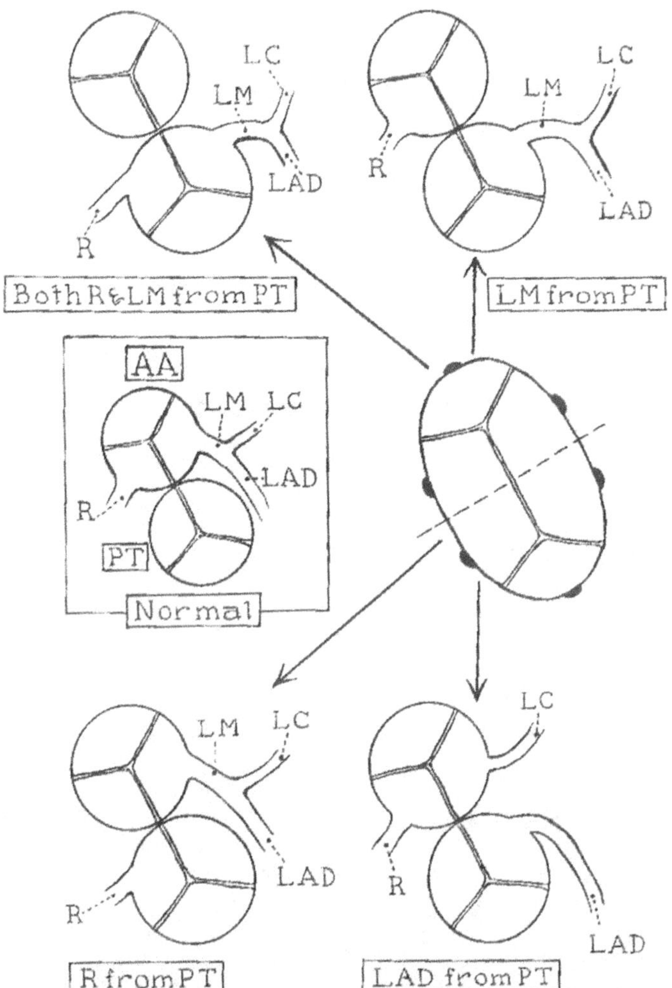

FIGURE 1. Diagram illustrating the common arterial trunk arising from the heart in its early development with 6 potential coronary arterial ostia and the possible coronary anomalies resulting when inappropriate ostia do not regress. AA = ascending aorta; LAD = left anterior descending coronary artery; LC = left circumflex coronary artery; LM = left main coronary artery; PT = pulmonary trunk; R = right coronary artery.

angina pectoris. The electrocardiogram (3 limb leads only) disclosed marked T-wave inversions, and chest radiograph showed marked enlargement of the cardiac silhouette. The clinical diagnosis in the infant was "congenital idiopathic hypertrophy of the heart." The coronary anomaly was discovered at necropsy.

Frequency

This anomaly was observed only once among 357 patients with congenital heart disease studied at necropsy by Fontana and Edwards[4] from January 1920 through June 30, 1954, dates that precede cardiopulmonary bypass operations. Fontana and Edwards[4] also found published reports describing 58 necropsy patients with origin of the left main from the pulmonary trunk. More than half of the 58 patients died between ages 3 and 6 months; 46 patients (79%) were dead by 13 months of age; the remaining 12 patients (21%) lived longer than 15 years. The major cause of death during the first year of life was congestive heart failure; 8 of the 12 adults died suddenly and unexpectedly. Edwards and Fontana[4] found no reports of death with this anomaly from age 13 months to 16 years. Thus, if a patient with this anomaly is able to survive the first year of life, the chances are good that the child will survive until adulthood. Origin of the left main from the pulmonary trunk occurs about equally often in both sexes. I have studied at necropsy 11 patients (7 females) in whom the left main arose from the pulmonary trunk: 9 were aged 1 to 18 months (mean 7); 1 was 3.5 years old, and 1 died suddenly at age 41 years. The latter patient was known to have a continuous precordial murmur but never had symptoms of cardiac dysfunction. Her sudden death was clearly the result of the coronary anomaly.

The frequency of this anomaly among adults having coronary arterial angiograms for suspected ischemic heart disease, of course, is quite low. Among 1750 adults having coronary angiograms as reported by Thomas and associates,[5] 2 had origin of the left main from the pulmonary trunk: 1 a 45-year-old woman and the other a 40-year-old woman. Among 9152 patients having coronary angiograms and reported by Donaldson and associates,[6] 6 had origin of the left main from the pulmonary trunk.

Flow in the Anomalous Artery

Why some patients with anomalous origin of the left main coronary artery from the pulmonary trunk die during the first year or so of life and why others survive into adulthood (without operative intervention) is related to the development of collaterals between the coronary artery attached to the ascending aorta (the right one) and the coronary artery attached to the pulmonary trunk (the left main).[7,8] At birth and during the first 2 months or so of life, the systolic and diastolic pressures in the ascending aorta and pulmonary trunk are similar, and consequently the left main coronary artery is perfused by blood within the pulmonary trunk. At about 2 months of life, the pressure in the pulmonary trunk falls, so that by about 12 months of life, the systolic pressure in the pulmonary trunk is about ¼ of that in the aorta. Survival is dependent on the development of collateral channels between the normally and abnormally arising coronary arteries so that flow in the anomalous left main coronary artery is retrograde, it being entirely supplied by blood from the normally arising right coronary artery. The anomalous artery "steals" blood from the normally arising artery (Fig. 2), placing considerable myocardium at risk of ischemia or necrosis (Fig. 3). It would appear that an extensive collateral system must develop for survival to occur. During the period of transition from antegrade to retrograde flow in the anomalously arising left main coronary artery, death is common.

Morphologic Features

The heart is quite different in the infant dying with this anomaly compared with that of the patient surviving to adulthood. In the infant, the cardiac mass is increased (this anomaly provides the best evidence available that chronic myocardial ischemia causes an increase in cardiac mass), and the ventricular cavities are dilated. The area occupied by the mitral valve appears small in comparison with the entire left ventricular cavity. The left ventricular papillary muscles appear to arise in the left ventricle about at the junction of the cephalad and middle thirds of the wall. Normally, the papillary muscles tend to arise about the level of the middle and caudal thirds of the left ventricle. The anterolateral papillary muscle is much smaller than the posteromedial papillary muscle. Additionally, the anterolateral papillary muscle is scarred, often calcified, and, in contrast, the myocardium of the posteromedial muscle is preserved. The endocardium of the left ventricle may be thickened such that it has the appearance of diffuse endocardial fibroelastosis. The margin of the anterior mitral leaflet often is thickened. The left atrium is dilated.

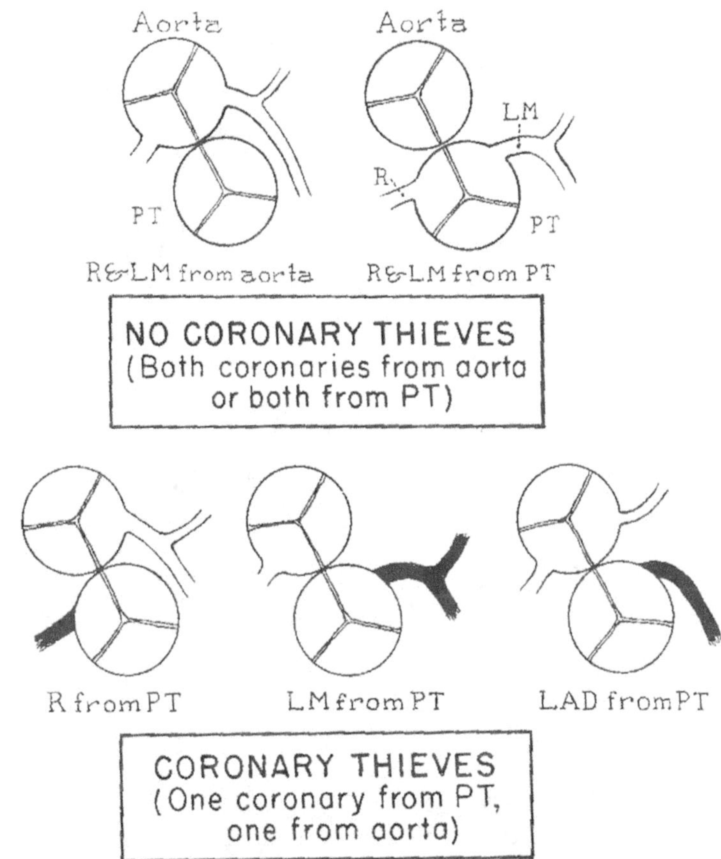

FIGURE 2. Diagram showing the coronary anomalies not associated with the "coronary steal" phenomena and those associated with this phenomena. Abbreviations as in Figure 1.

In contrast to the appearance in the infant's heart, the survivors of this anomaly into adulthood have hearts that are distinguished primarily by the appearances of the epicardial coronary arteries. The right one is dilated and tortuous. The branches of the left main, in contrast, are straighter, not as dilated, but have a thinner wall (like a vein). Vascular channels connecting the right coronary artery to the branches of the left main are visible on the surface of the heart. The mass of the heart usually is increased, and the ventricular cavities are usually dilated. The anterolateral papillary muscle usually is scarred and it also contains calcific deposits. One of 10 adults (aged 15 to 54 years [mean 31]) reported by Moodie and associates[9] had extensive left ventricular calcific deposits. Left ventricular endocardial fibroelastosis, which is commonly observed in the infants at necropsy, is usually absent in the adults with this anomaly.

Symptoms of Cardiac Dysfunction

Symptoms of cardiac dysfunction occur in about 80% of the infants in whom the left main arises from the pulmonary trunk, and the symptom complex is as reported by Bland and associates[3] and substantiated by others.[10-19] In adults or in children surviving the first year or so of life, the symptom complex is far more varied. Many patients with the adult form of anomalous left main from the pulmonary trunk are asymptomatic despite extremely active lives. A 29-year-old woman reported by Sabiston and associates[20] had had 5 full-term normal deliveries without difficulty.

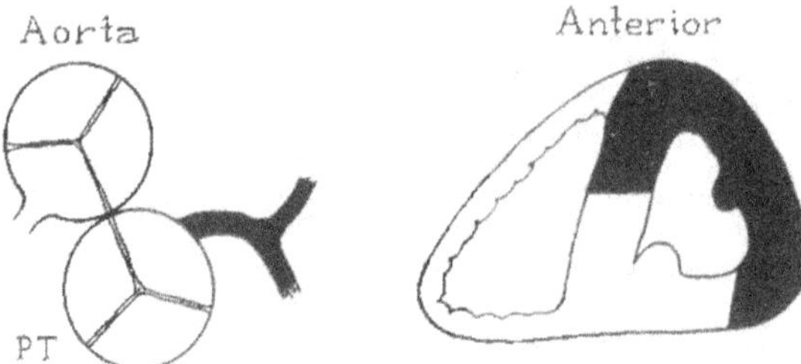

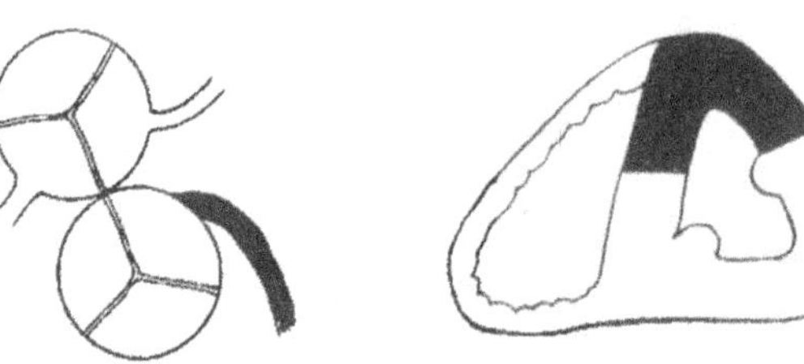

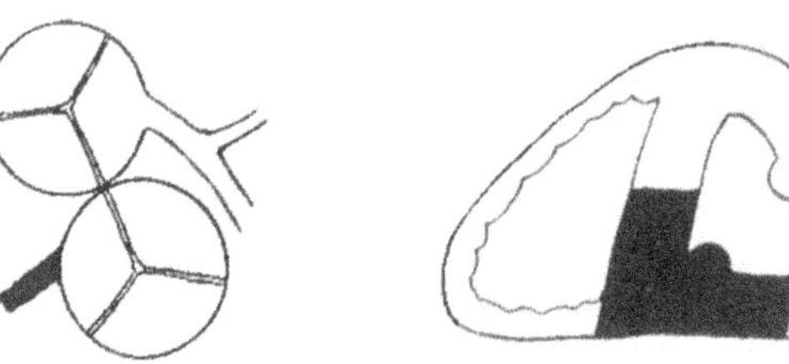

FIGURE 3. Diagram showing the portion of left ventricular myocardium at risk of ischemia or necrosis when the left main, left anterior descending, or right coronary artery arises from the pulmonary trunk (PT).

The 18-year-old boy reported by Harthorne and associates[16] was a star basketball player who eventually developed excessive dyspnea, chest pain, and finally syncope only with the strenuous exertion of athletic endeavors. The 18-year-old boy reported by Jurishica[10] was a star football player.

The asymptomatic older patients with this anomaly were usually brought to medical attention by the detection of a precordial murmur—often a continuous one—on precordial examination, by the finding of an abnormal electrocardiogram showing ischemic changes, and by the occurrence of sudden unexpected death. The latter, unfortunately, is common. Of 14 adults, aged 16 to 60 years (mean 36), with this anomaly reviewed by George and Knowlan,[11] 10 died suddenly and unexpectedly; and of the 10, sudden death was the initial clinical manifestation of the coronary anomaly in 8. The sudden death usually was associated with sudden physical exertion.

Other reported symptoms in adults with this anomaly have included angina pectoris, exertional dyspnea, and syncope. Clinical features consistent with acute myocardial infarction have not been described, to my knowledge, in adults with this anomaly. Likewise, overt evidence of congestive heart failure is rare in adults except possibly in those with clinical evidence of mitral regurgitation.[21,22]

Means of Diagnosis

The definitive diagnosis of this anomaly is by angiography with injection of contrast material into the lumen of the right coronary artery (or aortic root) with drainage via collaterals into the left main branches and visualization of the connection of the left main to the pulmonary trunk. Although angiography is the only definitive test, other procedures provide important clues to the diagnosis. The presence of a precordial continuous murmur is very helpful. In infants, the electrocardiogram showing ischemic myocardial changes (anterior wall) is most helpful.[19] In adults with this anomaly, unfortunately, the electrocardiogram is not as helpful. The ischemic changes in adults may or may not be present, and even if present, they could be attributed to coronary narrowing from atherosclerosis. Electrocardiographic evidence of left ventricular hypertrophy is common in adults with the anomaly.

The echocardiogram may provide clues to diagnosis. In each of 3 infants, Fisher and associates[23] demonstrated by cross-sectional echocardiography attachment of the left main coronary artery to the pulmonary trunk and markedly dilated poorly contracting left ventricles. Terai and associates[24] also in an infant demonstrated by cross-sectional echocardiography origin of the left main from the pulmonary trunk and also a very large right coronary artery arising from the ascending aorta. Robinson and associates[26] cautioned that the only reliable echocardiographic finding in the anomaly was the actual demonstration of the left main arising from the pulmonary trunk, not the absence of identification of origin of left main from the aorta. King and associates[27] by pulsed Doppler echocardiography demonstrated in a 2-month-old infant bidirectional Doppler flow in the proximal portion of the pulmonary trunk. The late systolic flow pattern on the Doppler flow tracing indicated a left-to-right shunt through the left main arising from the pulmonary trunk. Whether echocardiography will be useful in adults with this anomaly as in infants remains to be determined.

The presence of mitral regurgitation in a young person with ischemic changes on electrocardiogram might suggest the presence of the coronary anomaly. Mitral regurgitation may be the dominant clinical feature of this coronary anomaly. Usman and associates[21] and Burchell and Brown[22] each described a patient whose dominant clinical problem was mitral regurgitation.

Radionuclide angiography may be useful in distinguishing patients with origin of the left main from the pulmonary trunk from those with idiopathic dilated cardiomyopathy.[28] Origin of the left main from the pulmonary trunk cannot usually be seen by injecting contrast material into the pulmonary trunk. However, the left main can be seen arising from the pulmonary trunk if a balloon is inflated in the pulmonary trunk just distal to where contrast material is to be injected.[29]

Operative Treatment and Results

A number of operative procedures have been utilized for treatment of this anomaly:[5,9,14,16,19,20,23,30–46] (1) ligation of the left main coronary artery at its attachment to the pulmonary trunk; (2) obliteration of the left main ostium by covering it within the lumen of the pulmonary trunk by artificial or biologic material; (3) ligation of the left main artery or closure of its ostium plus insertion of a conduit, usually a reversed saphenous vein, from ascending aorta to left anterior descending coronary artery; (4) anastomosis of the left main to ascending aorta either directly or via an artificial (Gortex) or biologic graft with closure of the site of origin of the left main from the pulmonary trunk; (5) division of the left main artery close to its ostium in the pulmonary trunk and direct anastomosis of a subclavian or common carotid artery to the left main in an end-to-end fashion. In the procedures where a conduit has been interposed between aorta and left main coronary artery, the conduit has been located posterior to the pulmonary trunk, within the pulmonary trunk as a tunnel, and anterior to the pulmonary trunk. Despite the multiple different procedures utilized for treatment, the best one is unclear. Good results have been obtained by most.

An early operative procedure for this anomaly was simply ligation of the left main coronary artery. This procedure has produced good long-term results in infants, children, and adults. Shrivastava and associates[41] followed 2 infants and 2 children (aged 6 and 7 years) for > 10 years after simple left main ligation, and all were asymptomatic postoperatively although the electrocardiogram remained abnormal in 2. Wilson and associates[42] from polling many cardiovascular surgeons collected data on 13 patients who had left main ligation only when they were aged 13 years or older. The mean age at last follow-up was 37 ± 9 years, and the mean follow-up period was 9 years. Although there had been no deaths at operation or in the early postoperative period, 3 patients died later (2, 6, and 7 years after operation). These same authors also described results in 16 patients who had had left main ligation plus insertion of a saphenous vein between ascending aorta and left anterior descending coronary artery at age 13 years or older. At a mean age of last follow-up of 38 ± 11 years and a mean of 5 ± 3 years after operation, there was only 1 death and that was in the early postoperative period. Wilson and associates[42] concluded that the probability of survival was similar following either left main ligation alone or left main ligation plus aorta–left anterior descending grafting. About half the patients in both their operative groups were improved symptomatically by the operation.

Moodie and associates[9] described operative results in 10 patients aged 15 to 54 years (mean 31) at the time of closure of the left main ostium from within the pulmonary trunk plus aorta–left anterior descending grafting (6 patients), isolated closure of the left main ostium from inside the pulmonary trunk (3 patients), and transfer of the left main ostium with a cuff of pulmonary trunk directly to the ascending aorta (1 patient). The 10 patients were followed 4 months to 16 years (mean 6 years): 6 were asymptomatic postoperatively, 3 were functional class II (each was class III preoperatively [New York Heart Association classification]), and 1 died late. Postoperative stress electrocardiograms showed no evidence of myocardial ischemia in 6 of 6 patients and normal stress thallium tests in 8 of 8 patients.

The presently commonly employed operative procedures for this anomaly, namely left main ligation with aorta–left anterior descending grafting or connection of the left main to the aorta either directly or via a graft, appear to have similar effects on the sizes of the collaterals between the branches of the right coronary artery and the branches of the left anterior descending and left circumflex coronary arteries and the size of the right coronary artery postoperatively. Early after operation, and as long as 3 years postoperatively, the sizes of the collaterals and right coronary artery postoperatively may be similar to the sizes preoperatively. By 3 years after operation, however, the collaterals are usually much smaller or have disappeared, and the lumen of and the tortuosity of the right coronary artery are much less than preoperatively. However, in a patient reported by Chaitman and associates,[37] and evaluated at age 36, > 8 years after left main ligation and aorta–left anterior descending grafting via a saphenous vein, large collaterals were still present between the left main branches and the right coronary artery.

The operations have variable effects on the degree of mitral regurgitation postoperatively if mitral regurgitation had been present preoperatively. This valvular lesion may disappear or be unchanged, or it may lessen postoperatively. If electocardiographic evidence of left ventricular hypertrophy is present preoperatively, it usually persists after operation. Left ventricular function, however, is usually improved by operation. Bagger and associates[46] described a 19-year-old woman who had left main ligation and saphenous vein grafting between aorta and left anterior descending; evaluation 6 months postoperatively disclosed disappearance of the collaterals, normal left ventricular contractions compared with preoperative studies, a 100% increase in coronary sinus blood flow and a 128% increase during pacing, whereas preoperatively pacing did not increase the coronary sinus blood flow.

RIGHT CORONARY ARTERY FROM PULMONARY TRUNK

Historic Background

The first report of origin of the right coronary artery from the pulmonary trunk was by Sir John Brooks, an anatomist, who studied 2 cadavers and postulated in 1885 that blood flow in the anomalously arising right coronary artery was reversed: blood from the aorta entered the left main coronary artery, passed through collaterals to the right coronary artery, and then drained into the pulmonary trunk.[47] Monckelberg[48] in 1914 studied at necropsy a 30-year-old man who had died shortly following an epileptic seizure and found the right coronary artery anomaly. Schley[49] in 1925 described the anomaly in a 61-year-old man who died of syphilis. Jordan and associates[50] also found the anomaly in a patient at necropsy, as did Cronk and associates.[51] The latter patient had lived 90 years before he died shortly following seizures. These latter authors described severe atherosclerosis in the branches of the left main coronary artery and no atherosclerosis in the right coronary artery, a finding that proves that the pressure in the right coronary artery was venous and that in the left coronary arteries, arterial. Cronk and associates[51] also noted that the intramural coronary arteries in the right ventricular wall were numerous and in the left ventricular free wall, relatively sparse. The left coronary artery—probably the left anterior descending—had a maximal diameter of 20 mm, and the right coronary artery had a maximal diameter of 6 mm. The first patient with this anomaly treated operatively and reported was by Tingelstad and associates[52] in 1972.

Frequency

This anomaly is far less common than is origin of the left main from the pulmonary trunk. In their 1962 book, Fontana and Edwards[4] found reports of only 4 necropsy cases of origin of the right coronary artery from the pulmonary trunk while at the same time finding reports of 58 necropsy cases of origin of the left main from the pulmonary trunk. From review of the necropsy reports at Yale-New Haven Hospital from 1952 to 1968, Ogden[53] found 4 cases of origin of the right coronary artery from the pulmonary trunk and 39 cases of origin of the left main from the pulmonary trunk. By 1979, Lerberg and associates[54] found reports describing 14 patients with origin of the right coronary artery from the pulmonary trunk and reports describing 140 patients with origin of the left main from the pulmonary trunk.

Flow in the Anomalous Artery

Flow in the anomalous artery, be it right, left main, left anterior descending, or left circumflex from the pulmonary trunk, should be similar and variable depending on the patient's age. Although flow through the anomalously arising left main has been demonstrated to be antegrade early in life and retrograde after a year or so (sometimes earlier) of life, antegrade flow has not been demonstrated in infancy when the right coronary artery has arisen from the pulmonary trunk and the left main has arisen from the aorta. The reason, of course, is that diagnosis of origin of the right coronary artery from the pulmonary trunk has not been made during infancy; indeed, the youngest child in whom this diagnosis has been established was 6-year-old, and that patient was described by Lerberg and associates.[54] Retrograde flow through the anomalous right coronary artery has been established both by angiogram and visualized at operation.

Morphologic Features

Whereas increase in ventricular mass, left ventricular scarring, anterolateral papillary muscle fibrosis and calcification, right ventricular and left ventricular dilatation, and diffuse left ventricular endocardial fibroelastosis (of variable degree) might be expected in cases of origin of the left main from the pulmonary trunk, none of these morphologic findings appear to be the consequence of origin of the right coronary artery from the pulmonary trunk. Indeed, the only predictable morphologic finding is an increase in size of the left main coronary artery and its branches and an increase (but less so) in size of the right coronary artery with thinning of its wall (compared with normal).

Clinical Manifestations

This anomaly usually produces no symptoms of cardiac dysfunction and no evidence of myocardial ischemia. Of 9 necropsy cases reported up to 1979, and summarized by Lerberg and associates,[54] 1 patient, a 2-year-old boy, was found dead in his crib without preceding evidence of any illness. Another, an 11-year-old girl, had cardiac arrest; and another, a 72-year-old man, had evidence of chronic congestive cardiac failure. None of the 3 patients had another condition that could be responsible for their deaths. All the remaining 6 necropsy patients were either free of clinical evidence of cardiac dysfunction or they had another cardiac disorder (aortic regurgitation or systemic hypertension or mitral stenosis) that could readily explain any cardiac dysfunction. These 6 patients were aged 30 to 90 years (mean 62). Five other patients up to 1979 had the anomaly diagnosed by angiography, and each of them had operative therapy.[54] Their ages at operation were 11, 12, 25, 42, and 64 years, and 3 were female.[54–58] Three were asymptomatic and were found to have a continuous precordial murmur (left sternal border), 1 (age 64 years) presented with evidence of congestive cardiac failure,[56] and 1 (age 25 years) had cardiac arrest with successful resuscitation.[58] A year earlier, however, the latter patient had had 1 syncopal episode. Thus, anomalous origin of the right coronary artery from the pulmonary trunk is a cause of cardiac arrest, and this fact by itself justifies operative intervention if this coronary anomaly is known to be present even though the individual may be asymptomatic.

Recently, Mintz and associates[59] reported a 47-year-old man with angina pectoris for 2 months. The resting electrocardiogram and the chest radiography were normal. Thallium-201 myocardial perfusion disclosed a decrease in perfusion in the 4-hour study. Total anterograde left main coronary flow was 1440 to 1680 ml/minute, but only 240 to 280 ml/minute supplied the myocardium and the remainder passed to the pulmonary trunk via the right coronary artery. Thus, a 5:1 intercoronary shunt was present. This case was the first to quantitate the degree of the "coronary steal" in this anomaly (see Fig. 2).

In contrast to its usefulness when the left main coronary artery arises from the pulmonary trunk, the electrocardiogram in origin of the right coronary artery from the pulmonary trunk is usually of no benefit. Ischemic changes are usually absent, and signs of ventricular hypertrophy are usually absent or only borderline. The chest radiogram usually shows mild enlargement of the cardiac silhouette, but the cardiac size may be entirely normal. Cross-sectional echocardiography may be useful for diagnosis. Origin of the right coronary artery from the pulmonary trunk must be demonstrated—not absence of origin of the right coronary artery from the aorta.[51] The finding of a large left main coronary artery or a large right coronary artery by echocardiography might be the initial suspicion of this anomaly. Certain diagnosis is established by angiography with injection of contrast material in the left main coronary artery arising from the aorta with visualization of the right coronary artery via collaterals from the left main branches and finally the appearance of contrast material in the pulmonary trunk.

Operative Treatment and Results

The operation of choice for this anomaly appears to be transsection of the right coronary artery from the pulmonary trunk and direct anastomosis of the right coronary artery to the aorta (end-to-side). Tingelstad and associates[52] were the first to report this technique. Their patient was a 12-year-old asymptomatic boy who was found to have a continuous precordial murmur. The left-to-right shunt from the left main to the right coronary artery was calculated to have been 1.7 to 1. Others[53,54,56–61] have also successfully utilized this technique. The patient operated on by Bregman and associates[58] had presented with cardiac arrest that was successfully resuscitated. The patient was asymptomatic 2 years postoperatively.

LEFT ANTERIOR DESCENDING CORONARY ARTERY FROM PULMONARY TRUNK

At least 8 patients have been reported in whom the left anterior descending arose from the pulmonary trunk and both right and left circumflex arteries arose from the aorta, and the findings in them were summarized by Roberts and Robinowitz.[62] At the time of their 1984 report, 1 patient (a 7-month-old girl) had died of an anterior wall acute myocardial infarct; the other 7 (6 women) were aged 18 to 55 years (mean 34). The patient reported by Roberts and Robinowitz[62] is the only male thus far described. Of the 7 adults, 6 were symptomatic: 5 with angina pectoris, 1 of whom also had an anterior wall acute myocardial infarct, and 1 with severe fatigue attributed to severe mitral regurgitation from papillary muscle dysfunction. The angina at some time in all 5 patients was stable, but 3 of the 5 had unstable angina just before cardiac operation. The age at onset of symptoms of myocardial ischemia in the 6 adults ranged from 18 to 37 years (mean 27). Precordial murmurs were described in 5 of 6 adults. (No information was provided in the "addendum case" of Donaldson and coworkers.[63]) The murmur apparently was present only in systole in 4 patients, and also in diastole in 2. The intensity of the murmurs was mentioned in 3 patients: "soft" in 1, grade 2/6 in 1, and grade 3/6 in 1. Findings on the electrocardiogram at rest were described in 5 adults: 4 had poor R-wave progression in leads V_1 to V_3, and at least 2 had ST–T wave changes of ischemia in more than 1 lead. In 1 patient, the electrocardiogram was normal. Exercise stress tests in 2 patients disclosed ST segment ischemic changes in each. Chest x-rays in 6 of the 7 adults disclosed normal-sized cardiac silhouettes in 3 and cardiac enlargement in 3: mild in 2 and severe in 1. Right-sided cardiac catheterization, performed in at least 6 patients, disclosed normal pressures in each and oxygen step-up in the pulmonary trunk in 2. Coronary angiography with injection of contrast material in the right and left circumflex coronary arteries in all 7 adults disclosed that each of these 2 arteries in all 7 patients was large, occasionally also tortuous, and that the left anterior descending was filled by extensive collateral vessels from both the right and left circumflex coronary arteries. Injection of contrast material into the pulmonary trunk did not cause filling of

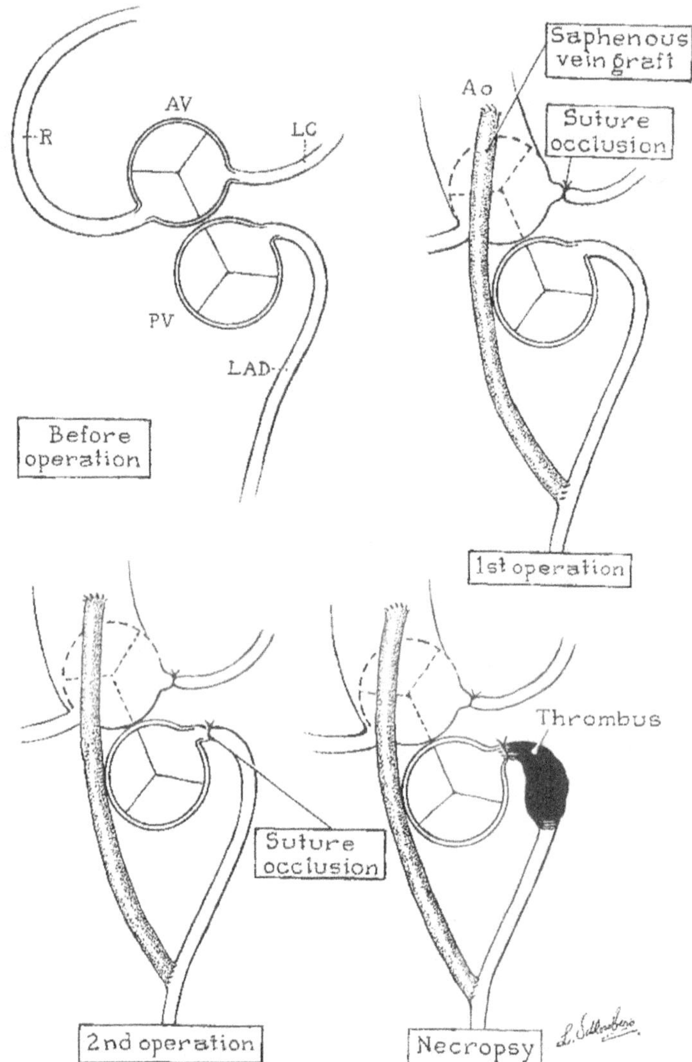

FIGURE 4. Diagram showing sequence of events in a 32-year-old man in whom the left anterior descending coronary artery arose from the pulmonary trunk. Before operation, he was asymptomatic but had a precordial continuous murmur. At the first operation, the left circumflex coronary artery was inadvertently ligated rather than the left anterior descending. At the second operation, performed 3 days after the first one, a conduit was inserted between ascending aorta and left anterior descending. The patient died suddenly soon after jogging 9 months after the cardiac operations. Obviously, if operation is to be performed for this anomaly, the anomalously arising artery must be clearly identified before ligation. Ao = aorta; AV = aortic valve; LAD = left anterior descending coronary artery; LC = left circumflex coronary artery; PV = pulmonic valve; r = right coronary artery. From Roberts WC, Robinowitz M. Am J Cardiol 1984; 54:1381–1383, with permission.

the left anterior descending; when the left anterior descending, however, was filled by injections into either the right or left circumflex coronary artery, contrast material did enter the pulmonary trunk through the left anterior descending, which was filled by collateral vessels.

Of the 8 reported adults, operative treatment was carried out in 6, four of whom preoperatively had angina: in 2 patients, the pulmonary trunk was opened and the ostium of the left anterior descending was obliterated by sutures; and in 2, the left anterior descending was ligated just proximal to its entrance into the pulmonary trunk and a reversed saphenous vein inserted from the ascending aorta to the left anterior descending. One patient, a 32-year-old asymptomatic man reported by Roberts and Robinowitz,[62] inadvertently had suture occlusion of the left circumflex rather than of the left anterior descending with insertion of a saphenous vein from aorta to left anterior descending at the first operation (Fig. 4). At the second operation 3 days later, the left anterior descending was ligated proximally (see Fig. 4). This patient died suddenly while jogging 9 months postoperatively. Of the 5 symptomatic patients who had operative treatment, angina disappeared in 3 and persisted in 1. Two patients had repeat coronary and left ventricular angiography 24 and 36 months, respectively, after operation; in each, the right and left circumflex coronary arteries were much smaller than they had been preoperatively, and the collateral vessels between the right and left circumflex coronary arteries and the left anterior descending coronary artery had disappeared; 1 patient had persistent angina postoperatively and the distal portions of both the right and left circumflex coronary arteries (36 months postoperatively) were quite narrowed; the cause of narrowing was unclear. Left ventricular angiograms, performed in 5 adults, were normal in 3, and in the other 2 the apical portion of the left ventricle was akinetic in 1 and aneurysmal in 1. Repeat left ventricular angiography in these latter 2 patients disclosed better overall contractions in 1 and no change in 1.

The presence of both subjective and objective evidence of myocardial ischemia in 6 of the 8 reported adults and the disappearance of angina and of the collateral vessels between the 2 coronary arteries arising from the aorta and the left anterior descending arising from the pulmonary trunk supports the view that operative treatment is proper for patients with this coronary anomaly. Whether left anterior descending ligation alone is enough or whether ligation plus insertion of a conduit between the aorta and left anterior descending is preferable is unclear. Direct connection of the left anterior descending to aorta in this situation appears technically inadvisable. Four of the 6 patients in whom operation was performed had angina pectoris. Two patients were asymptomatic preoperatively. Obviously, no data are available on the advisability of operation in an asymptomatic person in whom the left anterior descending arises from the pulmonary trunk, but it appears reasonable to believe that the operative therapy in this circumstance is proper. If operation is to be performed, however, clear identification of the anomalous artery before ligation is mandatory.

LEFT CIRCUMFLEX CORONARY ARTERY FROM THE PULMONARY TRUNK

Effler and associates[64] mentioned an 8-year-old boy (their case 7) who by angiogram had a left circumflex coronary artery attached to a pulmonary artery (which one was not mentioned); the correct diagnosis was not confirmed anatomically. Honey and associates[65] described a 13-year-old boy who had aortic isthmic coarctation, right aortic arch, bicuspid aortic valve, and origin of the left circumflex coronary artery from the right main pulmonary artery. Chaitman and associates[66] described a 14-year-old asymptomatic girl in whom the left circumflex apparently arose from the pulmonary trunk. Ott and associates[67] described an 8-year-old girl also with a bicuspid aortic valve in whom the left circumflex coronary artery arose from the right main pulmonary artery. No adults have been reported with origin of the left circumflex coronary artery from any pulmonary artery.

ACCESSORY CORONARY ARTERY FROM PULMONARY TRUNK

The most common accessory coronary artery arising from the pulmonary trunk is a conus artery (Fig. 5). Origin of this small coronary artery from the pulmonary trunk is of no functional significance.

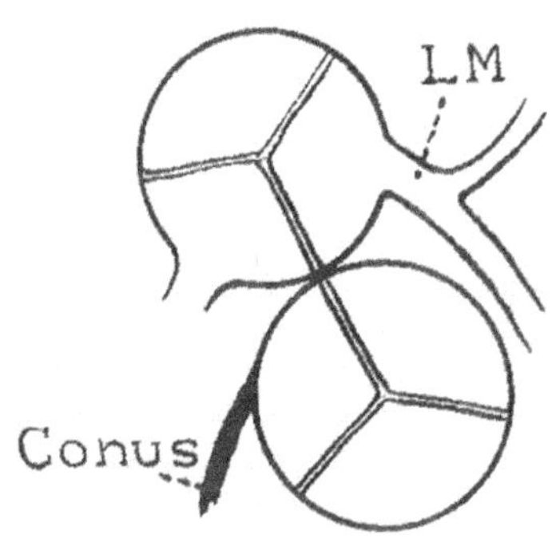

FIGURE 5. Diagram showing origin of the conus artery from the pulmonary trunk (PT). LM = left main coronary artery.

BOTH RIGHT AND LEFT MAIN CORONARY ARTERIES (OR SINGLE CORONARY ARTERY) FROM THE PULMONARY TRUNK WITHOUT A CORONARY ARTERY FROM THE AORTA

At least 12 patients with origin of both left main and right coronary arteries from the pulmonary trunk have been reported and all died during the first month of life usually in the first 1 or 2 days.[68-77] Thus, nearly all of these infants had patent ductus arteriosus. Most had other major anomalies of the heart or great arteries. At least 2 patients have been described in whom a single coronary artery arose from the pulmonary trunk and no coronary artery arose from the aorta.[78,79] Feldt and associates[78] described a 7-year-old girl who had a ductus closed at age 6 and a ventricular septal defect closed just before death. At necropsy, a single coronary arose from the pulmonary trunk and the mitral valve was stenotic. Monselise and associates[79] described a 1-year-old boy with a ventricular septal defect and a single coronary artery arising from the pulmonary trunk. Survival in these 2 patients was made possible by the presence of the associated congenital anomalies, which allowed systemic pressure in the pulmonary trunk.

ANOMALOUS ORIGIN OF 1 OR MORE CORONARY ARTERIES FROM THE AORTA

BOTH *LEFT MAIN* AND RIGHT CORONARY ARTERIES FROM THE *RIGHT* AORTIC SINUS

Classification of the Anomaly

This condition has been reviewed recently by Barth and Roberts.[80] Anomalous origin of the left main coronary artery from the right sinus of Valsalva can be classified into 4 major groups according to the course taken by the left main in relation to the aorta and pulmonary trunk enroute to the left side of the heart. The left main may course anterior to the pulmonary trunk, posterior to the aorta,[81] within the ventricular septum beneath the right ventricular infundibulum,[82] or between the aorta and pulmonary trunk (Fig. 6). When the left main passes anterior to the pulmonary trunk over the right ventricular infundibulum, symptoms of myocardial ischemia have not been reported unless significant coronary arterial narrowing due to atherosclerotic plaque was present. With the exception of the 12-year-old girl with this anomaly described by Murphy and associates,[83] symptoms of myocardial ischemia have not been reported when the left main arises from the right sinus of Valsalva and courses posterior to the aorta.

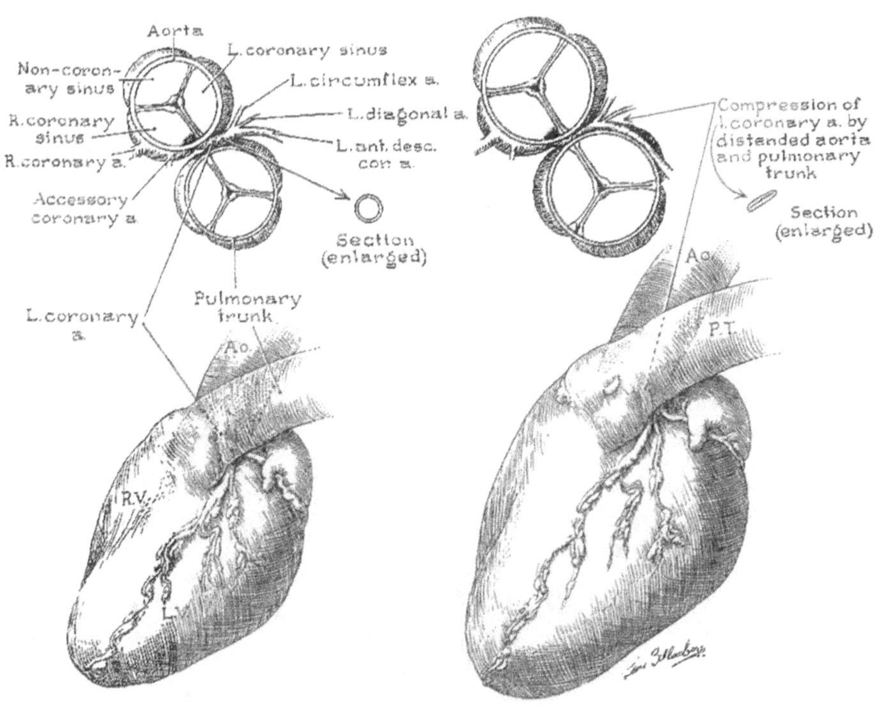

FIGURE 6. Diagram showing a proposed mechanism by which origin of the left (L) main coronary artery (a.) from the right sinus of Valsalva causes nonfatal or fatal cardiac dysfunction. From Roberts WC, et al.,[104] with permission.

Review of Published Reports

At least 43 necropsy patients have been reported with origin of the left main coronary artery from the right sinus of Valsalva with coursing between the aorta and pulmonary trunk[80,81,84–96] In 9, death was unrelated to the anomaly and symptoms of myocardial ischemia were absent during life. In the other 34 patients, death was of coronary origin. Of the 34 patients, 26 (76%) died before age 20 years and the other 8 (24%), from age 49 to 82 years (mean 64). Of the 26 patients who died young, 25 (96%) died suddenly during or shortly after vigorous exertion and 1 died of acute myocardial infarction, having survived for 19 hours after initial collapse, which likewise occurred shortly after exertion. Of the 14 patients where information was provided, 10 had had symptoms before the final collapse: exertional syncope in 6, angina in 4, and exertional dyspnea in 1. Of the 26 young patients, 24 (92%) were male. At necropsy, 5 of the 26 patients had histologic evidence of myocardial necrosis: 1 patient apparently had atherosclerotic narrowing in the anomalous left main coronary artery.

Mechanism of Death in Older Patients With the Anomaly

Of the 8 patients who died after age 20 years, 7 were men. Four died of consequences of acute myocardial infarction: 1 died suddenly; 1 died of a noncardiac cause (alcoholism) (Fig. 7); the mode of death in the other 2 was not described. Symptoms of cardiac dysfunction were described in only 1 of the 8 patients. Histologic evidence of myocardial necrosis or fibrosis was present in 5, absent in 1, and not discussed in 2 patients. Of the 8 older patients, 6 apparently had significant coronary narrowing

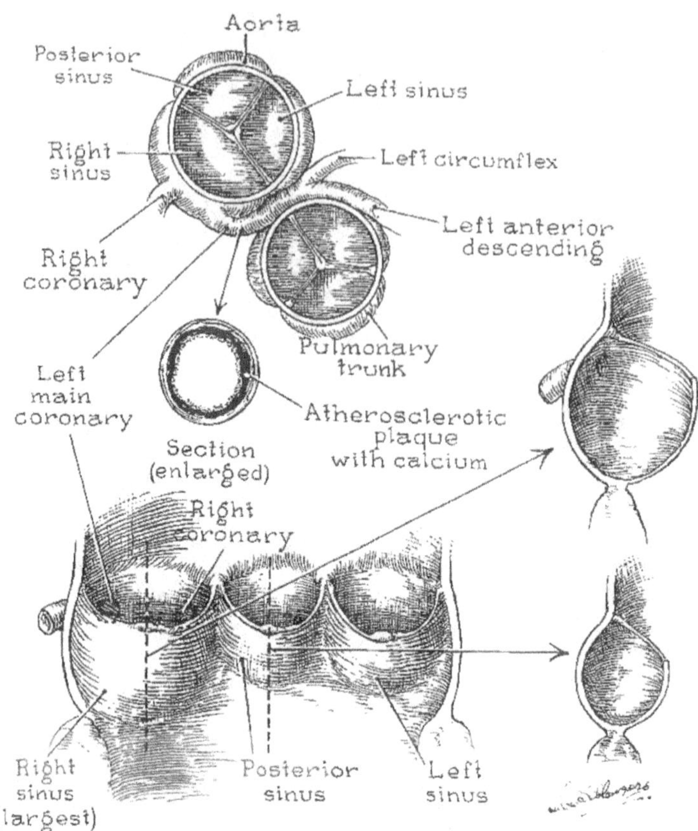

FIGURE 7. Drawing of an anomalously arising left main coronary artery from the right sinus of Valsalva in an 81-year-old man (DCMEO No. 80-04-332) who never had evidence of cardiac dysfunction and who died of a noncardiac condition. The wall of the anomalously arising left main coronary artery is heavily calcified. From Barth CW III, Roberts WC. J Am Coll Cardiol 1986; 7:366–373, with permission.

by atherosclerotic plaque in the abnormal and/or normal coursing arteries. One patient lacked the circumflex branch of the left main artery.

While it is clear from current necropsy information that this anomaly can cause sudden death at a young age, the role the anomaly plays in those who have survived past age 20 years is less clear. One of the 2 older patients reported by Barth and Roberts[80] appears to be the only 1 thus far reported in whom fatal myocardial ischemia could be attributed entirely to the coronary anomaly. Why this patient had fatal myocardial ischemia late in life after decades without symptoms is unclear. Possibly, the excessive cardiac weight (500 gm) was a factor. Why other older patients survive into the ninth decade free of symptoms of cardiac dysfunction is not clear either.

Pathogenesis of Myocardial Ischemia

The precise mechanism by which anomalous origin of the LM coronary artery from the right sinus of Valsalva with coursing between pulmonary trunk and aorta causes myocardial ischemia is unclear. In each of the 5 patients reported by Barth and Roberts,[80] the normal right coronary artery arose at an angle more or less perpendicular to the center of the aortic lumen, and it coursed directly away from the aorta; in contrast, the left main coronary artery arose from the aortic lumen at roughly a 180-degree angle to the center of the aorta. After takeoff, the anomalously arising left main was adherent to the wall of the aorta for roughly 1.5 cm as it coursed to the left side of the heart between pulmonary trunk and aorta. Additionally, the ostium of the anomalously arising left main was slit-like with the largest diameter in a cephalad-caudal direction; in contrast, the ostium of the normally arising right coronary artery was circular and larger. The firmly anchored root of the pulmonary trunk appears to present a potential barrier against which the left main could be compressed by expansion of the aortic root that occurs during increased intra-aortic pressure associated with exertion. The left main coronary artery, of course, is equivalent to 2 arteries in the sense that it is responsible for supplying coronary blood flow to the major portion of left ventricle and, therefore, significant reduction of flow through it is particularly perilous. While it is likely that the narrowed left main orifice has the potential to diminish flow through it, an actual reduction appears to be significant only during or immediately following exertion in those individuals without associated atherosclerosis.

Association of Death with Exertion

The association of death with exertion can be explained by 3 factors: (1) myocardial oxygen requirements increase with exertion and, therefore, any obstruction to coronary flow is more likely to result in myocardial ischemia; (2) it is likely that outward expansion of the roots of both aorta and pulmonary trunk during exertion causes further compression of the ostial lumen of the left main; (3) the left main as it courses between the aorta and pulmonary trunk could be compressed against the root of the pulmonary trunk where it is firmly anchored to the infundibular septum when the aortic root and pulmonary trunk dilate during exertion. The fact that sudden exertional death and nonfatal myocardial ischemia have been seen in persons in whom the left main originates from the proximal right coronary artery and then courses between the great arteries[81,85] and who therefore do not have the abnormal oblique take-off of the left main or the slit-like ostium in the right sinus of Valsalva suggests that hemodynamic compression (hemodynamic vice) of the left main between the great arteries cannot be excluded as an additional mechanism of myocardial ischemia. Davis and coworkers[97] described a 14-year-old boy who had 2 "exertionally related myocardial infarctions" due to this anomaly, underwent surgical enlargement of the narrowed left main ostium, and is asymptomatic during heavy labor 9 years later. This case lends further support to the theory that the primary mechanism causing myocardial ischemia is related to the narrowed left main ostium.

Usefulness of Exercise Electrocardiograph in Diagnosis

The usefulness of stress electrocardiography in identifying the ischemic nature of this anomaly in young persons has received little attention. The fact that 1 patient reported by Barth and Roberts,[80] a 14-year-old boy, had a normal stress test 1 month before death prompted them to review previous experience with stress electrocardiography in young patients with isolated anomalous origin of the left main from the right sinus of Valsalva with coursing of the left main between the aorta and pulmonary trunk. Results of stress electrocardiography in 7 patients,[6,81,91,98] disclosed that 3 had abnormal stress electrocardiograms (electrocardiographic evidence of ischemia or ventricular arrythmia), and 4 had normal stress electrocardiograms. In 3 of the latter 4, however, the test was not a maximal effort. Two of the 7, both of whom had normal submaximal stress electrocardiography, subsequently died suddenly. The other 5 patients had surgery. It is clear that the stress electrocardiogram, particularly that which is submaximal in effort, is not a reliable screening test for this anomaly in young patients who present with exertional syncope, angina, and even acute myocardial infarction.

Differential Diagnosis and Means of Diagnosis

Young patients with this anomaly often present with exertional syncope, dizziness, and angina, but other cardiovascular abnormalities, such as hypertrophic cardiomyopathy and aortic valve stenosis, can present in a similar manner and therefore must be distinguished. The diagnostic approach taken with these young patients must take into account the fallibilities of the various noninvasive tests in identifying this potentially fatal coronary anomaly. The resting electrocardiogram is normal in almost all young persons with this anomaly, and therefore it is not helpful. Physical examination may provide important clues to the noncoronary causes of these symptoms, that is, murmurs and peripheral pulses characteristic of aortic stenosis or hypertrophic cardiomyopathy. Echocardiography also is helpful in assessing for or confining aortic stenosis or hypertrophic cardiomyopathy. Liberthson and associates[99] reported a 54-year-old woman with angina pectoris in whom cross-sectional echocardiography identified anomalous origin of the left main coronary artery from the proximal right coronary artery with coursing of the left main between aorta and pulmonary trunk. Echocardiography, while potentially useful, has not been reported to have successfully identified origin of the left main directly from the right sinus of Valsalva. Continuous ambulatory electrocardiography may identify significant arrhythmias but provides no help in identifying the cause of the arrhythmias. If the noncoronary causes of exertional syncope and angina are not identified, then more extensive evaluation is dictated to exclude the possibility of anomalous origin of the left main. As has been demonstrated, stress electrocardiography does not always identify myocardial ischemia in young patients with this coronary anomaly who are at risk for sudden death, but it should be done and it should be carried to maximal effort if evidence of myocardial ischemia is not identified at lower levels of exercise. If stress electrocardiography is abnormal, then angiographic assessment of coronary anatomy is dictated.[100,101] If maximal stress electrocardiography is normal, then coronary angiography must still be considered in boys with clear cut exercise-induced symptoms. The usefulness of thallium stress electrocardiography for diagnosis of this anomaly is uncertain. The patient reported by Mustafa and associates[98] had normal thallium stress electrocardiography. Finally, the specific case of exertional syncope at a young age, particularly in males, coronary angiography should be done after a second episode of syncope. It should be considered, however, after a single episode if no other clear cause of exertional syncope is evident by noninvasive testing.

Management of Patients with the Anomaly

Once the origin of both left main and right coronary arteries from the right sinus with coursing of the left main between the great arteries has been diagnosed, at least in younger individuals, operative therapy appears warranted for the the prevention of sudden death and for relief of exercise-induced symptoms of myocardial ischemia. Various operative approaches for revascularization have been described. Aortocoronary conduits, either saphenous vein or mammary artery, or both, to the left anterior descending and left circumflex coronary systems has resulted in relief of symptoms and in relief of objective evidence of myocardial ischemia in several patients.[99,102,103] Other surgical approaches also have been successful. Davia and associates[97] described a 14-year-old boy who had 2 myocardial infarcts who underwent surgical enlargement of the narrowed left main coronary ostium by extending an incision from the ostium through the common wall of the aorta and the anomalous artery over the intercoronary commissure. He was free of symptoms and active 9 years later, despite the presence of mild aortic regurgitation due to the procedure. Four patients, aged 12 and 36 years, have undergone an operation of a similar nature to re-establish the normal anatomic location of the left main origin to the left sinus of Valsalva by incising along the course of the left sinus of Valsalva and joining the intima of the vessel to the aorta, resulting in a new ostium.[6,98] No evidence of ischemia was present in the follow-up period of 10 to 36 months.

BOTH LEFT MAIN AND *RIGHT* CORONARY ARTERIES FROM THE *LEFT* AORTIC SINUS

Origin of the right coronary artery from the left sinus of Valsalva until recently has been considered a minor congenital anomaly of no clinical significance.

Frequency

This anomaly is probably missed as frequently at necropsy as it is observed. Its true occurrence at necropsy therefore is really not known. It appears, however, that this anomaly is more frequent than origin of both right and left main coronary arteries from the right sinus with subsequent coursing of the left main between aorta and pulmonary trunk. At necropsy, I have seen 5 cases of origin of both left main and right coronary arteries from the right sinus and 16 cases of origin of both coronary arteries from the left sinus of Valsalva with coursing of either the left main or right coronary arteries between aorta and pulmonary trunk.

Angiographically, origin of both coronary arteries from the left sinus is more frequent than origin of both from the right sinus because patients with the former are more likely to have evidence of myocardial ischemia. Liberthson and associates[92] during the same time period observed at coronary angiography 9 patients in whom both left main and right coronary arteries arose from the right sinus and 9 in whom both arose from the left sinus of Valsalva with either left main or right coronary arteries passing between aorta and pulmonary trunk.

Evidence of Myocardial Ischemia

Of patients in whom both coronary arteries arise from the left aortic sinus with the right coronary artery passing between aorta and pulmonary trunk, it is unclear how many during life have evidence of myocardial ischemia and how many do not. Roberts and associates[104] collected reports describing at necropsy 26 patients with origin of both coronary arteries from the left sinus, and not a single patient had had symptoms of cardiac dysfunction and in none could death be attributed to the anomaly. In contrast, analysis of published data on 34 other patients in whom this congenital anomaly was detected by coronary angiography disclosed that at least 12 had had symptoms of cardiac dysfunction unassociated with significant coronary atherosclerosis or a noncoronary cardiac condition.[81,92,105–111] Of the 12, three had had acute myocardial infarcts; 7, angina pectoris; 1, syncope; and 1 had nonfatal ventricular fibrillation. Of the 12 necropsy patients with this coronary anomaly reported by Roberts and associates,[104] 3 died suddenly, 2 clearly during exertion, and 2 of them previously had had either angina or syncope. One of the 3 patients, a 23-year-old woman, became symptomatic only after she became a long-distance runner; she had frequent episodes of ventricular tachycardia. At necropsy, 2 of these 3 symptomatic patients had grossly visible left ventricular scars. Subsequently, Hanzlick and associates[112–114] reported a 26-year-old marathon runner who was training for the Ironman Triathalon. He collapsed and died just past the finish line of a 13.5-mile race. This patient previously had had 2 episodes of abnormally severe dyspnea after long runs. Brandt and associates[111] reported a 35-year-old man who had at that age developed periodic substernal chest pain, 1 episode being acute myocardial infarction. He underwent operation with placement of a cephalic vein between ascending aorta and right coronary artery. Doppler probe studies in him objectively confirmed that the coronary anomaly caused left ventricular function impairment and that it impaired coronary artery reserve. Coronary reserve was returned to normal by the operation, and the patient had been asymptomatic during the entire 9-month period after operation. Isner and associates[115] reported a 23-year-old man who developed severe chest pain after ingestion of a heavy meal, went to bed, and later was found dead in bed. This patient had occasional episodes of chest pain before his sudden death.

Mechanism of Myocardial Ischemia

The mechanism appears to be the same as in patients in whom both coronary arteries arise from the left sinus of Valsalva just as long as 1 of the major coronary arteries courses between aorta and pulmonary trunk. There are 3 possibilities: (1) the slit-like orifice of the anomalously arising coronary artery is compressed closed or nearly so as the aorta dilates with exertion; (2) the anomalous artery itself is compressed by the aorta and pulmonary trunk as it courses between these 2 arteries which dilate with exertion, or (3) both factors 1 and 2 (Fig. 8). The upright nature of the slit-like orifice of the anomalous artery prevents blood within the aortic lumen from flowing

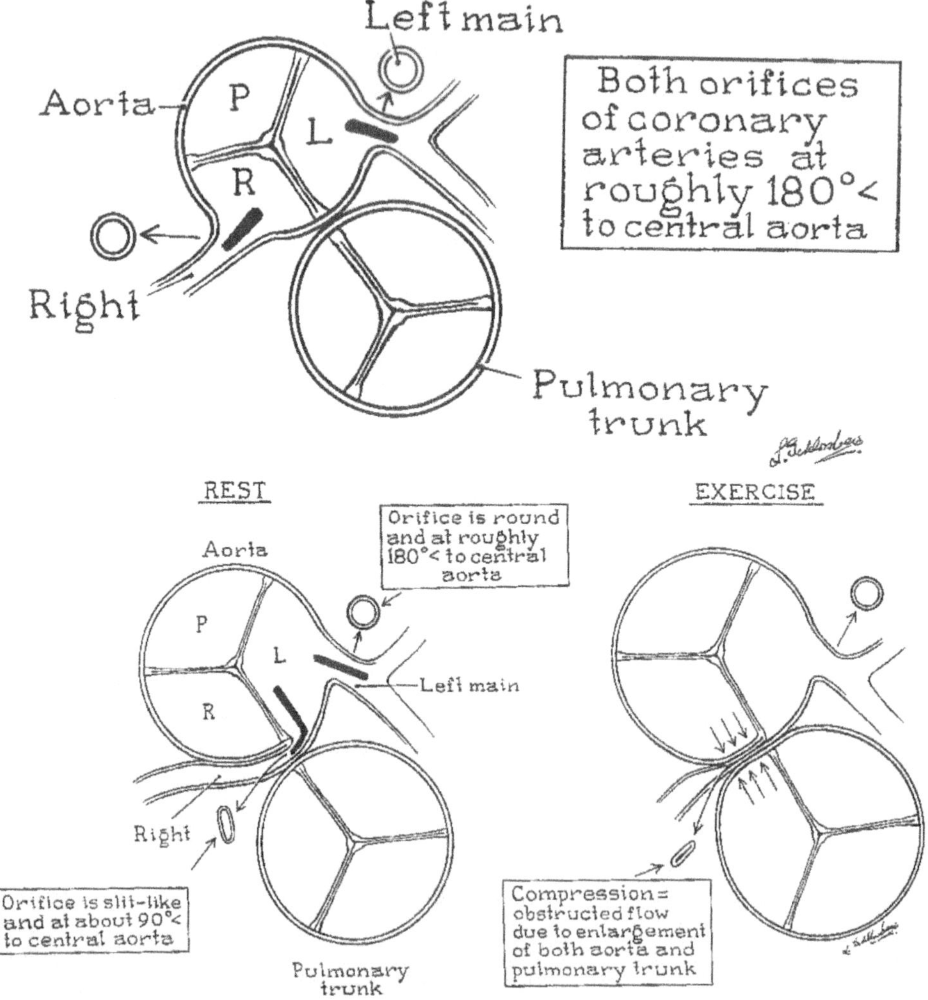

FIGURE 8. Diagram showing mechanism by which origin of the right coronary artery arising from the left sinus of Valsalva might cause fatal or nonfatal cardiac dysfunction (*lower*), and comparison with normal (*upper*). From Roberts WC, et al.,[104] with permission.

into the right coronary artery during ventricular diastole without a peculiar direction of flow. In a 60-year-old man with this coronary anomaly, Keren and associates[110] demonstrated angiographically significant narrowing of the right coronary artery as it coursed between the 2 great arteries during ventricular *systole*.

Treatment

In contrast to the situation when both coronary arteries arise from the right aortic sinus, therapy in the situation when both coronary arteries arise from the left aortic sinus is not as clear-cut. In the former group of patients, operative intervention is indicated even in the asymptomatic patient to prevent fatal or nonfatal myocardial ischemia. In that situation, however, it is the left main coronary artery that has a slit-like orifice and that courses between aorta and pulmonary trunk. The left main, of course, is not 1 but really 2 major coronary arteries. When both coronary arteries arise from the left aortic sinus, only 1 major coronary artery, the right coronary artery, arises from a slit-like orifice and courses between aorta and pulmonary trunk. In the latter situation, there appears no justification for operative intervention unless the patient has developed clinical signs or symptoms of myocardial ischemia. Sudden death as the initial manifestation of this coronary anomaly is extremely rare. Sudden death in almost all reported patients has been preceded by other symptoms of myocardial ischemia. If symptoms or signs of myocardial ischemia have occurred, however, operative therapy is clearly warranted.

BOTH LEFT MAIN AND RIGHT CORONARY ARTERIES FROM THE POSTERIOR AORTIC SINUS

To my knowledge, origin of both left main and right coronary arteries from the posterior sinus of Valsalva has never been reported.

BOTH RIGHT AND LEFT CIRCUMFLEX CORONARY ARTERIES FROM THE RIGHT AORTIC SINUS (OR ORIGIN OF THE LEFT CIRCUMFLEX FROM THE RIGHT CORONARY ARTERY) AND THE LEFT ANTERIOR DESCENDING CORONARY ARTERY FROM THE LEFT AORTIC SINUS

Initial Description

The first description of this anomaly was by Antopol and Kugel[116] in 1933. These authors described 4 cases in adults (1 a man; sex in other 3 not stated) at necropsy. In 3, the left circumflex arose from the right sinus of Valsalva, and in 1, from the right coronary artery. In all 4, the right coronary artery coursed retrograde to the aorta before reaching the left atrioventricular sulcus. The left anterior descending arose from the left sinus of Valsalva, and it coursed directly to its usual location. The left main was absent. When, however, the left circumflex arises as the first branch of the right cornary artery, the initial portion of the right coronary artery then is equivalent to the normal left main coronary artery[117] (Fig. 9). When the left circumflex arises directly from the right sinus of Valsalva or as the first branch of the right coronary artery, the left circumflex always follows a retroaortic course to the left atrioventricular sulcus (Fig. 10).

Frequency

Origin of the left circumflex from the right aortic sinus or from the right coronary artery is the most common anomaly of coronary arterial origin. Among 600 hearts

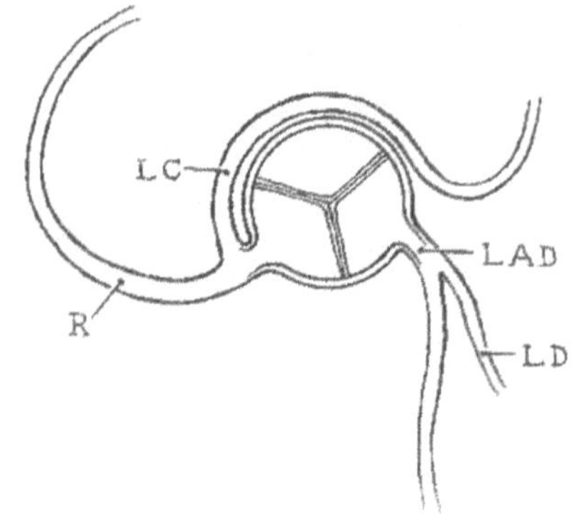

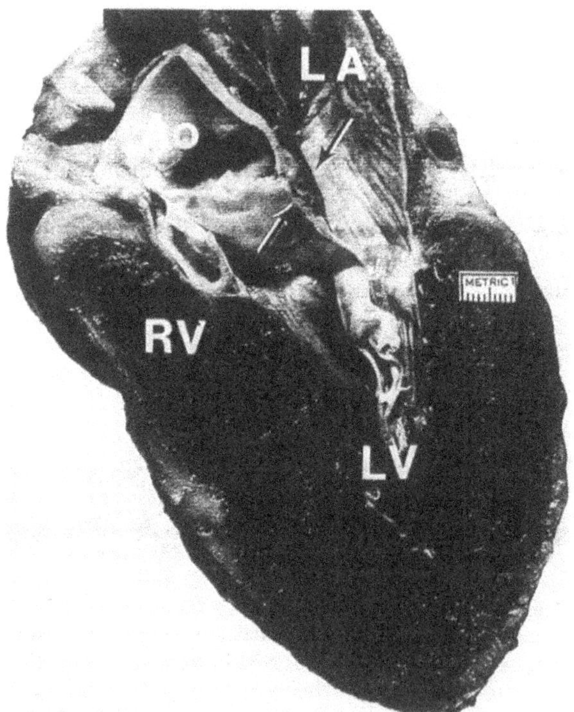

FIGURE 9. Diagram showing origin of left circumflex (LC) coronary artery arising as the first branch of the right (R) coronary artery and then coursing posterior to the aorta before reaching the left atrioventricular sulcus. The left anterior descending (LAD) coronary artery arises from the left sinus of Valsalva. LD = left diagonal.

of patients aged 30 to 89 years (100 hearts in each of the 6 decades), White and Edwards[118] found 2 cases of this anomaly—both were men, one aged 76 and one aged 81 years. Thus, a frequency of 1 per 300 adults at necropsy was reported. Odgen[53] found this anomaly in 14 necropsy patients studied in a 16-year period at the Yale-New Haven Hospital. I have seen this anomaly at necropsy in 14 patients (10 men) aged 22 to 71 years (mean 49): 11 had no associated anomalies and 3 had valvular heart disease (rheumatic heart disease in 2 and a normally functioning bicuspid aortic valve in 1 [Fig. 11]). In 13 patients, the coronary anomaly clearly was of no clinical significance; in 1, a 22-year old man who died suddenly while playing basketball, the anomaly may have been important. In 7 patients, the left circumflex arose directly from the right aortic sinus, and in 7 patients, it arose as the first branch of the right coronary artery.

FIGURE 10. Anteroposterior longitudinal view of the heart showing the course of an anomalously arising left circumflex coronary artery (arrows) between the aorta (Ao) and the left atrium (LA) before reaching the left atrioventricular sulcus. The left circumflex arose as the first branch of the right coronary artery. RV = right ventricle; LV = left ventricle.

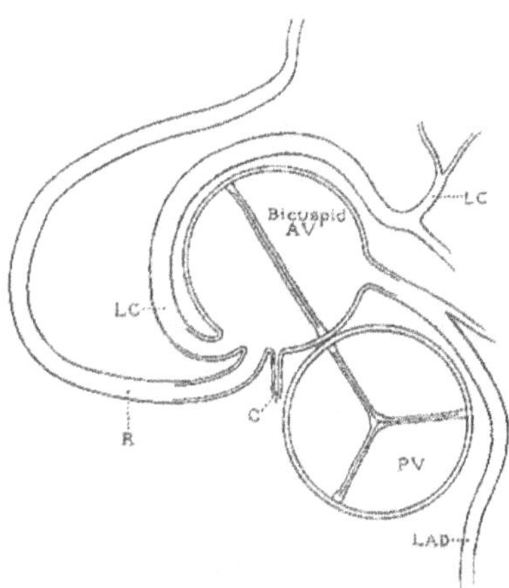

FIGURE 11. Origin of left circumflex (LC) coronary artery directly from the right anterior aspect of the aorta with retroaortic coursing to the left atrioventricular sulcus in a 43-year-old man (A81-5757) who died of complications of severe coronary atherosclerosis. Although congenitally bicuspid, the aortic valve (AV) appeared to have functioned normally. C = conus coronary artery; LAD = left anterior descending coronary artery; PV = pulmonic valve; R = right coronary artery.

Of 2996 patients having selective coronary angiography, Page and associates[119] found that 20 (16 men) had origin of the left circumflex from the right sinus of Valsalva or as the first branch of the right coronary artery. In none of the 20 patients could cardiac dysfunction be attributed to the presence of this coronary anomaly (1 of the 20 also had origin of the left anterior descending from the pulmonary trunk). Among 3750 coronary arteriograms reviewed by Chaitman and associates,[105] 31 adults had anomalies of coronary origin, the most common (17 patients) being origin of the left circumflex from the right sinus of Valsalva or as the first branch of the right coronary artery. The sex of the 17 patients was not stated. Of 200 coronary angiograms reviewed by Ray and associates,[120] 2 men aged 60 and 62 years, had origin of the left circumflex from the right coronary artery. Baltaxe and Wixson[121] reviewed 1000 consecutive coronary arteriograms, performed mainly because of angina pectoris, and various coronary anomalies were found in 9: two, a 51-year-old woman and a 56-year-old man, had origin of the left circumflex as the first branch of the right coronary artery. Of 7000 patients having coronary angiograms, Kimbiris and associates[106] found anomalous aortic origin of 1 or more coronary arteries in 45; origin of the left circumflex from the right sinus of Valsalva or as the first branch of the right coronary artery was the most common of the 5 anomalies found, occurring in 26 patients (58%). The sex of the 26 patients was not stated. Of 21 cases of anomalous coronary origin reported by Liberthson and associates[122] (9 obtained at necropsy in a cardiovascular registry and 11 by selective coronary angiography), 11 were origin of the left circumflex from the right sinus of Valsalva or as the first branch of the right coronary artery. The mean age of the 11 patients was 54 years, and 8 were men.

Clinical Significance

There is no clinical significance, unless cardiac surgery is performed. If coronary perfusion during coronary bypass is limited to the artery arising from the left sinus of Valsalva, then the myocardium in the distribution of the left circumflex coronary artery is not perfused. If perfusion is to the artery arising from the right sinus of Valsalva and if the left circumflex arises as the first branch of the right coronary artery, the tip of the perfusing canula might be past the origin of the left circumflex, and again the myocardium dependent on the left circumflex is deprived. If both right and left circumflex coronary arteries arise from the right sinus of Valsalva, 1 artery would be deprived by cannulation of only 1 of the coronary ostia in this sinus. If this anomaly is present in the patient who has replacement of both mitral and aortic valves, the fixation rings of the prostheses may compress the lumen of the left circumflex coronary artery, which courses in a path between the prosthetic anuli[123] (Fig. 12).

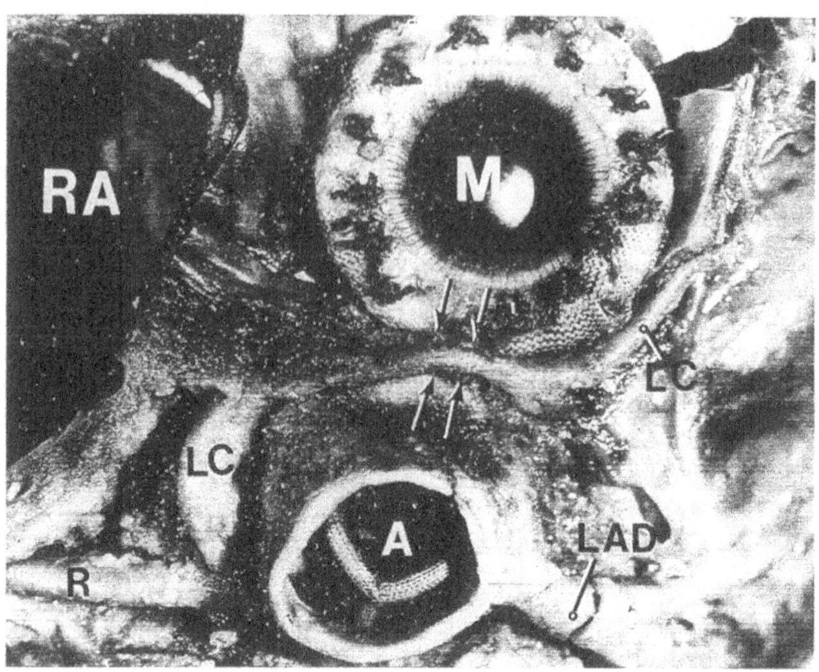

FIGURE 12. Compression (arrows) of an anomalously arising left circumflex (LC) coronary artery from the right (R) coronary artery by the rings of prosthetic valves in both the aortic (A) and mitral (M) valve positions. LAD = left anterior descending coronary artery; RA = right atrium. From Roberts WC, et al.,[123] with permission.

BOTH RIGHT AND LEFT ANTERIOR DESCENDING FROM THE RIGHT AORTIC SINUS (OR LEFT ANTERIOR DESCENDING FROM THE RIGHT CORONARY ARTERY) AND LEFT CIRCUMFLEX CORONARY ARTERY FROM THE LEFT AORTIC SINUS

This is a rare anomaly in hearts without other congenital anomalies of the heart or great anterior. Several varieties have been recognized or are possible: (1) Origin of the left anterior descending from the right sinus or from the right coronary artery with coursing to the left side of the heart anterior to the right ventricular infundibulum (Fig. 13). (2) Origin of the left anterior descending from the right sinus of Valsalva or directly from the right coronary artery with coursing to the left side of the heart between the aorta and pulmonary trunk. To my knowledge, this pattern has not been observed but is theoretically possible. (3) Origin of the left anterior descending from the right aortic sinus or directly from the aorta with coursing to the left side of the heart in the ventricular septum beneath the right ventricular infundibulum.

RIGHT CORONARY ARTERY FROM THE POSTERIOR AORTIC SINUS AND THE LEFT MAIN CORONARY ARTERY FROM THE LEFT AORTIC SINUS

This is an extremely rare anomaly in hearts without other congenital anomalies. Vlodaver and associates[124] found this anomaly in only 1 heart among their huge collection. That patient was a 72-year-old man who died from atherosclerotic coronary artery disease. I have seen this anomaly once (Fig. 14). The patient was a 19-year-

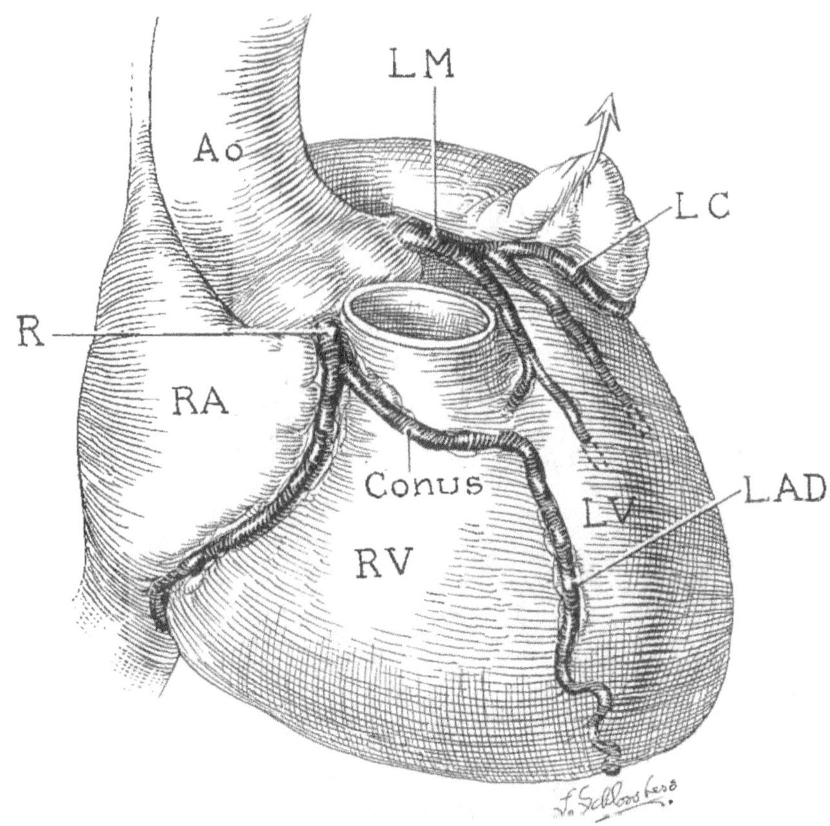

FIGURE 13. Origin of the left anterior descending (LAD) from the right (R) coronary artery with coursing anterior to the right ventricular (RV) outflow tract in a 60-year-old man (A81-63) who died of consequences of severe coronary atherosclerosis. From Roberts WC, et al.,[82] with permission.

old boy who died suddenly while playing basketball (DCMEO NO. 83-09-602). It seemed unlikely that the anomaly was associated with the boy's sudden death because the heart weighed 450 gm, a weight that is clearly abnormal. The cause of the cardiomegaly, however, is unknown. I have observed 1 heart in which the ostium of the right coronary artery was located just cephalad to the most cephalad extension of the commissures between the right and posterior aortic valve cusps (GT NO. 85A-143). This patient was a 79-year-old man who died from consequences of atherosclerosis.

LEFT MAIN CORONARY ARTERY FROM THE POSTERIOR AORTIC SINUS AND RIGHT CORONARY ARTERY FROM THE RIGHT AORTIC SINUS

To my knowledge this anomaly has not been reported in a patient without other anomalies of the heart or great vessels. I have examined a heart, however, in which the ostium of the left main coronary artery arose just above the commissure between the left and posterior aortic valve cusps (SGAH NO. A82-1). The patient was a 54-year-old man who died from atherosclerotic coronary artery disease. The anomaly did not appear to have clinical significance.

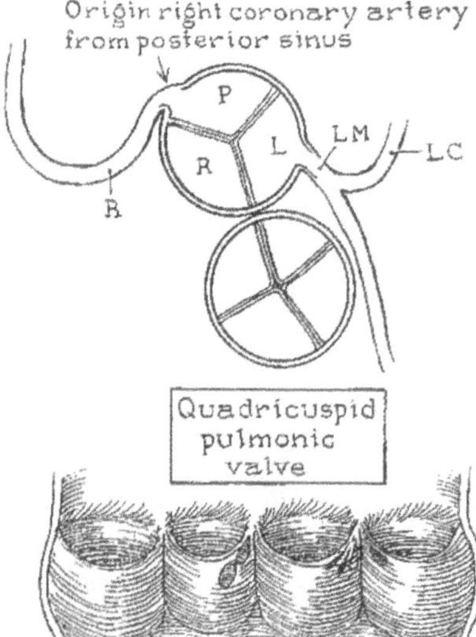

FIGURE 14. Origin of the right (R) coronary artery from the posterior (P) aortic sinus in a 19-year-old man (DCMEO No. 83-09-602) who died suddenly while playing basketball. The pulmonic valve was quadricuspid. The cause of sudden death was not determined. Whether the coronary anomaly played a role in the sudden death is unclear.

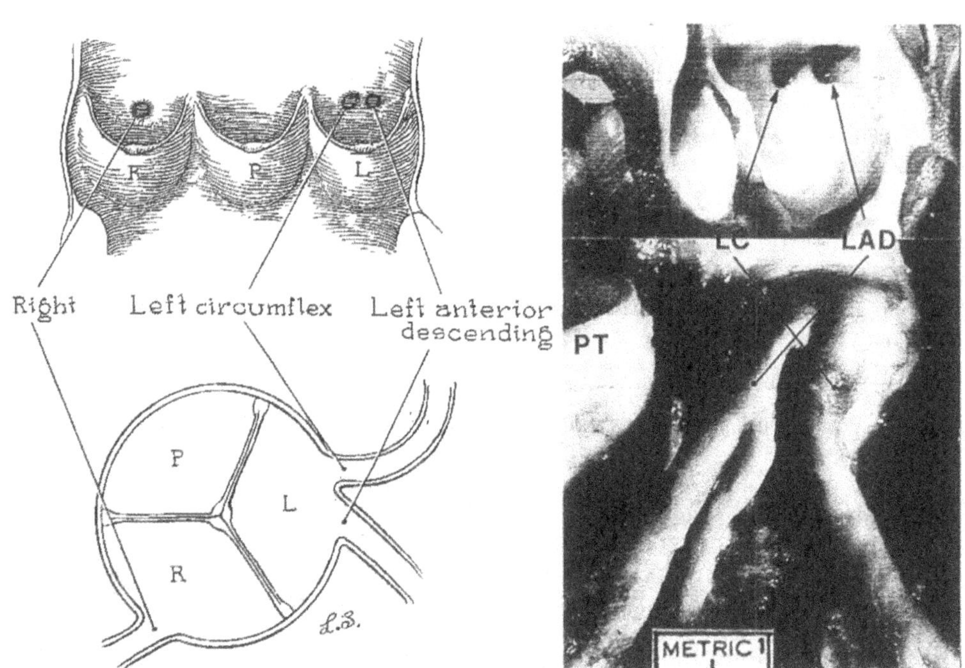

FIGURE 15. Drawing *(left)* of aorta showing origin of each of the left circumflex (LC) and left anterior descending (LAD) coronary arteries from a separate ostium in the left (L) sinus of Valsalva. *Upper right,* Interior of the left sinus showing each ostium (SH No. A81-49). *Lower right,* Exterior view showing both LC and LAD coronary arteries arising separately. PT = pulmonary trunk. From DiCicco BS, et al.,[125] with permission.

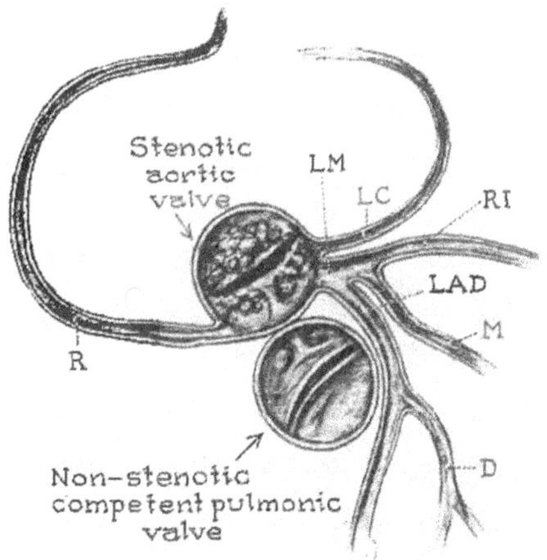

FIGURE 16. Drawing showing origin of both left-sided coronary arteries directly from the left anterior side of the aorta in a 60-year-old man (A82-79) in whom both semilunar valves were congenitally biscuspid and the aortic valve also stenotic. D = diagonal; LAD = left anterior descending; LC = left circumflex; LM = "left main"; M = marginal; R = right; RI = ramus intermedius.

BOTH LEFT ANTERIOR DESCENDING AND LEFT CIRCUMFLEX CORONARY ARTERIES FROM A SEPARATE OSTIUM IN THE LEFT AORTIC SINUS WITH THE RIGHT CORONARY ARTERY FROM THE RIGHT AORTIC SINUS

This anomaly is fairly common. Ogden[53] found this anomaly in 6 necropsy patients in a 16-year period. I have observed it at necropsy in 9 patients (7 men) aged 35 to 82 years (mean 60), all seen in a 7-year period. Two of the 9 patients were reported previously[125] (Fig. 15). In none of the 9 patients was the anomaly of clinical significance. One of the 9 patients was a 60-year-old man (A82-79) who also had congenitally biscuspid pulmonic and aortic valves; both left anterior descending and left circumflex arose from a separate ostium to the left of the raphe or in the location of the normal left aortic sinus of Valsalva (Fig. 16). Zumbo and associates[126] found this anomaly in 21 of 2089 hearts at necropsy.

ORIGIN OF ONLY 1 CORONARY ARTERY FROM THE AORTA WITHOUT ORIGIN OF A CORONARY ARTERY FROM THE PULMONARY TRUNK (SINGLE CORONARY OSTIUM IN AORTA)

HISTORY

According to Smith,[127] "single coronary artery" (a misnomer in my view—"single aortic coronary ostium without a pulmonary artery coronary ostium" is better) was first described by Banchi[128] in 1716.

CLASSIFICATION

Several authors have suggested classifications for single coronary ostium. Smith[127] in 1950 suggested 3 groups: (1) A single coronary artery that follows the course of the right coronary artery with continuation into the left circumflex, which continues as the left anterior descending, *or* a single left main that branches into the left anterior descending and left circumflex, the latter of which extends across the crux to form the right coronary artery; (2) After its origin from a single aortic ostium, the main trunk branches quickly into a right and left main coronary artery or into a right, left anterior descending, and left circumflex coronary artery, which reach their usual location a relatively short distance from the aortic ostium; (3) The single coronary artery branches so atypically that there is little similarity to the normal coursing of the 3 major (right, left anterior descending, and left circumflex) coronary arteries. In Smith's review of previously reported necropsy cases, there were 9 in group I unassociated with other major cardiovascular anomalies (aged 33 to 66 years; 6 men); 15 in group II (aged 35 to 65; 10 men); and only 2 in group III (aged 22 and 38; 1 man). Smith actually found 15 patients in group III, but 13 of them had various other congenital anomalies of the heart and great arteries.

Ogden and Goodyear[129] in 1970 suggested a classification employing 5 types subdivided by the letters "R" and "L" to indicate whether the single coronary ostium was in the right or left aortic sinus of Valsalva. These authors followed this letter by numbers 1 to 5 to indicate the pattern of anatomic distribution of the branches according to their initial divisions. In cases of single right coronary ostium, types 1 to 5, the letters "a," "b," and "c" were added to indicate the course of the branches. This classification has logic, but it is incomplete.

Lipton and associates[130] proposed a classification based on their angiographic studies, and it employed features of the classification of both Smith[127] and Ogden and Goodyear.[129] These authors used the latter authors' "R" and "L" and "a" and "b" systems but incorporated these letters into the 3 groups proposed by Smith. Thus, group I was designated R1 and L1; group II, R2-a and L2-a, R2-b and L2-b, and R2-p and L2-p; group III included cases in which the left circumflex and left anterior descending arose separately from a single trunk arising from the right aortic sinus. The letter "a" indicated that the "transverse" branch from the single coronary artery passed "anterior" to the right ventricular infundibulum; "b" that it passed "between" the aorta and PT, and "p" that it passed retroaortic. This classification provides more easily memorable numbers and letters than that proposed by Ogden and Goodyear. I like this newer classification, but their group III is incomplete.

A purely descriptive classification of "single coronary artery" is presented in Table 1.

TABLE 1. Congenital Coronary Arterial Anomalies

I. Origin of 1 or more coronary arteries from the pulmonary trunk and 1 or more coronary arteries from the aorta
  A. Left main from pulmonary trunk
  B. Right from pulmonary trunk
  C. Left anterior descending from pulmonary trunk
  D. Left circumflex from pulmonary trunk
  E. Accessory coronary artery from pulmonary trunk
II. Origin of 1 or more coronary arteries from the pulmonary trunk without origin of a coronary artery from the aorta.
  A. Right and left main from pulmonary trunk
  B. "Single coronary artery" from pulmonary trunk
III. Anomalous origin of 1 or more coronary arteries from the aorta
  A. Left main and right from right aortic sinus
  B. Left main and right from left aortic sinus
  C. Left main and right from the posterior aortic sinus
  D. Right and left circumflex from right aortic sinus (or left circumflex from right) and left anterior descending from left sinus
  E. Right and left anterior descending from right aortic sinus (or left anterior descending from right) and left circumflex from left sinus
  F. Right from posterior aortic sinus and left main from left sinus
  G. Left main from posterior aortic sinus and right from right sinus

      H. Left anterior descending and left circumflex from a separate ostium in the left aortic sinus and right from right aortic sinus

IV. Origin of only 1 coronary artery from the aorta without origin of a coronary artery from the pulmonary trunk (single coronary ostium)

  A. From right aortic sinus

    1. Right crosses crux and continues as the left circumflex, which continues as the left anterior descending

    2. Left main from right

      a. Coursing of left main posterior to aorta before dividing into left anterior descending and left circumflex

      b. Coursing of left main between aorta and pulmonary trunk before branching into left anterior descending and left circumflex

      c. Coursing of left main anterior to pulmonary trunk

      d. Coursing of left main in ventricular septum beneath right ventricular infundibulum

    3. Left anterior descending and left circumflex from right with coursing of left circumflex posterior to aorta and left anterior descending anterior to right ventricle

    4. Left anterior descending from right with coursing anterior to right ventricle with right crossing crux to form left circumflex

    5. Left anterior descending from right with coursing between aorta and pulmonary trunk with right crossing crux to continue as left circumflex

    6. Left anterior descending from right with coursing between aorta and pulmonary trunk and left circumflex from right with retroaortic course

    7. Left anterior descending from right coursing anterior to right ventricle, left circumflex from right coursing between aorta and pulmonary trunk

    8. Left anterior descending from right coursing retroaortic with right crossing crux to continue as left circumflex

    9. Left anterior descending from right with coursing to left side in ventricular septum beneath right ventricular outflow tract and left circumflex from right with retroaortic course to left atrioventricular sulcus

  B. From left aortic sinus

    1. Left anterior descending and left circumflex from single coronary artery with left circumflex crossing crux to continue as right

    2. Right, left anterior descending, and left circumflex from single coronary artery

      a. Right posterior to aorta

      b. Right between aorta and pulmonary trunk

      c. Right anterior to right ventricle

    3. Right and left circumflex from single coronary artery and left anterior descending from right

      a. Right between aorta and pulmonary trunk

      b. Right posterior to aorta

    4. Right and left anterior descending from single coronary artery and of left circumflex from left anterior descending

      a. Right between aorta and pulmonary trunk

      b. Right posterior to pulmonary trunk

  C. From posterior aortic sinus

    1. Single coronary artery between aorta and pulmonary trunk with trifurcation into right, left anterior descending, and left circumflex

    2. Single coronary artery to left of pulmonary trunk with trifurcation into right, left anterior descending, and left circumflex

    3. Single coronary artery to right and when anterior to aorta giving rise to right and left main, which subdivides into left anterior descending and left circumflex

V. Coronary arterial aneurysm

VI. Coronary arterial fistula

VII. High take off coronary artery

VIII. Tunneled major coronary artery (myocardial bridge)

IX. Congenital absence, atresia, or hypoplasia of a coronary artery

FREQUENCY

"Single coronary anomaly" is rare, particulary in the absence of other anomalies of the heart and great vessels. In 1968, Ogden (quoted by Ogden and Goodyear[129]) compiled 142 cases including 10 of his own. The male-to-female ratio was 1.4 to 1. The single coronary artery arose from the right aortic sinus in 70 cases (49%) and from the left aortic sinus in 64 cases (45%). Unfortunately, Ogden included 4 cases in which a single left main coronary artery arose from the pulmonary trunk. The ages of the 142 patients ranged from 7 months to 20 years, and 41 (68%) of them had associated anomalies of the heart or great vessels; of the 82 patients aged 20 years or older, only 5 (6%) had associated anomalies of the heart or great arteries. Of the 46 cases with associated anomalies of the heart or great vessels, 17 (37%) had transposition of the great arteries, 10 (22%) had coronary artery fistula, and 7 (15%) had biscuspid aortic valves; the remaining 12 patients (26%) had a variety of anomalies.

I have studied 5 adults at necropsy with a single coronary ostium unassociated with other congenital cardiovascular defects: in 2, both men aged 39 and 73 years, a single left main pattern was present (Fig. 17); in 1, a 60-year-old man, the left main was congenitally atretic and the coronary pattern was of the single right coronary artery type (Fig. 18); in 1, a 65-year-old man, the single artery arose in the left aortic sinus, but the right coronary artery coursed to the right between the aorta and pulmonary trunk after taking origin from the left main (Fig. 19); and in 1, a 69-year-old man with cardiovascular features of the Marfan syndrome but without the skeletal features of this syndrome, the single ostium was in the right aortic sinus with immediate origin of the left circumflex with retroaortic course from the right coronary artery and immediate origin of the left anterior descending from the right coronary artery with coursing anterior to the right ventricular outflow tract.

Of the 142 cases analyzed by Ogden and Goodyear,[129] 31 (23%) had a single artery that did not branch (their type I); 21 (15%) had 2 major branches with one coursing posterior to the aorta (type 2); 15 (11%) had 2 major branches with 1 branch coursing between the aorta and pulmonary trunk (type 3); 18 (13%) had 2 major branches with 1 branch coursing anterior to the pulmonary trunk (type 4); and 7 patients (5%) had 3 major branches, all with origin of the single coronary artery in the right aortic sinus (type 5).

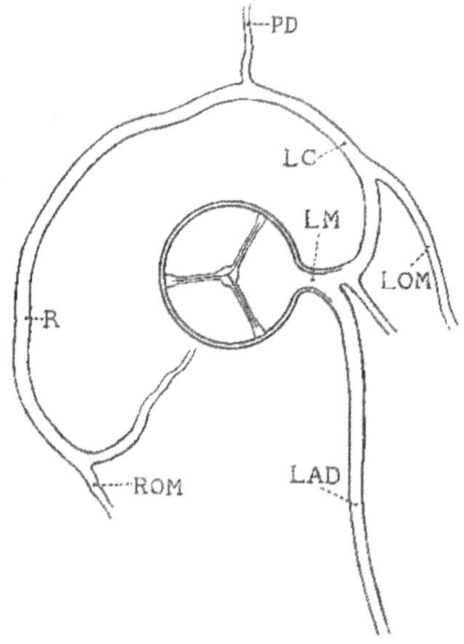

FIGURE 17. Drawing of single coronary ostium arising in the left aortic sinus with no coronary ostium in the other 2 aortic sinuses or in the aorta above the sinuses of Valsalva. The left circumflex (LC) continues across the crux as the right (R) coronary artery. This drawing was from the heart of a 39-year-old-man (DCMEO No. 81-06-416) who died from a gunshot wound. He never had evidence of cardiac dysfunction.

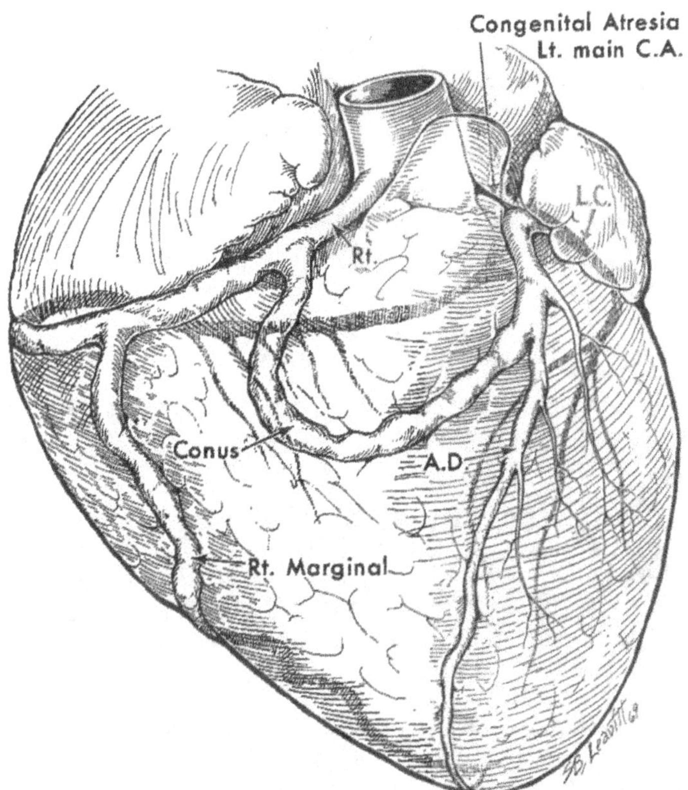

FIGURE 18. Diagram of epicardial coronary arteries in a 61-year-old man who died suddenly as a consequence of severe coronary narrowing by atherosclerotic plaques but in whom the left (Lt) main coronary artery (CA) was congenitally atretic. This anomaly is equivalent to single coronary ostium with the single ostium in the right sinus of Valsalva. From Fortuin NJ, Roberts WC. Congenital atresia of the left main coronary artery. Am J of Med 1971; 50:385–389, with permission.

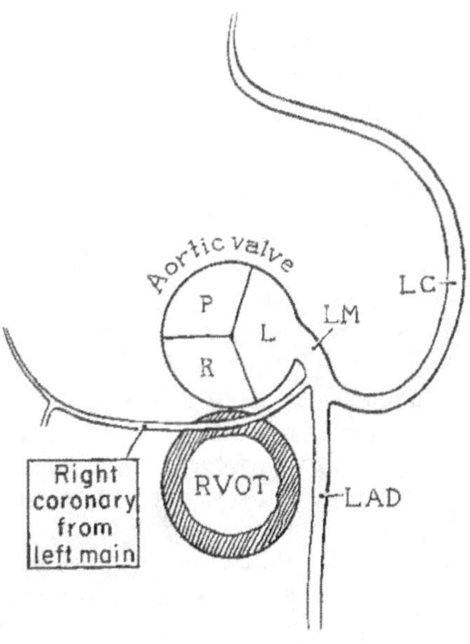

FIGURE 19. Single coronary ostium with origin of the right coronary artery from the left main (LM) and coursing of the right coronary artery between aortic valve and right ventricular outflow tract (RVOT) on its way to the right atrioventricular sulcus in a 65-year-old man (DCVAH No. 84A-112) who never had signs or symptoms of cardiac dysfunction. L = left aortic sinus; LAD = left anterior descending; LC = left circumflex; P = posterior aortic sinus; R = right aortic sinus. From Barbour DJ, Roberts WC. Origin of the right from the left main coronary artery. (Single coronary ostium in aorta.) Am J Cardiol 1985; 55:609, with permission.

Of the 10 cases of single coronary artery diagnosed angiographically by Lipton and associates,[130] 5 had group IIR (a in 1, b in 2, and p in 1), 1 had group IIL, and 4 had group IIL (b in 3 and p in 1). None of these 10 patients had other associated congenital cardiovascular anomalies; they ranged in age from 39 to 64 years, and 8 were men.

CLINICAL SIGNIFICANCE

Although some patients have been described in whom symptoms of myocardial ischemia have occurred, the symptomatic patients nearly always have had associated atherosclerotic coronary disease, or valvular heart disease or other major congenital anomalies of the heart or great arteries. Of course, severe atherosclerotic narrowing of the single coronary artery before it divides or narrowing of its ostium in the aorta may have particularly devastating consequences.

ORIGIN OF THE LEFT MAIN OR BOTH ANTERIOR DESCENDING AND LEFT CIRCUMFLEX CORONARY ARTERY FROM THE RIGHT CORONARY ARTERY WITH INTRAMYOCARDIAL COURSING TO THE LEFT SIDE OF THE HEART OF THE LEFT MAIN OR LEFT ANTERIOR DESCENDING IN THE VENTRICULAR SEPTUM BENEATH THE RIGHT VENTRICULAR INFUNDIBULUM

At least 13 necropsy patients (10 men) have been described in whom a single aortic coronary ostium, located in the right aortic sinus, gave rise to the right coronary artery, which in turn gave rise to the left main coronary artery, which coursed in the ventricular septum beneath the right ventricular infundibulum for about 5 cm before emerging in the epicardium, just anterior to the ventricular septum, where it gave off the left anterior descending and left circumflex branches (Fig. 20). These cases have been summarized by Roberts and associates.[82] In none of the 13 patients was death, or myocardial dysfunction, if present, related to the coronary anomaly. These cases in which the left main coronary artery was in an intramyocardial location for about 5 cm indicate that tunneling of a major coronary artery—indeed, an artery equivalent to 2 major coronary arteries—in myocardium has no functional significance. Saner and associates[131] and Schulte and associates[132] reported single cases (a 73-year-old man and a 71-year-old woman) in whom the left anterior descending arose either from the right aortic sinus or from the right coronary artery and coursed in the ventricular septum beneath the right ventricular infundibulum before emerging just anterior to the ventricular septum. In neither patient had there been clinical evidence of myocardial ischemia.

CORONARY ARTERIAL ANEURYSM

DEFINITIONS

Dilatation of coronary arteries can be *diffuse* or localized. Very elderly individuals often have dilated coronary arteries, as do younger individuals with huge hearts (most commonly from chronic aortic regurgitation or hypertrophic cardiomyopathy). Patients with supravalvular aortic stenosis have hugely dilated coronary arteries because in this condition these vessels fill mainly in ventricular systole rather than in diastole.[133] Patients with severe cyanotic congenital heart disease who survive well into adulthood also usually have very large coronary arteries that dilate in response to the severe systemic arterial desaturation[134] (Fig. 21, Table 2). An occasional

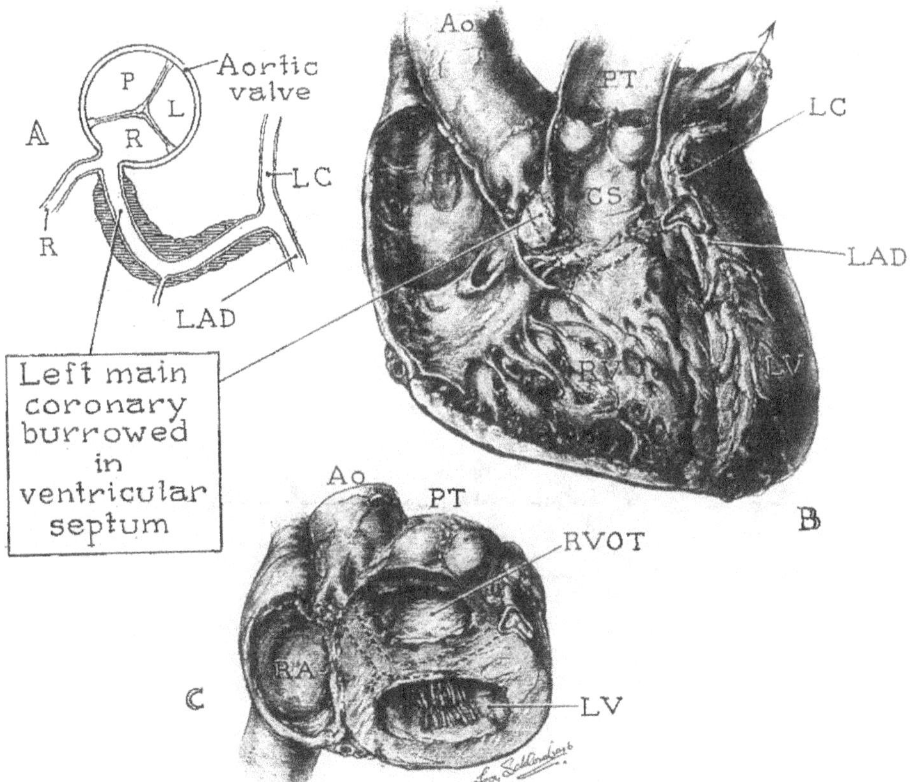

FIGURE 20. Drawing of the heart in which the left main coronary artery arose from the right (R) aortic sinus and then the left main coursed behind the right ventricular outflow tract and within the crista supraventricularis (CS) myocardium before entering the epicardium just anterior to the ventricular septum. The left main then divided into the left anterior descending (LAD) and left circumflex (LC) coronary arteries. This anomaly caused no cardiac dysfunction. Ao = ascending aorta; L = left aortic sinus; LV = left ventricle; P = posterior aortic sinus; PT = pulmonary trunk; LV = left ventricle; R = either right aortic sinus or right coronary artery; RA = right atrium; RV = right ventricle. From Roberts WC, et al.,[82] with permission.

adult has considerable diffuse dilation of 1 coronary artery unassociated with any of the aforementioned conditions. Of course, diffuse dilatation nearly always occurs in a coronary artery serving as part of an arteriovenous or arteriocameral fistula.

Localized dilatation of 1 portion of 1 or more epicardial coronary arteries, in contrast to diffuse dilation, is rare. Probably its most common cause is that occurring as a part of the *mucocutaneous lymph-node syndrome* (Kawasaki disease)[135] (Fig. 22). The next most common cause is *atherosclerosis*. Other extremely rare causes are *infection*, particularly as a result of a septic embolus (mycotic aneurysm); *trauma;* and *congenital.* The atherosclerotic coronary aneurysms are seen only in older individuals (usually > age 50 years), they nearly always contain intra-aneurysmal thrombus which may narrow or completely obstruct the lumen, and they are associated with extensive atherosclerosis in the portions of coronary artery that are not aneurysmal. In contrast, the congenital aneurysms are mainly in younger individuals, they are not associated with atherosclerotic plaquing in the aneurysmal or nonaneurysmal portions of the coronary arteries, and they may not contain intra-aneurysmal thrombus.

SIZE OF CORONARY ARTERY:
RELATIONSHIP TO AGE AND ARTERIAL OXYGEN SATURATION

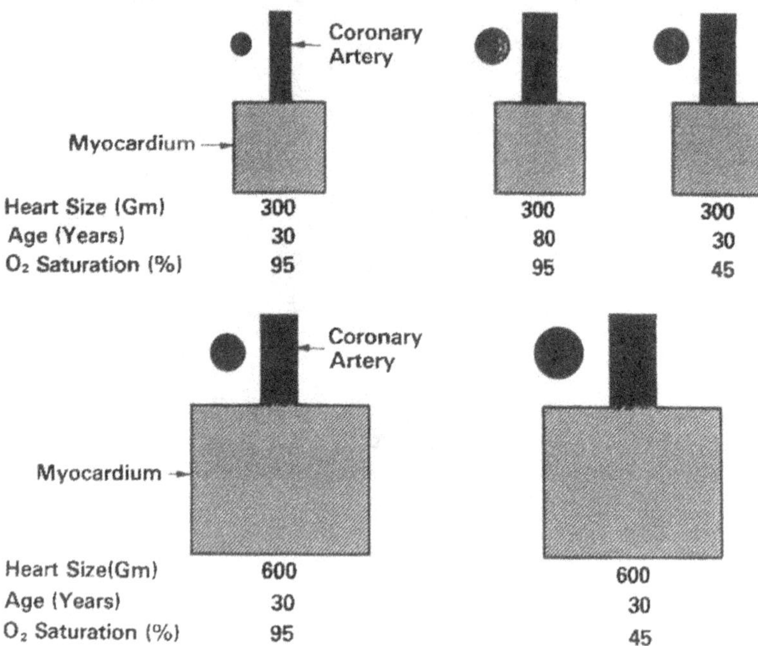

FIGURE 21. Diagram showing the relation between the sizes of the coronary arteries and the arterial oxygen saturation.

TABLE 2. Dilatation of the Epicardial Coronary Arteries (CA) in Cyanotic Congenital Heart Disease (25 Necropsy Patients > Age 20 Years)

DEGREE OF CA DILATATION (1⁺–4⁺)	NUMBER PATIENTS	AGES	PERCENT SYSTEMIC ARTERIAL OXYGEN SATURATION
4⁺	1	40	40
3⁺	3	33, 38, 49 (40)	61, 62, 70 (64)
2⁺	8	21–48 (28)	61–81 (72)
1⁺	13	21–46 (29)	69–87 (77)

FREQUENCY

Daoud and associates[136] described 10 cases of atherosclerotic coronary aneurysm and found 79 previously reported cases of coronary aneurysm. Of the total 89 cases (67 male), these authors considered 14 to be of congenital origin. The 14 cases, however, ranged in age from 23 to 74 years (mean 51) and 9 were men. These authors, however, did not provide definitions for "atherosclerotic" or "congenital." Kalke and Edwards[137] described coronary aneurysm in 8 patients at necropsy: in 6, the cause was atherosclerotic; 1, polyarteritis nodosa (probably today this case would have been called mucocutaneous lymph node syndrome because their patient was a 13-year-old boy); and 1 was congenital. The latter patient was a 30-year-old man with a congenitally bicuspid aortic valve that had become infected. The aneurysm involved the proximal portion of the right coronary artery. I have observed 10 adults

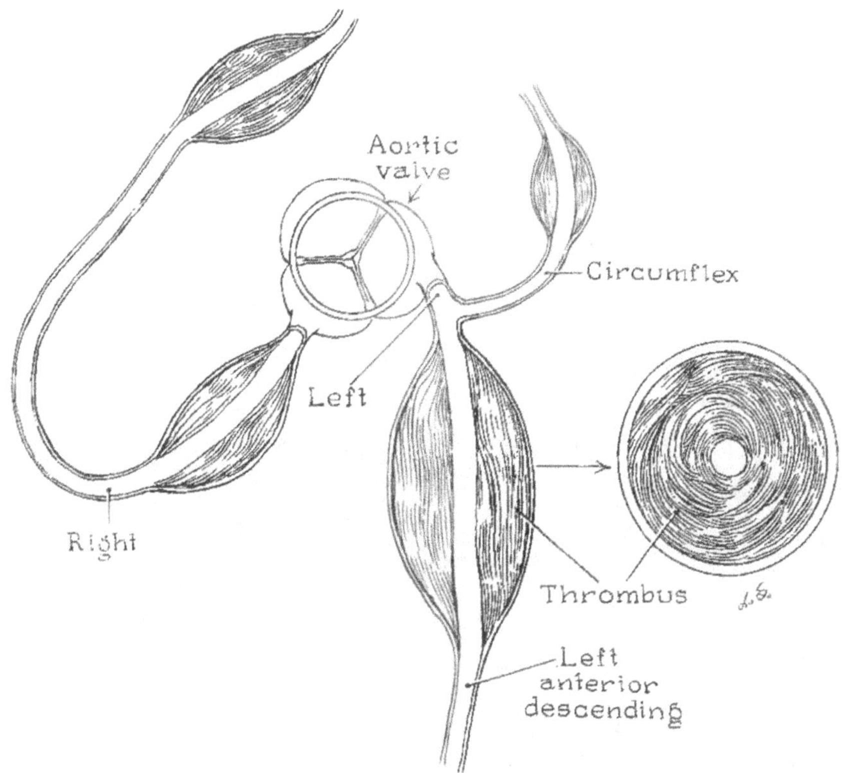

FIGURE 22. Diagram of multiple coronary arterial aneurysms in a 30-month-old boy who was known to have coronary aneurysms since age 6 months. He died suddenly at age 30 months and had been asymptomatic before that time. At necropsy, the anterior left ventricular wall was scarred, and all coronary aneurysms contained thrombus. The child had other features consistent with the mucocutaneous lymph-node syndrome.

at necropsy in a 25-year period with 1 or more localized aneurysms: in 9, the etiology was clearly atherosclerotic, and in 1, congenital. In the latter patient, a 70-year-old man who died as a consequence of trauma, the aneurysm involved the left circumflex coronary artery (Fig. 23). Both the aneurysmal and nonaneurysmal portions of the epicardial coronary arteries were devoid of atherosclerotic plaques and of thrombi.

CLINICAL SIGNIFICANCE

Some patients with aneurysms, be they congenital or atherosclerotic in origin, are asymptomatic, and others have clear evidence of myocardial ischemia. Symptoms appear to be related primarily to the presence of luminal narrowing produced by the intra-aneurysmal thrombus or due to compression by the coronary aneurysm of an adjacent coronary vessel or chamber (to produce, for example, right ventricular outflow obstruction). Scott[138] described what appears to have been multiple congenital coronary aneurysms, the largest of which measured 10 cm in size, and yet no symptoms of cardiac ischemia or dysfunction resulted. Many single case reports, however, have described patients with apparent congenital coronary aneurysms that caused severe myocardial ischemia.

Ebert and associates[139] described a 31-year-old woman with an 8 × 5 cm left circumflex aneurysm unassociated with angiographic narrowing of the left main, left anterior descending, or right coronary arteries, and she had clinical evidence of an acute myocardial infarct. The aneurysm was resected and flow re-established by an

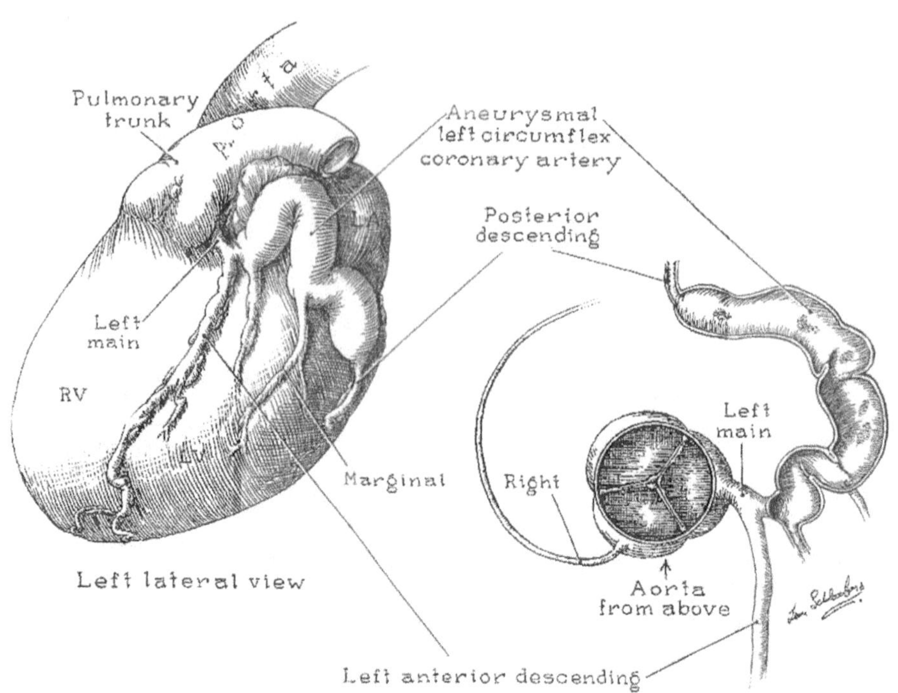

FIGURE 23. Drawing of a congenital coronary aneurysm unassociated with fistula in a 70-year-old man (DCMEO No. 80-04-293) who died from a head injury. The coronary aneurysm was a surprise finding at necropsy. There were never signs or symptoms of cardiac dysfunction. The aneurysm is devoid of thrombus, and few atherosclerotic plaques were present in any of the coronary arteries. The right coronary artery was hypoplastic. LV = left ventricle; RV = right ventricle.

end-to-end reversed saphenous vein. Ghahramani and associates[140] described a 32-year-old woman who had an acute myocardial infarction followed by angina. A large calcified aneurysm involving the left anterior descending was found, and a conduit was inserted between aorta and distal left anterior descending with good results. Dawson and Eillison[141] described a 30-year-old man who was asymptomatic, but chest radiograph disclosed a calcified coronary aneurysm that was operatively excised and flow re-established by a reversed saphenous vein. Mattern and associates[142] described a 26-year-old man with congenital aneurysms of both the right and left main coronary arteries with resulting acute myocardial infarction and angina pectoris. A bypass to the right coronary artery was performed. Seabra and associates[143] described 2 symptomatic patients, a 4-year-old boy and a 23-year-old woman, both treated operatively. Wilson and associates[144] reported a 15-year-old boy who collapsed and died shortly after participation in a basketball game. Multiple aneurysms of the right coronary artery and single aneurysms of the left main, left anterior descending, and left circumflex coronary arteries were found. (This case in retrospect suggests the etiology to be Kawasaki disease rather than a congenital etiology.) Lim and associates[145] described a 15 × 10 × 15 cm right coronary artery aneurysm that was successfully excised in a 32-year-old man. Gray and McMartin[146] described a 54-year-old woman in whom a right coronary artery aneurysm had eroded (acquired) through the right atrial wall, and it was successfully treated surgically. Gnepp and associates[147] described a 6 × 5 × 7 cm right coronary artery aneurysm that caused right ventricular outflow obstruction.

Thus, congenital coronary aneurysms present in several forms. If the aneurysm is found, it appears that operative intervention is warranted to prevent evidence of myocardial ischemia or outflow obstruction and to prevent the possibility of aneurysmal rupture or luminal occlusion by intra-aneurysmal thrombus.

CORONARY ARTERY FISTULA

FREQUENCY

Coronary artery fistula unassociated with a cardiac valve anomaly (mainly pulmonic valve atresia or aortic valve atresia), although rare, is one of the more common coronary arterial anomalies, especially those of clinical significance. Neufeld and Schneeweiss[148] observed 8 patients with coronary artery fistula among 3800 patients with congenital cardiac disease having had cardiac catheterization. About 300 cases of coronary artery fistula have been reported since the anomaly was first described in 1865.

SITES OF ORIGIN AND OF TERMINATION OF THE FISTULA

The fistula invovles the right coronary artery or 1 or more of its branches in about 60% of cases and either the left anterior descending or left circumflex or 1 or more of their branches in the other 40%.[148-154] Rarely, more than 1 coronary artery is part of the fistula, or a fistula may involve a single or an accessory coronary artery. The site of termination of the fistula in 90% of cases is the right side of the heart or vessels attached to it, most commonly the right ventricle followed by right atrium and pulmonary trunk (Figs. 24 and 25). The other 10% terminate in either the left atrium or left ventricle. The connection between the coronary artery fistula and the site of termination may be a single opening or multiple openings. Some of those with multiple openings may have telangiectatic-type connections.

MORPHOLOGIC CHARACTERISTICS OF THE FISTULA

The coronary artery that is part of the anomalous communication with a cardiac chamber or attached cardiac vein or artery nearly always is dilated, the dilatation

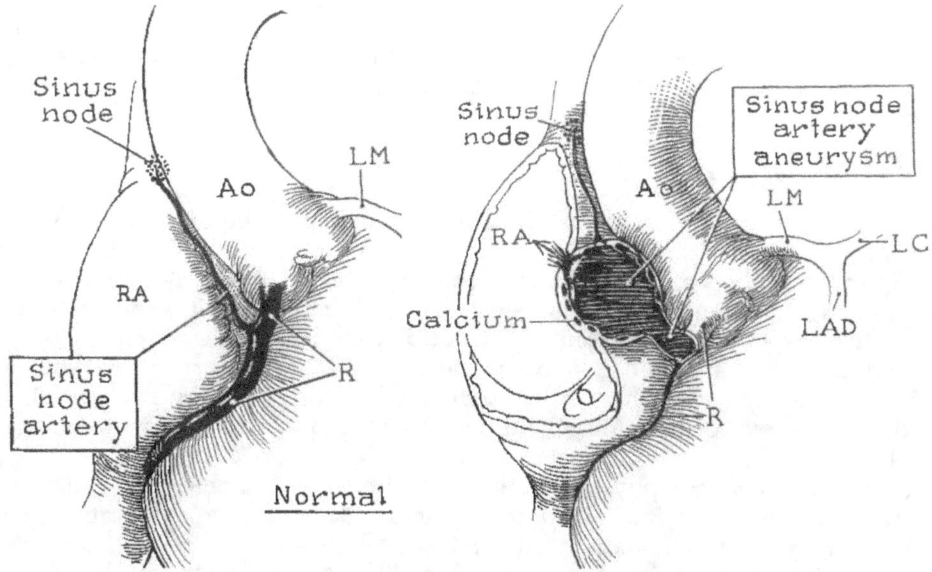

FIGURE 24. Drawings of heart in an older adult in whom an aneurysmal-sized sinus-node artery served as a fistula between the right (R) coronary artery and the right atrium (RA). The wall of the fistula contained calcific deposits. The normal for comparison is shown at the left. Ao = aorta; LAD = left anterior descending; LC = left circumflex; and LM = left main coronary arteries.

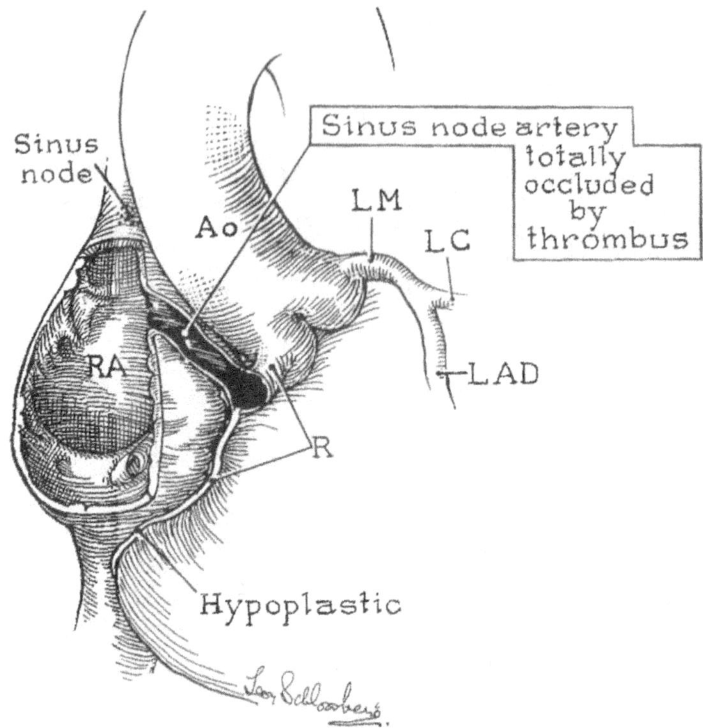

FIGURE 25. Thrombosed sinus-node artery that had served as a fistula between the right (R) coronary artery and right atrium (RA) in a 14-year-old girl who died of complications of regional ileitis. During life, she had no evidence of cardiac disease. The right coronary artery was hypoplastic. Ao = aorta; LAD = left anterior descending, LC = left circumflex, and LM = left main coronary artery.

being both transversely and longitudinally. The latter is manifest by tortuosity. The enlarged coronary artery often has focal outpouchings (saccular aneurysms superimposed on the fusiform aneurysm), and its wall may contain focal calcific deposits. On rare occasion, a coronary artery fistula is not dilated.

CLINICAL FEATURES

Symptoms appear to be determined mainly by the magnitude of the shunt via the coronary artery fistula. If the shunt is large, severe congestive heart failure and/or signs and symptoms of myocardial ischemia may result. The myocardial ischemia appears to result from the "coronary steal" effect whereby blood intended to be used to perfuse myocardium is "stolen" by the cardiac chamber or vessel proximal to its intended myocardial termination. Some individuals with coronary artery fistula are asymptomatic, and attention is called to the presence of a coronary artery fistula by a continuous precordial murmur. Symptoms may appear in infancy or not until older adulthood.

The most common physical finding is the presence of a precordial continuous murmur. The maximum intensity of the murmur is dependent on the location of the fistulous tract; most commonly, it is the left sternal border. If the termination site of the fistula is the left ventricle, the murmur is audible only during ventricular diastole. Occasionally, only a systolic precordial murmur is audible or no murmur is heard. The continuous murmur, of course, may be confused with that produced by patent ductus arteriosus, aorticopulmonary septal defect, or combined ventricular septal defect and aortic regurgitation.

TABLE 3. Observations in 187 Reported Patients with Coronary Artery Fistula Until May 1979

AGE AT DIAGNOSIS (YEARS)	No. PATIENTS	D No. (%)	AP No. (%)	Overt CHF No. (%)	AMI No. (%)	IE No. (%)	FR No. (%)	DEATH No. (%)	PREOPERATIVE SYMPTOMS AND/OR COMPLICATIONS	MEAN q^p/q^s	OPERATIVE LIGATION No. (%)
< 20 (mean 8)	99	9 (4%)	3 (3%)	6 (6%)	0	3 (3%)	0	1 (1%)	18 (18%)	1.6:1 (44 patients)	77 (77%)
≥ 20 (mean 43)	88	34 (39%)	22 (25%)	19 (22%)	7 (8%)	4 (5%)	1 (1%)	11 (12%)	58 (66%)	1.7:1 (36 patients)	48 (55%)
TOTALS	187	38 (20%)	25 (13%)	25 (13%)	7 (4%)	7 (4%)	1 (.5%)	12 (6%)	76 (41%)	1.6:1 (80 patients)	125 (67%)

AMI = acute myocardial infarction; AP = angina pectoris; CHF = congestive heart failure; D = dyspnea; FR = fistula rupture; IE = infective endocarditis; q^p/q^s = pulmonic to systemic flow ratio.

Modified from Liberthson et al.[153]

Findings on electrocardiogram, echocardiogram, and chest radiogram are usually dependent on the magnitude of the shunt through the coronary artery fistula. All cardiac chambers may be dilated or only the right-sided chambers, and the left ventricular wall may be thickened. Doppler echocardiography is useful for diagnosis.[155–157] The best review on this subject is by Liberthson and associates,[153] and findings in their patients and in those reported before 1979 are summarized in Table 3.

HIGH TAKE OFF CORONARY ARTERY

Normally, both coronary arterial ostia are located just caudal to an imaginary line separating the sinuses of Valsalva from that portion of aorta just above the sinuses, commonly referred to as the "tubular portion" of aorta. Occasionally, 1 and rarely both coronary arteries arise just cephalad to the sino-tubular junction and their origin may be called "high take off" (Figs. 26 and 27). High take off of a coronary artery is of no functional consequence.

TUNNELED MAJOR CORONARY ARTERY (MYOCARDIAL BRIDGE)

Much has been written on this subject. Any epicardial coronary artery can burrow into myocardium for a variable distance and then reappear in the epicardium again. Myocardial tunneling most commonly involves the left anterior descending, left diagonal, and left obtuse marginal coronary arteries. In about 20% of hearts, 1 or more of these arteries have a tunneled portion into left ventricular myocardium. Far less commonly, a portion of the right or left circumflex coronary artery burrows into atrial myocardium. Although there are reports suggesting that myocardial tunneling is of clinical importance, that is, causing symptomatic or even fatal myocardial ischemia, I am unconvinced that tunneling is of any clinical significance. Indeed, in patients with considerable coronary atherosclerosis, the tunneled portion of a coronary artery is nearly always devoid of atherosclerotic plaques (Fig. 28). It appears likely that the blood is "squeezed out" of the tunneled portion of coronary artery by the adjacent contracting myocardium and that these contractions prevent the deposition of atherosclerotic plaques. Of course, the coronary arteries fill primarily during ventricular diastole and thus any narrowing of them only during ventricular systole would not appear to be of functional significance.

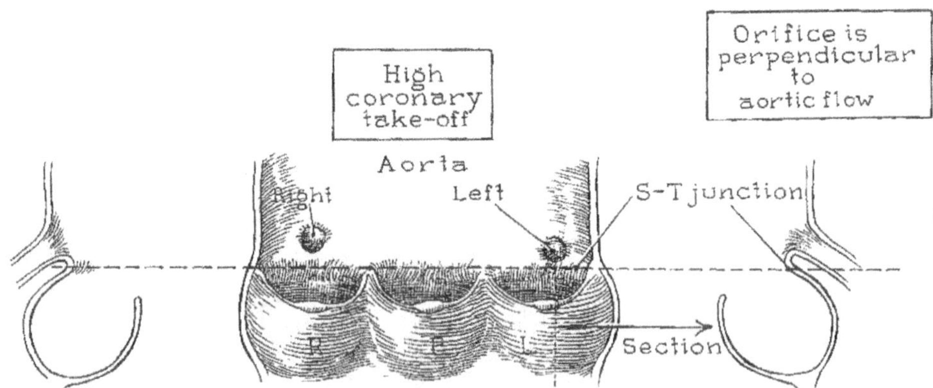

FIGURE 26. Diagram showing origin of both coronary arteries cephalad to the sino-tubular (S-T) junction. L, P, and R are the left, posterior, and right aortic cusps, respectively.

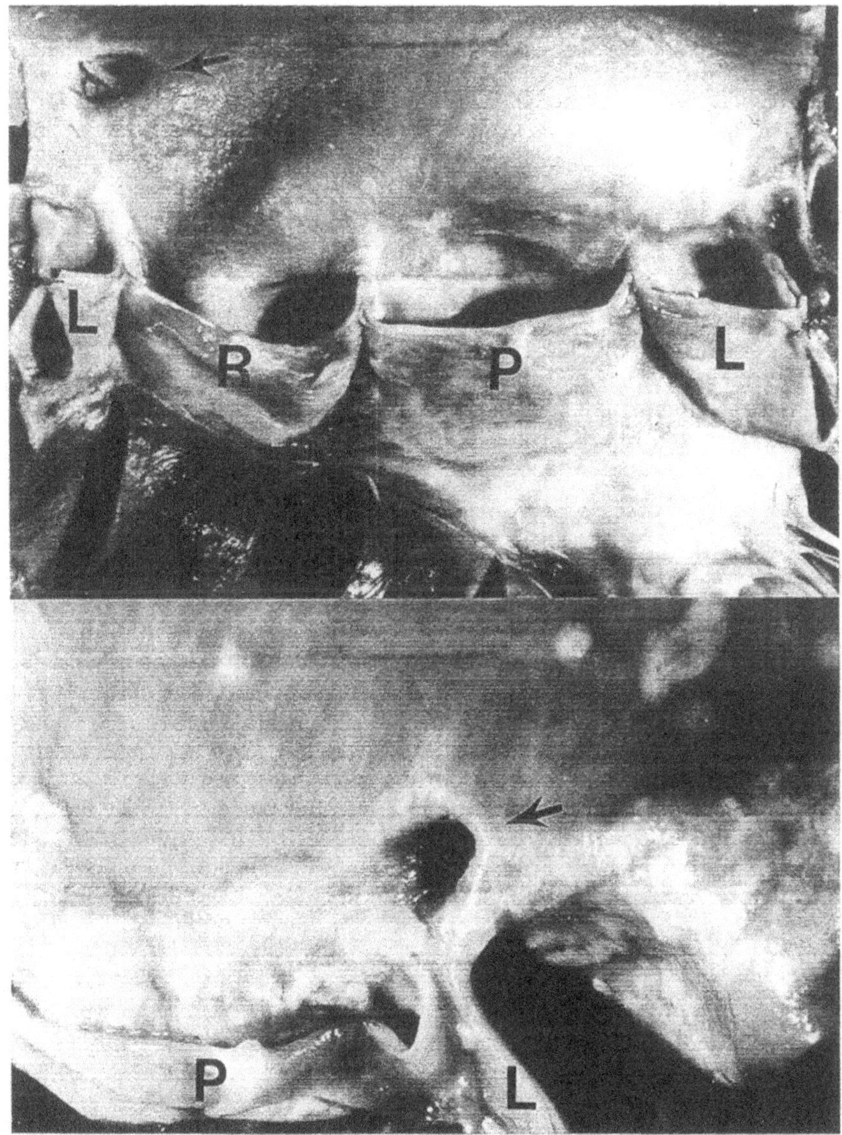

FIGURE 27. Opened aortas in each of 2 adults in whom 1 coronary artery arose above the sino-tubular junction. *Upper*, Origin of the right coronary artery ostium (arrow) directly above the commissure between the right (R) and left (L) cusps in a 68-year-old man (DCMEO No. 80-03-250) who died of burns. *Lower*, Ostium (arrow) of left main coronary artery located above commissure between the posterior (P) and left (L) cusps in a 54-year-old man (SGH No. A82-1) who died of consequences of coronary atherosclerosis.

CONGENITAL ABSENCE, ATRESIA, OR HYPOPLASIA OF A CORONARY ARTERY

This is a very rare occurrence. I have seen complete absence of a left circumflex coronary artery in a 60-year-old man who died of myocardial infarction secondary to severe coronary atherosclerosis. Atresia of a left main coronary artery, as mentioned earlier, is similar to single right coronary artery as long as the right coronary artery is large. Hypoplasia of the left circumflex is common with dominant right coronary

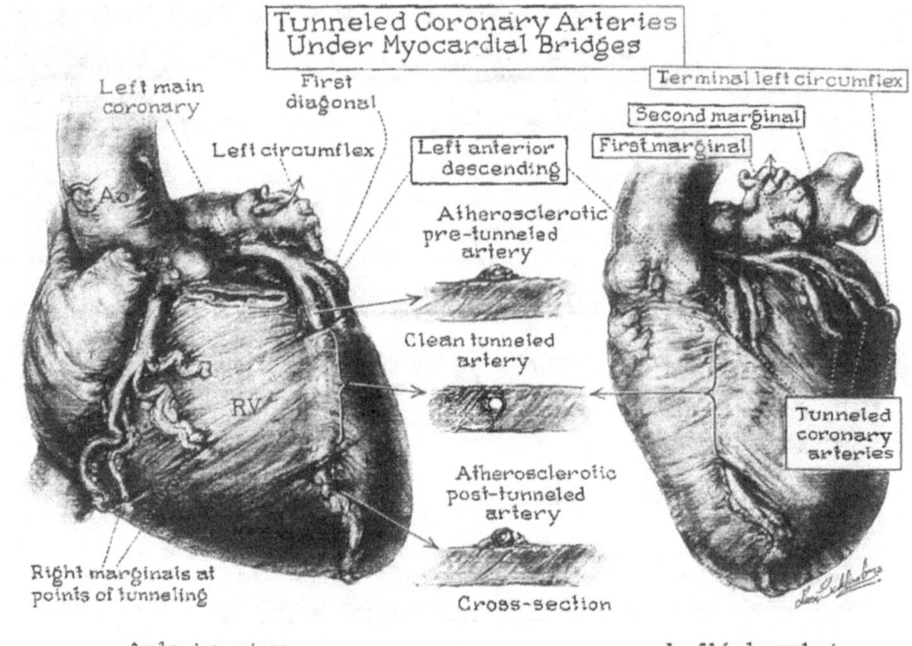

FIGURE 28. Drawing of a heart from a 71-year-old man (DCGH No. 80A-60) in whom several coronary arteries coursing over the left ventricle tunneled for varying lengths into myocardium. The non-tunneled portions of the coronary arteries contained atherosclerotic plaques distributed diffusely, but the tunneled portions of the same coronary arteries were devoid of atherosclerotic plaques. This patient died of colonic cancer and was severely cachetic, hence, the near absence of subepicardial adipose tissue which often hides coronary tunneling. The heart weighed only 260 gm.

circulation, and hypoplasia of the right coronary artery is common with a dominant left circulation. Hypoplasia of the left anterior descending has not been described to my knowledge.

REFERENCES

1. Abbott ME. Anomalous origin from the pulmonary arteries. In: Osler W, ed. Osler's Modern Medicine, Its Theories and Practice. Philadelphia: Lea and Febiger, 1908 (vol 4):420.
2. Abrikossoff A. Aneurysm des Linken Herzventrikels mit Abnormer Abganstelle der Linken Koronararterie von der Pulmonalis Bei Einem Funfmonatlichen Kinde. Virchow Arch Path Anat 1911; 203:413–420.
3. Bland EF, White PD, Garland J. Congenital anomalies of the coronary arteries: Report of an unusual case associated with cardiac hypertrophy. Am Heart J 1933; 8:787–801.
4. Fontana RS, Edwards JE. Congenital Cardiac Disease: A Review of 357 Cases Studied Pathologically. Philadelphia: WB Saunders, 1962:291.
5. Thomas CS, Campbell WB, Alford WC Jr, Burrus GR, Stoney WS. Complete repair of anomalous origin of the left coronary artery in the adult. J Thorac Cardiovasc Surg 1973; 66:439–446.
6. Donaldson RM, Raphael M, Radley-Smith R, Yacoub MH, Ross DN. Angiographic identification of primary coronary anomalies causing impaired myocardial perfusion. Cathet Cardiovasc Diagn 1983; 9:237–249.
7. Edwards JE. Anomalous coronary arteries with special reference to arteriovenous-like communications. Circulation 1958; 17:1001–1006.

8. Edwards JE. The direction of blood flow in coronary arteries arising from the pulmonary trunk. Circulation 1964; 29:163–166.

9. Moodie DS, Fyfe D, Gill CC, Cook SA, Lytle BW, Taylor PC, Fitzgerald R, Sheldon WC. Anomalous origin of the left coronary artery from the pulmonary artery (Bland-White-Garland syndrome) in adults patients: long-term follow-up after surgery. Am Heart J 1983; 106:381–388.

10. Jurishica AJ. Anomalous left coronary artery. Adult type. Am Heart J 1957; 54:429–436.

11. George JM, Knowlan DM. Anomalous origin of the left coronary artery from the pulmonary artery in an adult. New Engl J Med 1959; 261:993–998.

12. Lampe CFJ, Verheught APM. Anomalous left coronary artery. Adult type. Am Heart J 1960; 59:769–776.

13. Liebman J, Hellerstein HK, Ankeney JL, Tucker A. The problem of the anomalous left coronary artery arising from the pulmonary artery in older children. Report of three cases. New Engl J Med 1963; 269:486–494.

14. Talner NS, Halloran KH, Mahdavy M, Gardner TH, Hipona F. Anomalous origin of the left coronary artery from the pulmonary artery. A clinical spectrum. Am J Cardiol 1965; 15:689–695.

15. Likar I, Criley JM, Lewis KB. Anomalous left coronary artery arising from the pulmonary artery in an adult. A review of the therapeutic problem. Circulation 1966; 33:727–732.

16. Harthorne JW, Scannell JG, Dinsmore RE. Anomalous origin of the left coronary artery. Remediable cause of sudden death in adults. New Engl J Med 1966; 275:660–663.

17. Wesselhoeft H, Fawcett JS, Johnson AL. Anomalous origin of the left coronary artery from the pulmonary trunk. Its clinical spectrum, pathology, and pathophysiology, based on a review of 140 cases with seven further cases. Circulation 1968; 38:403–425.

18. Perry LW, Scott LP. Anomalous left coronary artery from pulmonary artery. Report of 11 cases; review of indications for and results of surgery. Circulation 1970; 41:1043–1052.

19. Askenazi J, Nadas AS. Anomalous left coronary artery originating from the pulmonary artery. Report on 15 cases. Circulation 1975; 51:976–987.

20. Sabiston DC Jr, Floyd WL, McIntosh HD. Anomalous origin of the left coronary artery from the pulmonary artery in adults. Surgical management. Arch Surg 1968; 97:963–968.

21. Usman A, Fernandez B, Uricchio JF, Nichols HT. Aberrant origin of left coronary artery combined with mitral regurgitation in an adult. Am J Cardiol 1961; 8:130.

22. Burchell HB, Brown AL Jr. Anomalous origin of coronary artery from pulmonary artery masquerading as mitral insufficiency. Am Heart J 1962; 63:388–393.

23. Fisher EA, Sepehri B, Lendrum B, Luken J, Levitsky S. Two-dimensional echocardiographic visualization of the left coronary artery in anomalous origin of the left coronary artery from the pulmonary artery. Pre- and postoperative studies. Circulation 1981; 63:698–704.

24. Terai M, Nagai Y, Toba T. Cross-sectional echocardiographic findings of anomalous origin of left coronary artery from pulmonary artery. Br Heart J 1983; 50:104–105.

25. Caldwell RL, Hurwitz RA, Girod DA, Weyman AE, Feigenbaum H. Two-dimensional echocardiographic differentiation of anomalous left coronary artery from congestive cardiomyopathy. Am Heart J 1983; 106:710–716.

26. Robinson PJ, Sullivan ID, Kumpeng V, Anderson RH, MaCartney FJ. Anomalous origin of the left coronary artery from the pulmonary trunk. Potential for false negative diagnosis with cross sectional echocardiography. Br Heart J 1984; 52:272–277.

27. King DH, Danford DA, Huhta JC, Gutgesell HP. Noninvasive detection of anomalous origin of the left main coronary artery from the pulmonary trunk by pulsed Doppler echocardiography. Am J Cardiol 1985; 55:608–609.

28. Gutgesell HP, Pinksy WW, DePuey EG. Thallium-201 myocardial perfusion imaging in infants and children; value in distinguishing anomalous left coronary artery from congestive cardiomyopathy. Circulation 1980; 61:596–599.

29. Shem-Tov AA, Hegesh J, Schneeweiss A, Neufeld HN. Visualization of left coronary artery in anomalous origin of left coronary artery from pulmonary artery. Am Heart J 1984; 108:621–622.

30. Sabiston DC Jr, Neill CA, Taussig HB. The direciton of blood flow in anomalous left coronary artery arising from the pulmonary artery. Circulation 1960; 22:591–597.

31. Rowe GG, Young WP. Anomalous origin of the coronary arteries with special reference to surgical treatment. J Thorac Cardiovasc Surg 1960; 39:777–780.

32. Roche AHG. Anomalous origin of the left coronary artery from the pulmonary artery in the adult. Report of uneventful ligation in two cases. Am J Cardiol 1967; 20:561–565.

33. Baue AE, Baum S, Blakemore WS, Zinsser HF. A later stage of anomalous coronary circulation with origin of the left coronary artery from the pulmonary artery. Coronary artery steal. Circulation 1967; 36:878–885.

34. Reis, RL, Cohen LS, Mason DT. Direct measurement of instantaneous coronary blood flow after total correction of anomalous left coronary artery. Circulation 1969; 39–40(Suppl I):I-229–I-234.

35. Somerville J, Ross DN. Left coronary artery from the pulmonary artery. Physiological considerations of surgical correction. Thorax 1970; 25:207–212.

36. Neches WH, Mathews RA, Park SC, Lenox CC, Zuberbuhler JR, Siewers RD, Bahnson HT. Anomalous origin of the left coronary artery from the pulmonary artery. A new method of surgical repair. Circulation 1974; 50:582–587.

37. Chaitman BR, Bourassa MG, Lesperance J, Grondin P. Anomalous left coronary artery from the pulmonary artery. An eight year angiographic follow-up after saphenous vein bypass graft. Circulation 1975; 51:552–555.

38. Pinsky WW, Fagan LR, Mudd JFG, William VL. Subclavian-coronary artery anastomosis in infancy for the Bland-White-Garland syndrome. A three-year and five-year follow-up. J Thorac Cardiovasc Surg 1976; 72:15–20.

39. Grace RR, Angelini P, Cooley DA. Aortic implantation of anomalous left coronary artery arising from pulmonary artery. Am J Cardiol 1977; 39:608–613.

40. Wilson CL, Dlabal PW, Holeyfield RW, Akins CW, Knauf DG. Anomalous origin of left coronary artery from pulmonary artery. Case report and review of literature concerning teenagers and adults. J Thorac Cardiovasc Surg 1977; 73:887–893.

41. Shrivastava S, Castaneda AR, Moller JH. Anomalous left coronary artery from pulmonary trunk. Long-term follow-up after ligation. J Thorac Cardiovasc Surg 1978; 76:130–134.

42. Wilson CL, Dlabal PW, McGuire SA. Surgical treatment of anomalous left coronary artery from pulmonary artery: follow-up in teenagers and adults. Am Heart J 1979; 98:440–446.

43. Donaldson RM, Raphael MJ, Yacoub MH, Ross DN. Hemodynamically signficant anomalies of the coronary arteries. Surgical aspects. Thorac Cardiovasc Surg 1982; 30:7.

44. Fisher J, McDonald G, Brinker J, Neill CA, Donahoo JS, Baughman KL. Transpulmonary artery correction of anomalous origin of the left coronary artery by saphenous vein graft. Cathet Cardiovasc Diagn 1983; 9:373–380.

45. Savage RW, Glover MU, Utley JR. Reoperation for correction of anomalous origin of left coronary artery from the pulmonary artery with return of left ventricular function. Cathet Cardiovasc Diagn 1984; 10:37–42.

46. Bagger JP, Vesterlund T, Nielsen TT. Cardiac metabolism and coronary hemodynamics before and after bypass surgery for anomalous origin of the left main coronary artery from the pulmonary trunk. Am J Cardiol 1985; 55:864–865.

47. Brooks H St J. Two cases of an abnormal coronary artery of the heart arising from the pulmonary artery: with some remarks upon the effect of this anomaly in producing cirsoid dilation of the vessels. J Anat Physiol 1885 and 1886; 20:26–29.

48. Monckelberg JG. Uber eine seltene Anomalie des Koronarterienabgangs. Zentralbl Herz Krankheiten 1914; 6:441–445.

49. Schley J. Abnormer Ursprung der rechten Kranzarterie aus der Pulmonalis bei einem 61-jahriger Mann. Frankfurt Z Path 1925; 32:1–7.

50. Jordan RA, Dry TJ, Edwards JE. Anomalous origin of the right coronary artery from the pulmonary trunk. Mayo Clin Proc 1950; 25:673–678.

51. Cronk ES, Sinclair JG, Rigdon RH. An anomalous coronary artery arising from the pulmonary artery. Am Heart J 1951; 42:906–911.

52. Tingelstad JB, Lower RR, Eldredge WJ. Anomalous origin of the right coronary artery from the main pulmonary artery. Am J Cardiol 1972; 30:670–673.

53. Ogden JA. Cogential anomalies of the cornary arteries. Am J Cardiol 1970; 25:474–479.

54. Lerberg DB, Ogden JA, Zuberbuhler JR, Bahnson HT. Anomalous origin of the right coronary artery from the pulmonary artery. Ann Thorac Surg 1979; 27:87–94.

55. Wald S, Stonecipher K, Baldwin BJ, Hutter DO. Anomalous origin of the right coronary artery from the pulmonary artery. Am J Cardiol 1971; 27:677–681.

56. Eugstes GS, Oliva PB. Anomalous origin of the right coronary artery from the pulmonary artery. Chest 1973; 63:294–296.

57. Achtel RA, Zaret BL, Iben AB, Hurley EJ. Surgical correction of congenital left coronary artery-main pulmonary artery fistula in association with anomalous right coronary artery. J Thorac Cardiovasc Surg 1975; 70:46–51.

58. Bregman D, Brennan FJ, Singer A, Vinci J, Parodi EN, Cassarella WJ, Edie RN. Anomalous origin of right coronary artery from the pulmonary artery. J Thorac Cardiovasc Surg 1976; 72:626–630.

59. Mintz GS, Iskandrian AS, Bemis CE, Mundth ED, Owens JS. Myocardial ischemia in anomalous origin of the right coronary artery from the pulmonary trunk. Proof of a coronary steal. Am J Cardiol 1983; 51:610–612.

60. Worsham C, Sanders SP, Bulger BM. Origin of the right coronary artery from the pulmonary trunk: diagnosis by two-dimensional echocardiography. Am J Cardiol 1985; 55:232–233.

61. van Meurs-van Woezik H, Serruys PW, Reiber JH, Bos E, deVilleneuve VH. Coronary artery changes 3 years after reimplantation of an anomalous right coronary artery. Eur Heart J 1984; 5:175–178.

62. Roberts WC, Robinowitz M. Anomalous origin of the left anterior descending coronary artery from the pulmonary trunk with origin of the right and left circumflex coronary arteries from the aorta. Am J Cardiol 1984; 54:1381–1383.

63. Donaldson RM, Thornton A, Raphael MJ, Sturridge MF, Emanuel RW. Anomalous origin of the left anterior descending coronary artery from the pulmonary trunk. Eur J Cardiol 1979; 10:295.

64. Effler DB, Sheldon WC, Turner JJ, Groves LK. Coronary arteriovenous fistulae: diagnosis and surgical management. Report of fifteen cases. Surgery 1967; 61:41–50.

65. Honey M, Lincoln JCR, Osborne MP, de Bono DP. Coarctation of the aorta with right aortic arch. Report of surgical correction in 2 cases: one with associated anomalous origin of left circumflex coronary artery from the right pulmonary artery. Br Heart J 1975; 37:937–945.

66. Chaitman BR, Bourassa MG, Lesperance J, Dominquez JLD, Saltiel J. Aberrant course of the left anterior descending coronary artery associated with anomalous left circumflex origin from the pulmonary artery. Circulation 1975; 52:955–958.

67. Ott DA, Cooley DA, Pinsky WW, Mullins CE. Anomalous origin of circumflex coronary artery from right pulmonary artery. Report of a rare anomaly. J Thorac Cardiovasc Surg 1978; 76:190–194.

68. Grayzel DM, Tennant R. Congenital atresia of the tricuspid orifice and anomalous origins of the coronary arteries from the pulmonary artery. Am J Pathol 1934; 10:791–794.

69. Limbourg M. Uber den Ursprung der Kranzarterien des Herzens aus der Arteria pulmonalis. Beitr Pathol Anat 1937; 100:191.

70. Williams JW, Johnson WS, Boulware JR Jr. Case of tetralogy of Fallot with both coronary arteries arising from pulmonary artery. J Fla Med Assoc 1951; 37:561.

71. Swan WC, Werthammer S. Aberrant coronary arteries: Experiences in diagnosis with report of three cases. Ann Intern Med 1955; 42:873–884.

72. Alexander RW, Griffith GC. Anomalies of the coronary arteries and their clinical significance. Circulation 1956; 14:800–805.

73. Schulze WB, Rodin AE. Anomalous origin of both coronary arteries. Report of a case with discussion of teratogenic theories. Arch Pathol 1961; 72:36–46.

74. Roberts WC. Anomalous origin of both coronary arteries from the pulmonary artery. Am J Cardiol 1962; 10:595–600.

75. Blake HA, Manion WC, Mattingly TW, Baroldi G. Coronary artery anomalies. Circulation 1964; 390:927–940.

76. Gonzales-Angulo A, Reyes HA, Wallace SA. Anomalies of the origin of coronary arteries (special reference to single coronary artery). Angiology 1966; 17:96–103.

77. Kecton BR, Keenan DJM, Monro JL. Anomalous origin of both coronary arteries from the pulmonary trunk. Br Heart J 1983; 49:397.

78. Feldt RH, Ongley PA, Titus JL. Total coronary arterial circulation from pulmonary artery with survival to age seven: report of case. Mayo Clin Proc 1965: 40:539–543.

79. Monselise MB, Vlodaver Z, Neufeld HN. Single coronary artery; origin from the pulmonary trunk in association with ventricular septal defect. Chest 1970; 58:613–616.

80. Barth CW III, Roberts WC. Left main coronary artery originating from the right sinus of Valsalva and coursing between aorta and pulmonary trunk. J Am Coll Cardiol 1986; 7:366–373.

81. Cheitlin MD, DeCastro CM, McCallister HA. Sudden death as a complication of anom-

alous left coronary origin from the anterior sinus of Valsalva. A not so minor congenital anomaly. Circulation 1974; 50:780–787.

82. Roberts WC, Dicicco BS, Waller BF, Kishel JC, McManus BM, Dawson SL, Hunsaker JC III, Luke JL. Origin of the left main from the right coronary artery or from the right aortic sinus with intramyocardial tunneling to the left side of the heart via the ventricular septum: the case against clinical significance of myocardial bridge or coronary tunnel. Am Heart J 1982; 104:303–305.

83. Murphy DA, Roy DL, Sohal M, Chandler BM. Anomalous origin of left main coronary artery from anterior sinus of Valsalva with myocardial infarction. J Thorac Cardiovasc Surg 1978; 74:282–285.

84. Sanes S. Anomalous origin and course of the left coronary artery in a child. Am Heart J 1937; 14:219–229.

85. Nicod JL. Anomalie coronaire et mort subite. Cardiologia 1952; 20:172–179.

86. Alexander RW, Griffith GC. Anomalies of the coronary arteries and their clinical significance. Circulation 1956; 14:800–805.

87. Jokl E, McClellan JT, Ross GD. Congenital anomaly of the left coronary artery in young athlete. JAMA 1962; 182:174–175.

88. Jokl E, McClellan JT, WIlliams WC, Gouze FJ, Bartholomew RD. Congenital anomaly of left coronary artery in young athletes. Cardiologia 1966; 49:253–258.

89. Benson PA, Lack AR. Anomalous aortic origin of the left coronary artery. Arch Pathol 1968; 86:214–216.

90. Benson PR. Anomalous aortic origin of coronary artery with sudden death: case report and review. Am Heart J 1970; 79:254–257.

91. Pedal I. Aortale ursprungsanomalie einer koronararterie. Dtsch Med Wochenschr 1976; 101:1601–1604.

92. Liberthson RR, Dinsomre RE, Fallon JT. Abberant coronary artery origin form the aorta. Report of 18 patients, review of the literature and delineation of natural history and management. Circulation 1979; 59:748–754.

93. Lynch P. Soldiers, sport and sudden death. Lancet 1980; 1:1235–1237.

94. Tsung SH, Huant TY, Chang HH. Sudden death in young athletes. Arch Pathol Lab Med 1982; 106:168–170.

95. Betend B, Gillet P, Moreau P, David L. Origine aortique anormale de l'artere coronaire gauche. A propos del la mort subite d'un adolescent. Arch Fr Pediatr 1983; 40:479–481.

96. Topaz O, Edwards JE. Pathologic features of sudden death in children, adolescent, and young adults. Chest 1985; 87:476–482.

97. Davia JE, Green DC, Cheitlin MD, DeCastro C, Brott WH. Anomalous left coronary artery origin from the right coronary sinus. Am Heart J 1984; 108:165–166.

98. Mustafa I, Gula G, Radley-Smith R, Durrer S, Yacoub M. Anomalous origin of the left coronary artery from the anterior aortic sinus: a potential cause of sudden death. J Thorac Cardiovasc Surg 1981; 82:297–300.

99. Liberthson RR, Zaman L, Weyman A, et al. Aberrant origin of the left coronary artery from the proximal right coronary artery: diagnostic features and pre- and postoperative course. Clin Cardiol 1982; 5:377–381.

100. Ishikawa T, Brandt PW. Anomalous origin of the left main coronary artery from the right anterior aortic sinus: angiographic definition of anomalous course. Am J Cardiol 1985; 55:770–776.

101. Kimbiris D. Anomalous origin of the left main coronary artery from the right sinus of Valsalva. Am J Cardiol 1985; 55:765–769.

102. Moodie DS, Gill C, Loop FD, Sheldon WC. Anomalous left main coronary artery originating from the right sinus of Valsalva. Pathophysiology, angiographic definition and surgical approaches. J Thorac Cardiovasc Surg 1980; 80:198–205.

103. Sacks JH, Londe SP, Rosenbluth A, Zalis EG. Left main coronary artery bypass for aberrant (aortic) intramural left coronary artery. J Thorac Cardiovasc Surg 1977; 73:733–737.

104. Roberts WC, Siegel RJ, Zipes DP. Origin of the right coronary artery from the left sinus of Valsalva and its functional consequences: analysis of 10 necropsy patients. Am J Cardiol 1982; 49:863–868.

105. Chaitman BR, Lesperance J, Saltiel J, Bourassa MG. Clinical, angiographic, and hemodynamic findings in patients with anomalous origin of the coronary arteries. Circulation 1975; 53:122–131.

106. Kimbiris D, Iskandrian AS, Segal BL, Bemis CE. Anomalous aortic origin of coronary arteries. Circulation 1978; 58:606–615.

107. Thompson SI, Vieweg WVR, Alpert JS, Hagan AD. Anomalous origin of the right coronary artery from the left sinus of Valsalva with associated chest pain. Report of 2 cases. Cathet Cardiovasc Diagn 1976; 2:397–402.

108. Benge W, Martins JB, Funk DC. Morbidity associated with anomalous origin of the right coronary artery from the left sinus of Valsalva. Am Heart J 1980; 99:96–100.

109. Bloomfield P, Erhlich C, Folland ED, Bianco JA, Tow DE, Parisi AF. Anomalous right coronary artery: a surgically correctable cause of angina pectoris. Am J Cardiol 1983; 51:1235–1237.

110. Keren A, Tzivoni D, Stern S. Functional consequences of right coronary artery originating from left sinus of Valsalva (letter). Am J Cardiol 1983; 51:1241.

111. Brandt B III, Martins JB, Marcus ML. Anomalous origin of the right coronary artery from the left sinus of Valsalva. New Engl J Med 1983; 309:596–598.

112. Hanzlick R, Stivers RR. Sudden death in a marathon runner with origin of the right coronary artery from the left sinus of Valsalva (letter). Am J Cardiol 1983; 51:1467.

113. Hanzlick RL, Stivers RR. Sudden death due to anomalous right coronary artery in a 26-year-old marathon runner. Am J Forensic Med Pathol 1983; 4:265–268.

114. Hanzlick R, Stivers RR. Anomalous right coronary artery (letter). Am J Forensic Med Pathol 1984; 5:285.

115. Isner JM, Shen EM, Martin ET, Fortin RV. Sudden unexpected death as a result of anomalous origin of the right coronary artery from the left sinus of Valsalva. Am J Med 1984; 76:155–158.

116. Antopol W, Kugel MA. Anomalous origin of the left circumflex coronary artery. Am Heart J 1933; 8:802–806.

117. Roberts WC, Waller BF, Roberts CS. Fatal atherosclerotic narrowing of the right main coronary artery: origin of the left arterior descending or left circumflex coronary artery from the right (the true "left main equivalent"). Am Heart J 1982; 104:638–641.

118. White NK, Edwards JE. Anomalies of the coronary arteries: report of four cases. Arch Pathol 1948; 45:766–771.

119. Page HL Jr, Engel JH, Campbell WB, Thomas CS. Anomalous origin of the left circumflex coronary artery. Recognition, angiographic demonstration and clinical significance. Circulation 1974; 50:768–773.

120. Ray PR, Saunders A, Sowton GE. Reveiw of variations in origin of left circumflex coronary artery. Br Heart J 1975; 37:287–292.

121. Baltaxe HA, Wixson D. The incidence of congenital anomalies of the coronary arteries in the adult population. Radiology 1977; 122:47–52.

122. Liberthson RR, Dinsmore RE, Bharati S, Rubenstein JJ, Caulfeld J, Wheeler EO, Harthorne JW, Lev M. Aberrant coronary origin from the aorta. Diagnosis and clincal significance. Circulation 1974; 50:774–779.

123. Roberts WC, Morrow AG. Compression of anomalous left circumflex coronary arteries by prosthetic valve fixation rings. J Thorac Cardiovasc Surg 1969; 57:834–838.

124. Vlodaver Z, Neufeld HN, Edwards JE. Coronary Arterial Variations in the Normal Heart and in Congenital Heart Disease. New York: Academic Press, 1975:171.

125. DiCicco BS, McManus BM, Waller BF, Roberts WC. Separate aortic ostium of the left anterior descending and left circumflex coronary arteries from the left aortic sinus of Valsalva (absent left main coronary artery). Am Heart J 1982; 104:153–154.

126. Zumbo O, Fani K, Jarmolych J, Daoud AS. Coronary atherosclerosis and myocardial infarction in hearts with anomalous coronary arteries. Lab Invest 1965; 14:571.

127. Smith JC. Review of single coronary artery with report of 2 cases. Circulation 1950; 1:1168–1175.

128. Banchi A. Morfologia della arteriae coronariae cordis. Arch Ital Anat e di Embriol 1903; 3:89.

129. Ogden JA, Goodyear AVN. Patterns of distribution of the single coronary artery. Yale J Biol Med 1970; 43:11–21.

130. Lipton MJ, Barry WH, Obrez I, Silverman J, Wexler L. Isolated single coronary artery: diagnosis, angiographic classification, and clinical significance. Radiology 1979; 130:39–47.

131. Saner HE, Saner BD, Dykoski RK, Edwards JE. Origin of anterior descending coronary artery from right aortic sinus. Intramyocardial tunneling to the left side of the heart. Arch Pathol Lab Med 1984; 108:642–643.

132. Schulte MA, Waller BF, Hull MT, Pless JE. Origin of the left anterior descending coronary artery from the right aortic sinus with intramyocardial tunneling to the left side of the

heart via the ventricular septum: a case against clinical and morphologic significance of myocardial bridging. Am Heart J 1985; 110:499–501.

133. Roberts WC. Valvular, subvalvular, and supravalvular aortic stenosis: morphologic features. Cardiovas Clin 1973; 5:97–126.

134. Perloff JK, Urschell CW, Roberts WC, Caulfield WH Jr. Aneurysmal dilatation of the coronary arteries in cyanotic congenital cardiac disease. Report of a forty-year-old patient with the Taussig-Bing complex. Am J Med 1968; 45:802–810.

135. Nakanishi T, Takao A, Nakazawa M, Endo M, Niwa K, Takahashi Y. Mucocutaneous lymph node syndrome: clinical, hemodynamic and angiographic features of coronary obstructive disease. Am J Cardiol 1985; 55:662–668.

136. Daoud AS, Pankin D, Tulgan H, Florentin RA. Aneurysms of the coronary artery. Report of ten cases and review of literature. Am J Cardiol 1963; 11:228–237.

137. Kalke B, Edwards JE. Localized aneurysms of the coronary arteries. Angiology 1968; 19:460–470.

138. Scott DH. Aneurysm of the coronary arteries. Am Heart J 1948; 36:403–421.

139. Ebert PA, Peter RH, Gunnells JC, Sabiston DC Jr. Resecting and grafting of coronary artery aneurysm. Circulation 1971; 43:593–598.

140. Ghahramani A, Iyengar R, Cunha D, Jude J, Sommer L. Myocardial infarction due to congenital coronary arterial aneurysm (with successful saphenous vein bypass graft). Am J Cardiol 1972; 29:863–867.

141. Dawson JE Jr, Ellison RG. Isolated aneurysm of the anterior descending coronary artery. Surgical treatment. Am J Cardiol 1972; 29:868–871.

142. Mattern AL, Baker WP, Mchale JJ, Lee DE. Congenital coronary aneurysms with angina pectoris and myocardial infarction treated with saphenous vein bypass graft. Am J Cardiol 1972; 30:906–909.

143. Seabra-Gomes R, Somerville J, Ross DN, Emanuel R, Parker DJ, Wong M. Congenital coronary artery aneurysms. British Heart J 1974; 36:329–335.

144. Wilson CS, Weaver WF, Zeman ED, Forker AD. Bilateral nonfistulous congenital coronary arterial aneurysms. Am J Cardiol 1975; 35:319–323.

145. Lim CH, Tan NC, Tan L, Seah CS, Tan D. Giant congenital aneurysm of the right coronary artery. Am J Cardiol 1977; 39:751–753.

146. Gray LA Jr, McMartin DE. Surgical treatment of coronary artery aneurysm with rupture into the right atrium. J Thorac Cardiovasc Surg 1977; 74:455–460.

147. Gnepp DR, Deglin SM, Bekheit S. Massive coronary arterial aneurysm. Am J Cardiol 1979; 44:184–187.

148. Neufeld HN, Schneeweiss A. Coronary Artery Disease in Infants and Children. Philadelphia: Lea & Febiger, 1983:189.

149. Neufeld HN, Lester RG, Adams P Jr, Anderson RC, Lillehei CW, Edwards JE. Congenital communication of a coronary artery with a cardiac chamber or the pulmonary trunk ("coronary artery fistula"). Circulation 1961; 24:171–179.

150. Upshaw CB Jr. Congenital coronary arteriovenous fistula. Report of a case with an analysis of seventy-three reported cases. Am Heart J 1962; 63:399.

151. Sakakibara S, Yokoyamo M, Takas A, Nogi M, Gomi H. Coronary arteriovenous fistula: Nine operated cases. Am Heart J 1966; 72:307.

152. de Nef JJE, Varghese PJ, Losekoot G. Congenital coronary artery fistula: Analysis of 17 cases. Br Heart J 1971; 33:857.

153. Liberthson RR, Sagar K, Berkoben JP, Weintraub RM, Levine FH. Congenital coronary arteriovenous fistula. Report of 13 patients, review of the literature and delineation of management. Circulation 1979; 59:849–854.

154. Urrutia-S CO, Falaschi G, Ott DA, Cooley DA. Surgical management of 56 patients with congenital coronary artery fistulas. Ann Thorac Surg 1983; 35:300–307.

155. Miyataka K, Okamoto M, Kinoshita N, Fusejima K, Sakakibara H, Nimura Y. Doppler echocardiographic features of coronary arteriovenous fistula. Complementary roles of cross sectional echocardiography and the Doppler techniques. Br Heart J 1984; 51:508–518.

156. Agatston AS, Chapman E, Hildner FJ, Samet P. Diagnosis of a right coronary artery–right atrial fistula using two-dimensional and Doppler echocardiography. Am J Cardiol 1984; 54:238–239.

157. Slater J, Lighty GW Jr, Winer HE, Kahn ML, Kronzon I, Isom OW: Doppler echocardiography and computed tomography in diagnosis of left coronary arteriovenous fistula. J Am Coll Cardiol 1984; 4:1290–1293.

Anomalous Origin of Either the Right or Left Main Coronary Artery from the Aorta with Subsequent Coursing Between Aorta and Pulmonary Trunk: Analysis of 32 Necropsy Cases

Amy H. Kragel, MD, and William C. Roberts, MD

Anomalous origin of either the left main coronary artery (LMCA) or right coronary artery (RCA) from the aorta with subsequent coursing between the aorta and pulmonary trunk is a rare and sometimes fatal coronary artery anomaly. Thirty-two cases of these anomalies were reviewed, with particular attention to the exact location and shape of the anomalistically positioned ostium and coronary dominance. The LMCA (7 cases) arose either from behind the right coronary sinus (6 cases) or as a single ostium with the RCA straddling the right-left commissure and right coronary sinus (1 case). In 5 of the 7 cases, the anomaly was fatal. In 6 cases of anomalous origin of the LMCA, the RCA was dominant and in 4 the anomaly was fatal. In only 1 case of anomalous origin of the LMCA was the left circumflex coronary artery dominant, and in this case the anomaly also was fatal. The RCA (25 cases) arose either from behind the left coronary sinus (8 cases), above the left coronary sinus (5 cases), from above the right-left commissure (10 cases) or as a single ostium with the LMCA above the right-left commissure and left coronary sinus (2 cases). In 8 of these 25 cases the anomaly was fatal. In 7 cases of anomalous origin of the RCA, the left circumflex coronary artery was dominant and in no case was the anomaly clinically significant. In 1 case, both the RCA and left circumflex coronary artery were hypoplastic and the anomaly was fatal. Coronary dominance, not ostial shape, was useful in separating the clinically significant from the clinically insignificant anomalies.

(Am J Cardiol 1988;62:771–777)

From the Pathology Branch, National Heart, Lung, and Blood Institute, National Institutes of Health, Bethesda, Maryland. Manuscript received May 5, 1988; revised manuscript received and accepted June 7, 1988.

Address for reprints: William C. Roberts, MD, Building 10, Room 2N258, Pathology Branch, National Heart, Lung, and Blood Institute, National Institutes of Health, Bethesda, Maryland 20892.

Before 1974 little information was available regarding patients in whom either the right (RCA) or left main (LMCA) coronary artery arose anomalously from the aorta. In 1974, Cheitlin et al[1] described certain clinical and necropsy findings in 13 patients in whom the LMCA arose from the right sinus of Valsalva and coursed between aorta and pulmonary trunk and they called attention to the frequency of sudden death as a consequence of this "not so minor congenital anomaly." Since 1974, other cases of anomalous origin of the LMCA from the right sinus of Valsalva have been reported and the danger of this anomaly has been confirmed.[2–5] Additionally, several reports have described the origin of the RCA from the left sinus of Valsalva with subsequent coursing of the anomalous arising artery between aorta and pulmonary trunk.[6–10] The number of necropsy cases of anomalous origin of either the LMCA from the right sinus or the RCA from the left sinus of Valsalva reported by any 1 group of investigators has been small and a diversity of clinical outcomes has been described in both types of anomaly. In this report we describe necropsy findings in 32 patients with one or the other of these anomalies. The major purpose of this analysis is to gain insight as to why 1 patient with the particular coronary anomaly has either fatal or nonfatal consequences from it and why others have no clinical consequences from it. The 3 major factors examined were coronary dominance, the precise location of the ostium of the anomalous artery in the aorta and the shape of that ostium.

METHODS

The records of the Pathology Branch, National Heart, Lung, and Blood Institute, National Institutes of Health, were searched for all cases of anomalous origin of the RCA or LMCA from the aorta. Cases associated with major congenital anomalies of the heart or great arteries or veins, other than isolated abnormalities of the aortic valve, were excluded. Such excluded cases included a 25-year-old woman who died suddenly. Twenty years before death she had closure of a large atrial septal defect; at autopsy there was anomalous origin of the right coronary artery from above the commissure between the right and left sinus of Valsalva with subsequent coursing between the aorta and pulmonary trunk.

A total of 45 hearts with isolated anomalous origin were studied from 1976 to 1988. One case was excluded

TABLE I Clinical and Morphologic Features of Patients with Anomalous Origin of the Left Main Coronary Artery

Pt	Age (yrs), Sex	Race	AP	SD	Cause of Death	Anomaly Group	Slit-Like Ostium	Dominant CA	CA Narrowed >75% in CSA by Plaque	LV		AV Abnormality	HW (g)
										Ne	Fi		
1	13, F	—	0	+	Coronary anomaly	1A	+	R	0	0	0	0	210
2	14, M	C	0	+	Coronary anomaly	1A	+	R	0	0	+	0	370
3	19, M	A	0	+	Coronary anomaly	1A	+	R	0	0	0	0	325
4	29, M	B	+	+	Coronary anomaly	1A	—	L	0	0	+	0	350
5	64, F	C	+	0	Coronary anomaly	1A	+	R	0	0	+	0	510
6	81, M	—	0	+	Trauma	1A	0	R	0	0	0	0	420
7	50, F	B	0	+	Renal disease	1B	0	R	+	0	+	0	650

A = Asian; AP = angina pectoris; AV = aortic valve; B = Black; C = Caucasian; CA = coronary artery; CSA = cross-sectional area; Fi = fibrosis; HW = heart weight; L = left coronary artery; LV = left ventricular; Ne = necrosis; R = right coronary artery; SD = sudden death.

because the heart was not available for reexamination and the case had not been adequately photographed. This patient was a 62-year-old man who died of cancer. An incidental autopsy finding was anomalous origin of the RCA from behind the left sinus of Valsalva. Twelve cases were excluded because the anomalistically arising RCA or LMCA did not course between aorta and pulmonary trunk, but coursed either anterior or posterior to both great arteries. These 12 cases will be described elsewhere.

The clinical summaries, general autopsy findings, heart specimens and photographs were reviewed in the remaining 32 cases. All were initially examined by one of us (WCR) and then 26 hearts were examined by

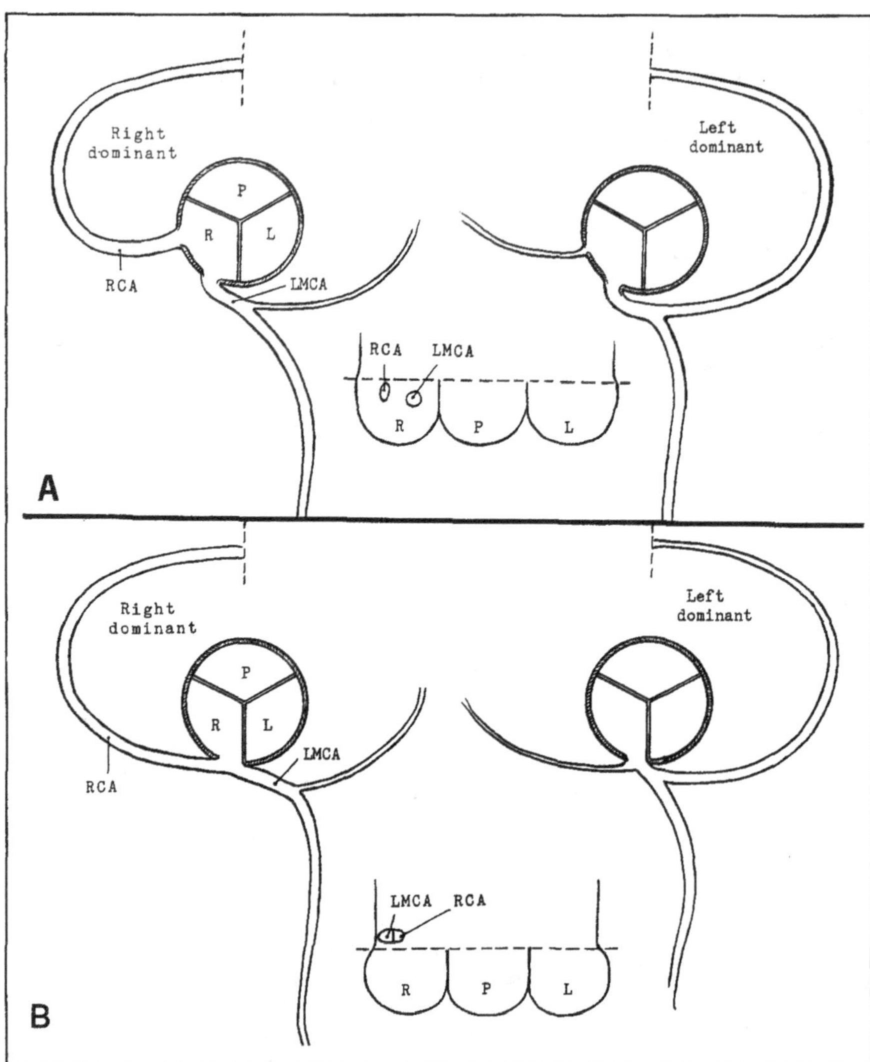

FIGURE 1. Coronary anatomy in cases of anomalous origin of the LMCA from the aorta illustrating both right and left circumflex coronary artery dominance. *A*, group 1A (patients 1–6, Table I). Anomalous origin of the LMCA from behind the right sinus of Valsalva. *B*, group 1B (patient 7, Table I). Anomalous origin of the LMCA from a common ostium above the right coronary sinus and R-L commissure. L = left coronary sinus; LMCA = left main coronary artery; P = posterior coronary sinus; R = right coronary sinus; RCA = right coronary artery.

TABLE II Clinical and Morphologic Features of Patients with Anomalous Origin of the Right Coronary Artery

Pt	Age (yrs), Sex	Race	AP	SD	Cause of Death	Anomaly Group	Slit-like Ostium	Dominant CA	CA Narrowed >75% in CSA by Plaque	LV Ne	Fi	AV Abnormality	HW (g)
1	17, M	B	0	+	Coronary anomaly	2A	+	R	0	0	0	0	425
2	29, F	B	0	+	Heroin overdose	2A	0	R	0	0	0	0	<350
3	42, M	B	—	+	Seizure disorder	2A	+	L	+	0	0	0	375
4	43, M	B	0	0	Renal disease	2A	—	L	0	0	0	0	885
5	48, M	B	0	+	Trauma	2A	+	R	0	0	0	0	350
6	49, M	B	+	+	Coronary anomaly	2A	+	R	0	0	+	+	482
7	51, M	C	+	0	Myocardial infarction	2A	+	R	+	+	+	0	540
8	74, M	C	0	0	Amyloidosis	2A	+	R	0	0	0	0	535
9	36, M	B	+	+	CAD	2B	0	R	+	0	+	0	450
10	41, M	B	0	+	Renal disease	2B	—	L	0	0	0	0	540
11	55, M	C	0	0	Aortic dissection	2B*	—	R	0	+	0	+	580
12	65, F	C	+	0	HC	2B	+	R	0	0	0	0	410
13	66, M	B	—	+	Trauma	2B	+	R	+	0	0	+	480
14	2, F	B	0	+	Panhypopituitism	2C	0	L	0	0	0	0	40
15	16, M	B	0	+	Coronary anomaly	2C	0	Neither	0	0	0	0	320
16	17, M	B	0	+	Coronary anomaly	2C	+	R	0	0	+	0	465
17	18, M	B	+	+	Coronary anomaly	2C	+	R	0	0	0	0	345
18	23, F	C	0	+	Coronary anomaly	2C	+	R	0	0	+	0	340
19	31, M	B	0	0	Infective endocarditis	2C	+	L	0	0	0	+	450
20	40, M	C	0	+	Coronary anomaly	2C	+	R	0	+	0	0	415
21	42, M	B	0	+	Trauma	2C	0	L	+	0	0	0	410
22	68, M	B	+	0	Cancer	2C	0	R	+	0	0	0	330
23	68, M	B	0	0	Burns	2C	—	R	+	0	0	0	360
24	33, F	—	0	+	Coronary anomaly	2D	0	R	0	0	0	0	23
25	19, M	C	0	0	Cancer	2D	+	L	0	0	0	0	260

* This is a congenitally bicuspid aortic valve in which the RCA arises above a position corresponding to what would be the left sinus of Valsalva in a tricuspid valve.
CAD = coronary artery disease; HC = hypertrophic cardiomyopathy; other abbreviations as in Table I.

both of us. In 6 cases, the hearts were not available for review but had been adequately photographed or described, or both, and so were included in this study. The signs and symptoms of cardiac disease and the mode of death were noted in each case. The anatomy of the 4 major epicardial coronary arteries was reviewed and the dominant coronary artery identified. The relation of the coronary ostia to the sinotubular junction and to the coronary sinuses was determined and the shape of the coronary ostia noted. A coronary ostium was considered to be above the sinotubular junction only if all of the ostium was clearly above the sinotubular junction.

The coronary anomaly was classified into 1 of 2 types: (1) anomalous origin of the LMCA from an aortic sinus other than the left one, from above an aortic sinus other than the left one or above an aortic valve commissure; and (2) anomalous origin of the RCA from an aortic sinus other than the right one, above an aortic sinus other than the right one or above an aortic valve commissure. The coronary arteries were examined and the presence or absence of >75% cross-sectional area narrowing of 1 or more of the 4 major epicardial coronary arteries was noted. The presence or absence of left ventricular necrosis or fibrosis was also recorded.

RESULTS

Anomalous origin of the left main coronary artery: In 7 (22%) of the 32 cases, the LMCA arose abnormally and then coursed between the aorta and pulmonary trunk. Five of these cases (patients 1–3, 5 and 6) have been reported previously.[5] Certain clinical and morphologic features of these 7 patients are listed in Table I. The ages ranged from 13 to 81 years (mean 38). Four were men and 3 were women. In 5 patients, the anomaly was considered the cause of death. All of these 5 patients had signs or symptoms of cardiac disease during life. Two had angina pectoris, 3 had 1 or more episodes of syncope (patients 1, 2 and 4), 1 (patient 3) had an abnormal electrocardiogram and 1 (patient 5) had congestive heart failure.

Both coronary ostia arose within the right sinus of Valsalva in 6 cases (group 1A, Figure 1) and as a single coronary ostium, which divided immediately to form the RCA and LMCA, which straddled the right sinus of Valsalva and the commissure between the right and left cusps in 1 case (group 1B, Figure 1). The ostium of the LMCA was slit-like in at least 4 cases. The RCA was dominant in 6 cases and the left circumflex coronary artery was dominant in 1 case. Grossly visible foci of left or right ventricular wall necrosis were absent in all 7 cases, but 4 had grossly visible left ventricular scars, only 1 of whom had significant coronary artery narrowing (>75% cross-sectional area narrowing of 1 or more major epicardial coronary arteries).

Anomalous origin of the right coronary artery: In 25 cases (78%), the RCA arose anomalistically and then coursed between the aorta and pulmonary trunk. Certain features in 10 of these cases (patients 1, 2, 5–7,

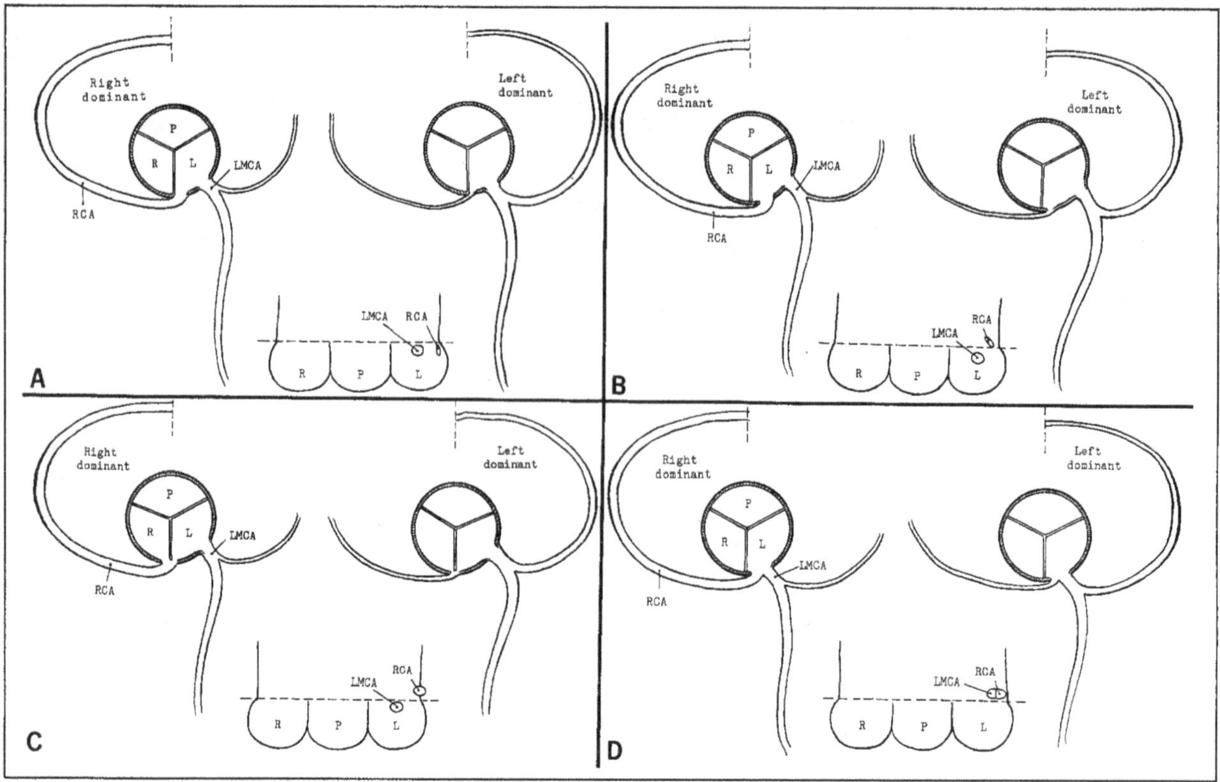

FIGURE 2. Coronary anatomy in cases of anomalous origin of the RCA from the aorta illustrating both right and left circumflex coronary artery dominance. *A,* group 2A (patients 1–8, Table II). Anomalous origin of the RCA from behind the left sinus of Valsalva. *B,* group 2B (patients 9–13, Table II). Anomalous origin of the RCA from above the left sinus of Valsalva. *C,* group 2C (patients 14–23, Table II). Anomalous origin of the RCA from above the commissure between the right and left sinus of Valsalva. *D,* group 2D (patients 24 and 25, Table II). Anomalous origin of the RCA from a common ostium with the LMCA straddling the left coronary sinus and the R-L commissure. Abbreviations as in Figure 1.

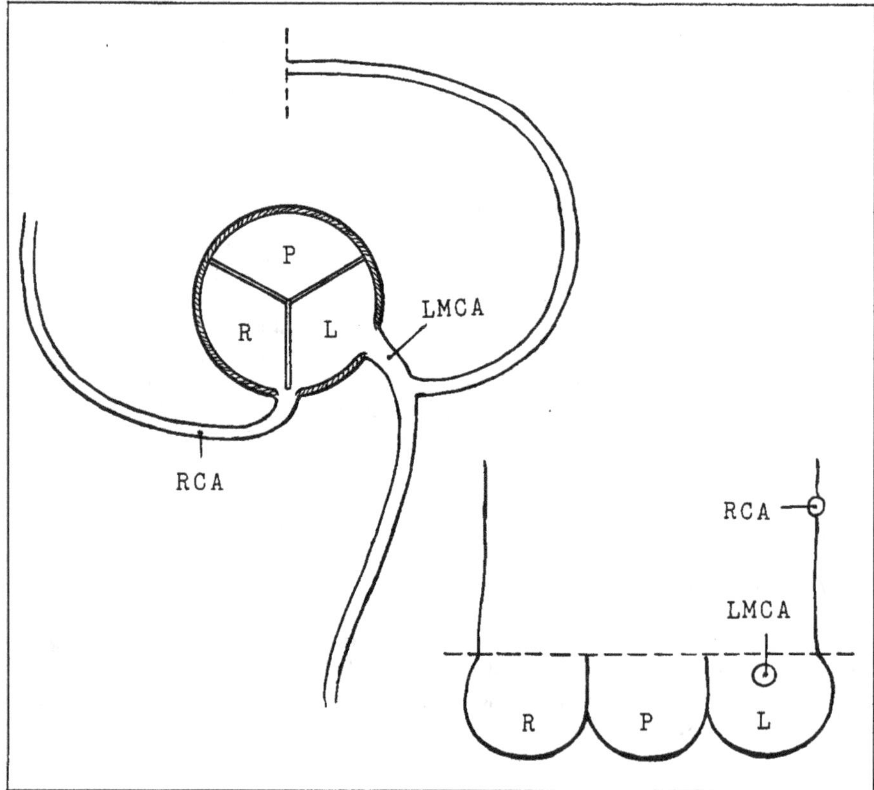

FIGURE 3. Coronary anatomy in a 2-year-old infant with panhypopituitarism (patient 14, Table II). The ostium of the RCA is high above the R-L commissure. Abbreviations as in Figure 1.

FIGURE 4. Coronary anatomy in a patient (patient 11, Table II) with a congenitally bicuspid aortic valve. The RCA arises from what would correspond to the left sinus of Valsalva in a tricuspid valve. Abbreviations as in Figure 1.

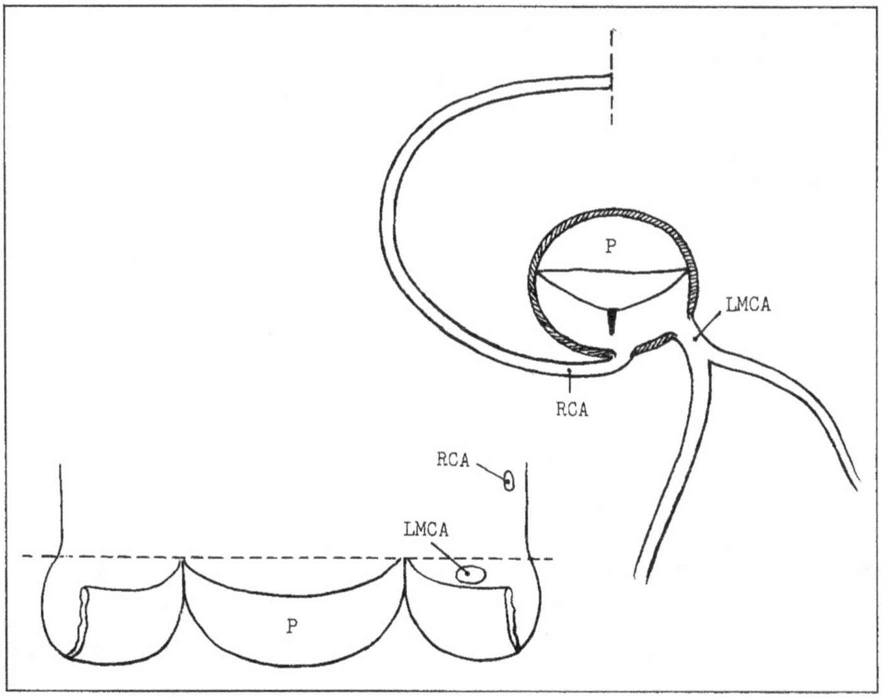

10, 18, 19, 24 and 25) have been reported previously.[6,9] Certain clinical and morphologic findings of these patients are listed in Table II. The ages of the 25 patients ranged from 4 months to 74 years (mean 39 years). Five were female and 20 were male. The anomaly was considered the cause of death in 8 patients. Of these, 5 (patients 1, 15, 16, 20 and 24) had no signs or symptoms of cardiac disease during life; 2 had angina pectoris; 2 (patients 17 and 18) had abnormal electrocardiograms and 1 (patient 18) had recurrent ventricular tachycardia with a nonfatal cardiac arrest later followed by a fatal cardiac arrest. Four others (patients 7, 9, 12 and 22) had evidence of myocardial ischemia disease during life; in 3, necropsy revealed >75% cross-sectional area narrowing of 1 or more major epicardial coronary arteries; 1 of the 4 patients had hypertrophic cardiomyopathy.

The ostium of the RCA arose from within the left sinus of Valsalva in 8 cases (group 2A, Figure 2), from above the left sinus of Valsalva in 5 cases (group 2B, Figure 2), directly above the commissure between the right and left cusps in 10 cases (group 2C, Figure 2 and Figure 3) and as a single ostium, which straddled the left sinus of Valsalva and the commissure between the right and left cusp, in 2 cases (group 2D, Figure 2). Of the 25 cases, the ostium of the RCA was slit-like in 14, oval in 7 and not determined in 4.

In 7 cases the left circumflex coronary artery was dominant, in 10 cases the RCA was dominant and in 1 case both the RCA and the left circumflex coronary artery were small and neither artery coursed to the crux of the heart. In no case where the anomaly was clinically significant was the left circumflex coronary artery dominant. Seven patients had >75% cross-sectional area narrowing by plaque of 1 or more major epicardial coronary arteries. Grossly visible foci of left ventricular

necrosis were present in 2 cases, 1 of which had significant coronary arterial atherosclerosis, and the other (patient 11) had evulsion of the RCA from the aorta from an aortic dissection. Grossly visible left ventricular scars were present in 5 patients, 2 of whom had 1 or more of the major epicardial coronary arteries significantly narrowed by plaque.

Abnormalities of the aortic valve were present in 4 patients: in patient 11 (Figure 4) the aortic valve was congenitally bicuspid, in patient 19 (Figure 5) all cusps were partially fused and in patients 6 and 13 (Figure 5) the commissure between the right and left cusps was fused.

DISCUSSION

Anatomic classification of anomalous origin of the LMCA and RCA from the aorta with subsequent coursing between the aorta and pulmonary trunk is complex. It is not sufficient, as has been done in the past, to classify the anomaly as "origin of the RCA from the left sinus of Valsalva" and "origin of the LMCA from the right sinus of Valsalva." The LMCA may arise from either behind the right sinus of Valsalva (group 1A) or from a common ostium with the RCA straddling the right-left commissure and the left sinus of Valsalva (group 1B). The RCA may arise from behind or above the left sinus of Valsalva (groups 2A and 2B, respectively), from above the commissure between the right and left cusps (group 2C) or from a common ostium with the LMCA which straddles the commissure between the right and left sinus of Valsalva and the left sinus of Valsalva (group 2D). Subclassification of the anomalies was not a predictor of clinical significance of the anomaly (Table III).

The *shape of the ostium* was not helpful in predicting the clinical significance of the anomaly. In cases in

	No. Cases	Clinically Important
Anomalous origin of LMCA		
From right sinus	6	5
From common ostium with RCA above right sinus and R-L commissure	1	0
Anomalous origin of RCA		
From left sinus	8	2
From above left sinus	5	0
From above commissure between	10	5
From common ostium with LMCA above left sinus and R-L commissure	2	1

anomaly was fatal. In 21 cases of anomalous origin of the RCA in which ostial shape was determined, the ostium was slit-like in 14 cases (67%) and in 6 of them (42%) the anomaly was fatal; in 7 cases (33%) the ostium was round and in 2 (29%) the anomaly was fatal. The numbers are too small to show a statistical difference.

Coronary dominance was important in separating clinically significant from clinically insignificant anomalies. In 7 cases of anomalous origin of the RCA from the left sinus of Valsalva, the left circumflex coronary artery was dominant and in none of them was the anomaly clinically significant. In 1 case (patient 15, Table II), both the left circumflex and right coronary arteries were hypoplastic (neither was dominant) and the anomaly was considered the cause of death. In our 7 patients with anomalous origin of the LMCA, the left circumflex coronary artery was dominant in only 1 (an anomaly that was clinically significant); in the other 6 cases, the left circumflex coronary artery was non-

which the anomaly was considered to be the cause of death, the anomalistically arising artery was in some instances slit-like and in others the ostium was round. When anomalous origin of the LMCA alone is considered, 4 of 6 cases had slit-like ostia and in all 4 the

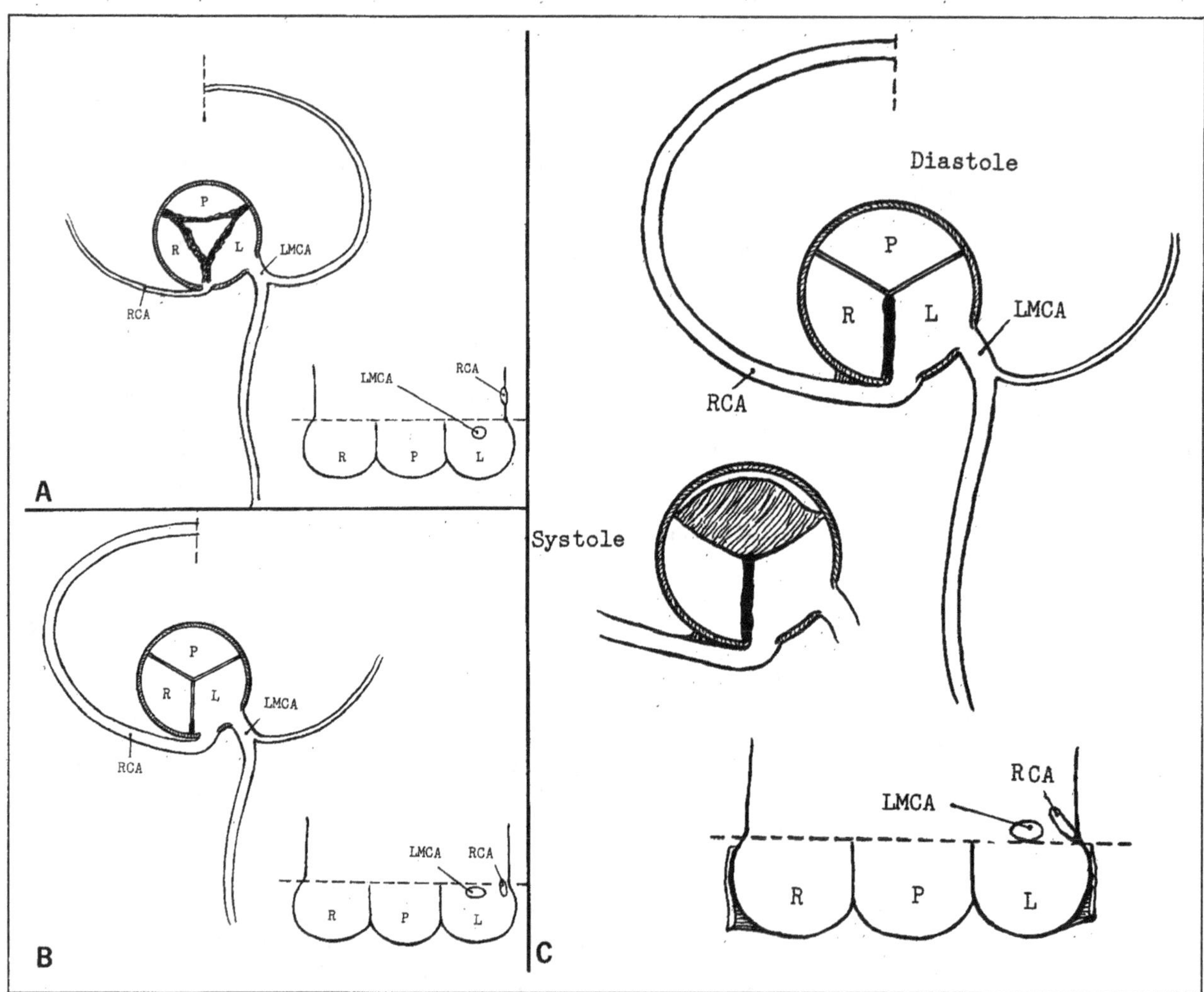

FIGURE 5. Coronary and aortic valve anatomy in cases of anomalous origin of the RCA with isolated aortic valve abnormalities present. *A*, patient 19, Table II. Partial fusion of all 3 commissures. Death was considered secondary to complications of infective endocarditis. *B*, patient 6, Table II. Partial fusion of the R-L commissure, clinically insignificant. *C*, patient 13, Table II. Complete fusion of the R-L commissure, clinically insignificant. Abbreviations as in Figure 1.

dominant (the RCA was dominant) and in 4 the anomaly was clinically significant while in 2 it was not. Thus, in the case of anomalous origin of the LMCA, left circumflex dominance is probably always clinically significant or at least potentially significant whereas RCA dominance is usually, but not always, clinically significant.

REFERENCES

1. Cheitlin MD, DeCastro CM, McAllister HA. Sudden death as a complication of anomalous left coronary origin from the anterior sinus of Valsalva. A not-so-minor congenital anomaly. *Circulation 1974;50:780–787.*
2. Liberthson RR, Dinsmore RE, Fallon JT. Aberrant coronary artery origin from the aorta, report of 18 patients, review of literature and delineation of natural history and management. *Circulation 1979;59:748–754.*
3. Ishikawa T, Brandt PWT. Anomalous origin of the left main coronary artery from the right anterior aortic sinus: angiographic definition of anomalous course. *Am J Cardiol 1985;55:770–776.*
4. Kimbiris D. Anomalous origin of the left main coronary artery from the right sinus of Valsalva. *Am J Cardiol 1985;55:765–769.*
5. Barth CW, Roberts WC. Left main coronary artery originating from the right sinus of Valsalva and coursing between the aorta and pulmonary trunk. *JACC 1986;7:366–373.*
6. Roberts WC, Siegel RJ, Zipes DP. Origin of the right coronary artery from the left sinus of Valsalva and its functional consequences: analysis of 10 necropsy patients. *Am J Cardiol 1982;49:863–867.*
7. Liberthson RR, Gang DL, Custer J. Sudden death in an infant with aberrant origin of the right coronary artery from the left sinus of Valsalva of the aorta: case report and review of the literature. *Ped Cardiol 1983;4:45–48.*
8. Isner JM, Shen EM, Martin ET, Fortin RV. Sudden unexpected death as a result of anomalous origin of the right coronary artery from the left sinus of Valsalva. *Am J Med 1984;76:155–158.*
9. Barth CW, Bray M, Roberts WC. Sudden death in infancy associated with origin of both left main and right coronary arteries from a common ostium above the left sinus of Valsalva. *Am J Cardiol 1986;57:365–366.*
10. Kucera RF, Bowden WD, Thomas HM, Blue PW. Anomalous origin of the right coronary artery from the left sinus of Valsalva: a case report. *Cathet Cardiovasc Diagn 1986;12:334–336.*

Anomalous Origin of Either the Right or Left Main Coronary Artery from the Aorta Without Coursing of the Anomalistically Arising Artery Between Aorta and Pulmonary Trunk

William C. Roberts, MD, and Amy H. Kragel, MD

Clinical and necropsy findings are described in 12 adults (10 men) in whom either the left main coronary artery or the right coronary artery arose abnormally from the aorta and the anomalistically arising artery coursed thereafter either normally or abnormally, but if abnormally not between the pulmonary trunk and ascending aorta. None of the 12 patients had symptoms of myocardial ischemia that unequivocally could be attributed to the anomalously arising coronary artery. One patient, a 19-year-old man, however, died suddenly and no abnormality other than the anomalistically arising right coronary artery from the posterior aortic valve sinus was found.

(Am J Cardiol 1988;62:1263–1267)

From the Pathology Branch, National Heart, Lung, and Blood Institute, National Institutes of Health, Bethesda, Maryland 20892. Manuscript received August 19, 1988, and accepted August 22.

Address for reprints: William C. Roberts, MD, Building 10, Room 2N258, Pathology Branch, National Heart, Lung, and Blood Institute, National Institutes of Health, Bethesda, Maryland 20892.

We recently reported clinical and necropsy findings in 32 patients in whom both right (RCA) and left main (LMCA) coronary arteries arose from the aorta but one arose anomalously and then coursed between pulmonary trunk and aorta.[1] While collecting these 32 cases for the previous report, we found 12 cases in whom either the RCA or the LMCA arose anomalistically from the aorta and thereafter did not course between pulmonary trunk and aorta. We then searched for reported cases in which the latter circumstance occurred and found few. Therefore, we believe it appropriate to describe clinical and necropsy features in these 12 patients in whom either the RCA or the LMCA arose anomalistically from the aorta without coursing of the anomalous arising coronary artery between pulmonary trunk and aorta.

METHODS

Sources of cases: The records of the Pathology Branch, National Heart, Lung, and Blood Institute, National Institutes of Health, were searched for all cases of anomalous origin of the RCA or LMCA from the aorta. Cases associated with other major congenital anomalies of the heart or great vessels including isolated anomalies of the aortic valve were excluded. In addition, all cases in which the anomalistically arising artery coursed between aorta and pulmonary trunk were excluded.

Examinations performed: The clinical summaries, general autopsy findings, photographs and hearts were reviewed in each case. All had been examined initially by one of us (WCR) and then reviewed by both of us. In each case the relation of the coronary ostia to the coronary sinuses and to the sinotubular junction was recorded. Whether the lumens of the major epicardial coronary arteries were narrowed >75% in cross-sectional area was noted. The presence or absence of left ventricular necrosis and fibrosis also was recorded.

RESULTS

Types of coronary anomalies observed: Certain clinical and necropsy findings in the 12 patients are summarized in Table I. Patients 1 to 5 had anomalous origin of the LMCA from the right sinus of Valsalva (Figures 1 through 3). In patient 1 the anomalously arising artery subsequently coursed anterior to the pulmonary trunk; in patients 2 and 3 it coursed posterior to the aorta; and in patients 4 and 5 it coursed within the ventricular septum to reach the subepicardial adipose tissue anterior to the septum.[2] Patient 6 had origin of the LMCA from above the commissure between the left and posterior cusps (Figure 4). Patient 7 had origin of the LMCA cephalad to the sinotubular junction above the posterior sinus of Valsalva (Figure 5). Patients 8 and 9 had origin of the RCA cephalad to the sinotubular junction above the right coronary sinus (Figure 6).

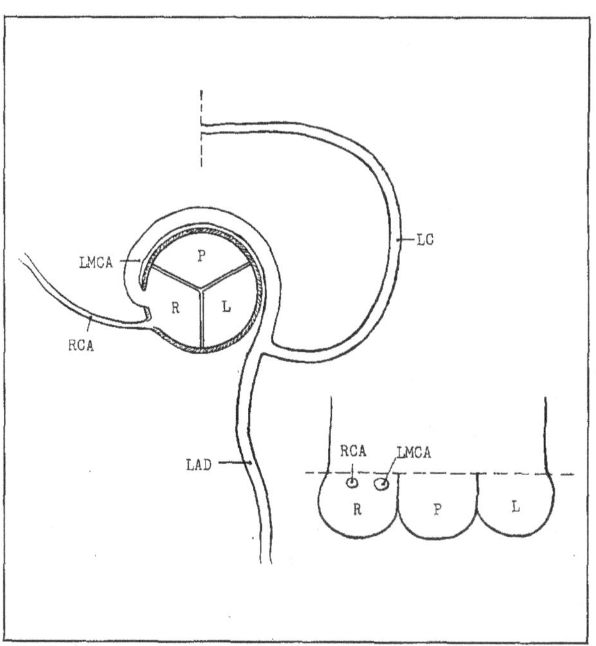

FIGURE 1. Patient 1 (Table I). Diagram showing origin of the left main coronary artery (LMCA) from the right (R) sinus of Valsalva and coursing of the anomalistically arising artery anterior to the pulmonary trunk before dividing into the left anterior descending (LAD) and left circumflex (LC) coronary arteries. A = anterior; L = left; P = posterior; R = right; RCA = right coronary artery.

FIGURE 2. Patient 2 (Table I). Diagram showing origin of the left main coronary artery (LMCA) from the right (R) sinus with coursing of the anomalistically arising artery posterior to the aorta before dividing into the left anterior descending (LAD) and left circumflex (LC) branches. Other abbreviations as in Figure 1.

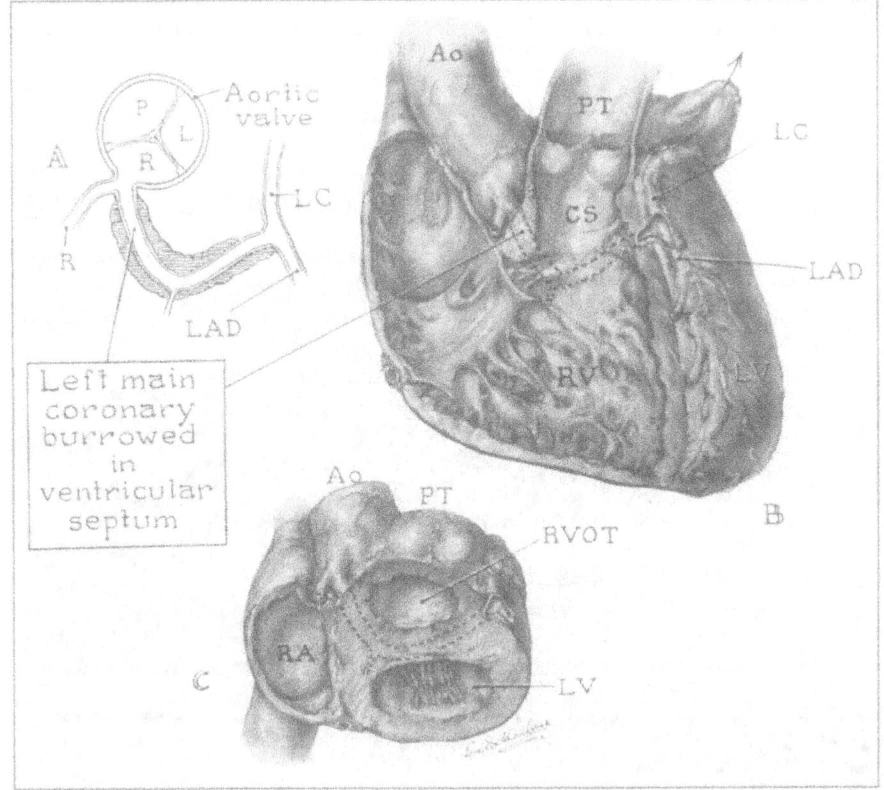

FIGURE 3. Patient 4 (Table I). Drawing of origin and course of the left main coronary artery from the right (R) sinus of Valsalva with its coursing within the ventricular septum beneath the right ventricular outflow tract (RVOT) and exiting in the subepicardial adipose tissue directly anterior to the septum and then subdividing into the left anterior descending (LAD) and left circumflex (LC) branches. Ao = aorta; CS = crista supraventricularis; PT = pulmonary trunk; L = left; LV = left ventricle; P = posterior; RA = right atrium; RV = right ventricle. Reproduced with permission from Roberts et al; Am Heart J.[2]

TABLE I Certain Clinical and Morphologic Features in 12 Patients With Anomalous Origin of Either the Right or Left Main Coronary Artery from the Aorta Without Subsequent Coursing Between Aorta and Pulmonary Trunk

Case No.	Autopsy No.	Coronary Anomaly	Age (yrs), Sex	SD	Associated Disorders	No. Major CAs >75% ↓ by Plaque	LV Scar	HW (g)
1	A78-140	LMCA from RSV coursing anterior	22, M	+	HC	0	+	870
2	82-02-240	LMCA from RSV coursing posterior	32, M	+	Trauma	0	0	330
3	79-10-813	LMCA from RSV coursing posterior	57, F	0	Alcoholism	0	0	300
4	82-03-291	LMCA from RSV coursing through VS	48, M	+	Trauma	0	0	550
5	81-09-750	LMCA from RSV coursing through VS	34, M	0	Trauma	0	0	330
6	SA 82-1	LMCA from above L-P commissure	54, M	0	CAD	1	+	550
7	88A-25	LMCA from above PSV	78, M	0	SH, CHF	0	0	580
8	79-07-571	RCA high take-off	30, M	0	Methemoglobi-nemia	0	0	330
9	A86-61	RCA high take-off	61, M	0	AMI	3	0	405
10	83-09-602	RCA from PSV	19, M	+	0	0	0	450
11	A86-13	RCA from above PSV	53, F	0	HC	0	0	550
12	85A-143	RCA from above R-P commissure	79, M	0	CAD, CVA, PVD	2	0	490

AMI = acute myocardial infarction; CA = coronary artery; CAD = atherosclerotic coronary artery disease; CHF = congestive heart failure; CVA = cerebrovascular accident; HC = hypertrophic cardiomyopathy; HW = heart weight; L = left; LV = left ventricular; LMCA = left main coronary artery; R = right; RCA = right coronary artery; PSV = posterior sinus of Valsalva; RSV = right sinus of Valsalva; P = posterior; PVD = peripheral vascular disease; SD = sudden death; SH = systemic hypertension; VS = ventricular septum; + = present; 0 = absent.

Patient 10, who died suddenly while playing basketball and who had been healthy previously without signs or symptoms of cardiac dysfunction or myocardial ischemia, had origin of the RCA from the posterior sinus of Valsalva and a quadricuspid pulmonic valve (Figure 7). Histologic study of sections of left ventricular wall in him disclosed patchy subendocardial replacement fibrosis. Patient 11 had origin of the RCA at and above the level of the sinotubular junction cephalad to the posterior sinus and just posterior to the commissure between right and posterior cusps (Figure 7). Patient 12 had anomalous origin of the RCA cephalad to the commissure between right and posterior cusps (Figure 8).

DISCUSSION

Clinical consequences of the coronary anomalies: Of the 12 aforementioned patients in whom either the LMCA or the RCA arose anomalistically from the aorta and thereafter did not course between the pulmonary trunk and aorta, none had evidence during life of cardiac dysfunction that unequivocally could be attributed to the anomalously arising coronary artery. Of the 12 patients, however, 5 had other types of cardiac disease that clearly accounted for their deaths (hypertrophic cardiomyopathy in 2, severe coronary atherosclerosis in 2 and chronic congestive heart failure secondary to systemic hypertension in 1). Six patients died from noncar-

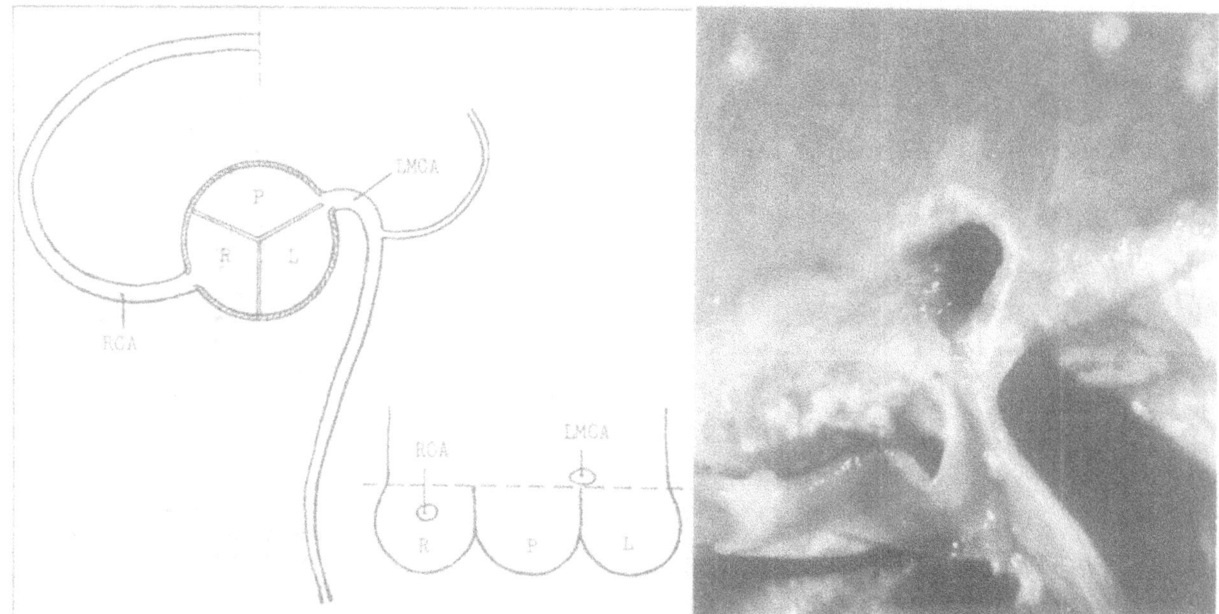

FIGURE 4. Patient 6 (Table I). Diagram (*left*) showing origin of the left main coronary artery (**LMCA**) directly cephalad to the commissure between the left (**L**) and posterior (**P**) aortic valve cusps, and photograph (*right*) of the opened aorta showing the ostium of the **LMCA** above the commissure. Other abbreviations as in Figure 1.

diac conditions and none of them during life had evidence of cardiac dysfunction or myocardial ischemia. The remaining patient (no. 10), a 19-year-old man, died suddenly and unexpectedly while playing basketball. He had not previously had clinical evidence of cardiac dysfunction or myocardial ischemia. No abnormalities in any organ were found at necropsy except the coronary anomaly and no toxic substances were found in the blood or tissues at necropsy. Whether or not the coronary anomaly was responsible for his sudden death

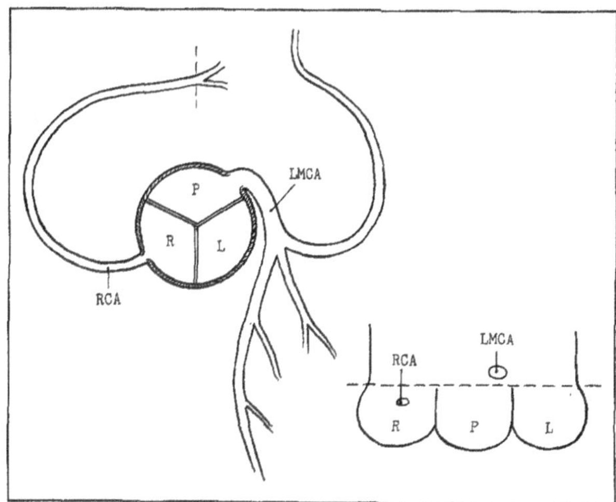

FIGURE 5 *(right).* **Patient 7 (Table I). Diagram showing origin of the left main coronary artery (LMCA) from the posterior (P) aortic valve sinus just posterior to the commissure between the left (L) and posterior cusps. R = right; RCA = right coronary artery.**

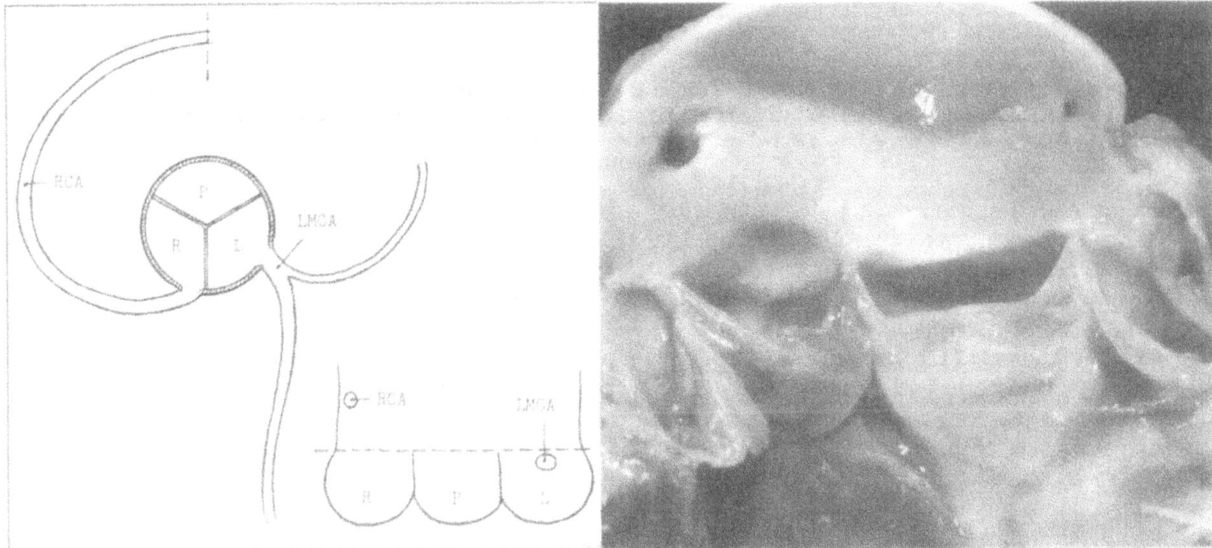

FIGURE 6. Patient 8 (Table I). Diagram *(left)* showing high take-off of the right coronary artery (RCA) above the right (R) sinus of Valsalva, and photograph *(right)* of the opened aortic valve and ascending aorta again showing the high take-off of the ostium of the RCA. Other abbreviations as in Figure 1.

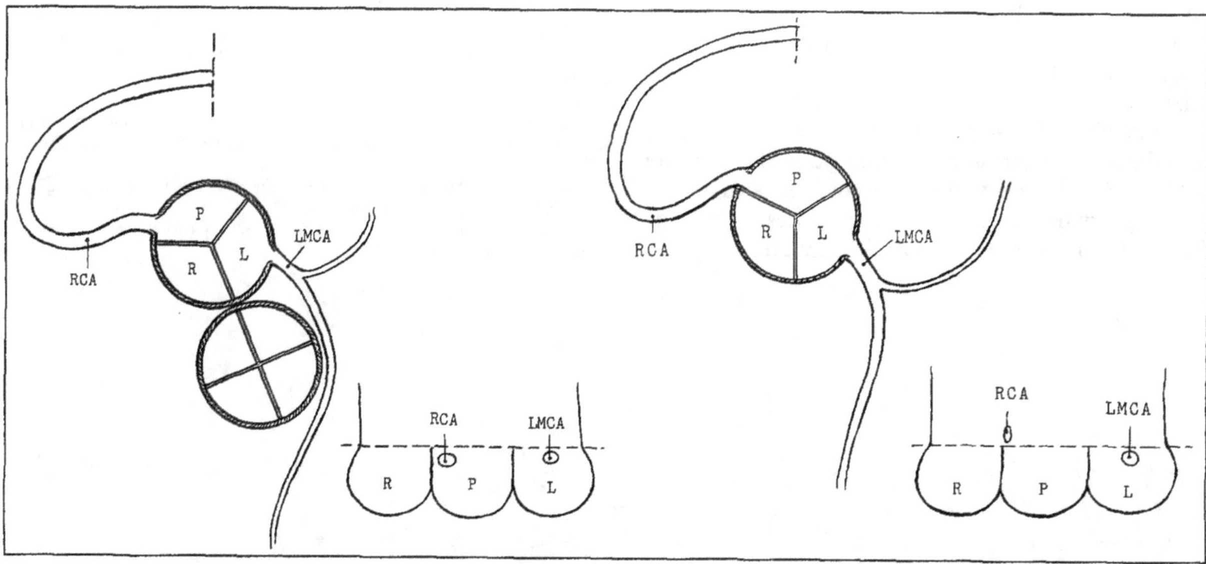

FIGURE 7. Patients 10 *(left)* and 11 *(right)* (Table I). The diagrams show origin of the right coronary artery (RCA) from behind the posterior aortic valve sinus *(left)* or just cephalad to *(right)* the posterior sinus of Valsalva. Other abbreviations as in Figure 1.

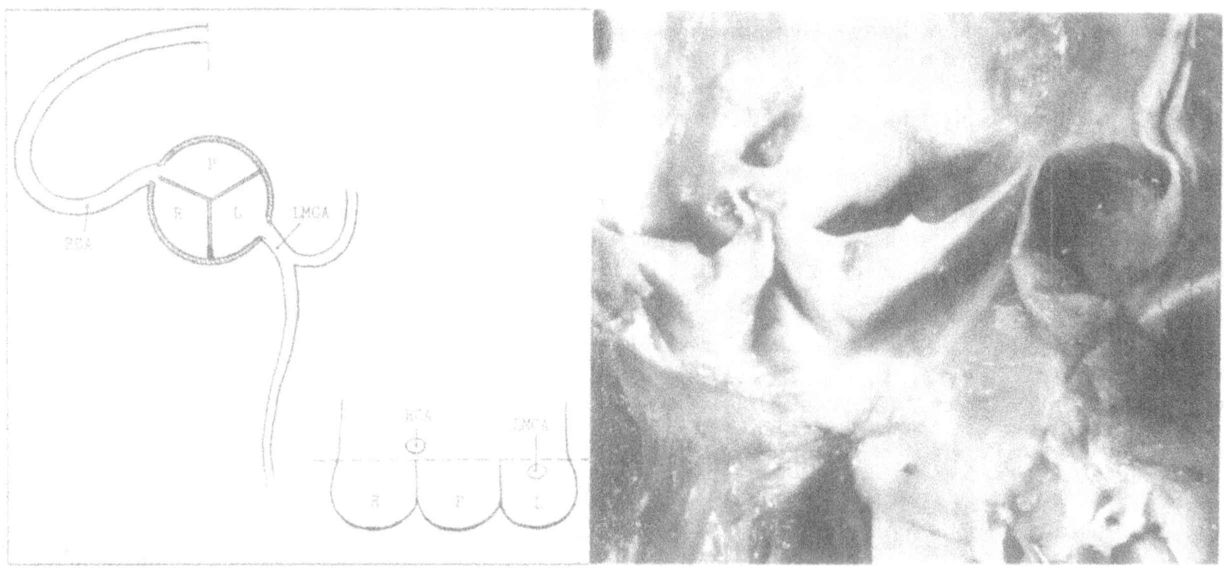

FIGURE 8. Patient 12 (Table I). Diagram (*left*) showing origin of the right coronary artery (RCA) cephalad to the commissure between the right (R) and posterior (P) aortic valve cusps, and photograph (*right*) of the opened aorta and aortic valve showing the ostium of the RCA above the commissure between the right and posterior aortic valve cusps. Other abbreviations as in Figure 1.

is uncertain. Small subendocardial left ventricular microinfarcts, however, were found, suggesting that myocardial ischemia had been present before death.

Previously published reports: We did not find any reports confirmed at necropsy of origin of the LMCA from the right sinus of Valsalva with coursing of the anomalistically arising artery either anterior to the pulmonary trunk or posterior to the aorta unassociated with major anomalies of the heart or great arteries. The earlier report by Roberts et al[2] described findings in 2 patients who had origin of the LMCA from the right sinus of Valsalva with subsequent coursing of the anomalous-arising artery within the ventricular septum to reach the subepicardial adipose tissue anterior to the ventricular septum. That report also mentioned 11 previously reported necropsy cases of origin of the LMCA from either the right aortic sinus of Valsalva or from the RCA with coursing of the anomalistically arising LMCA behind the aorta. No reports describing origin of the LMCA directly cephalad to the commissure between the left and posterior aortic valve cusps or cephalad to the sinotubular junction cephalad to the posterior aortic valve cusp have appeared, to our knowledge, in a medical journal. Several reports have described high take-off (cephalad to sinotubular junction) of the

RCA.[3-5] If, however, high take-off is defined as ≥ 1 cm cephalad to the sinotubular junction, high take-off of the RCA is rare. Vlodaver et al[4] described at necropsy a 72-year-old man in whom the RCA arose from behind the posterior sinus of Valsalva. We did not find other necropsy reports of origin of the RCA from behind the posterior sinus of Valsalva. Alexander and Griffith[6] described origin of the RCA directly cephalad to an aortic valve commissure in 5 patients at necropsy, but in none was it of clinical significance.

REFERENCES

1. Kragel AH, Roberts WC. Anomalous origin of either right or left main coronary artery from the aorta with subsequent coursing between aorta and pulmonary trunk: analysis of 32 necropsy cases. *Am J Cardiol 1988;62:771–777.*
2. Roberts WC, Dicicco BS, Waller BF, Kishel JC, McManus BM, Dawson SL, Hunsaker JC III, Luke JL. Origin of the left main from the right coronary artery or from the right aortic sinus with intramyocardial tunneling to the left side of the heart via the ventricular septum: the case against clinical significance of myocardial bridge or coronary tunnel. *Am Heart J 1982;104:303–305.*
3. Ogden JA. Congenital anomalies of the coronary arteries. *Am J Cardiol 1970;25:474–479.*
4. Vlodaver Z, Neufeld HN, Edwards JE. Coronary Arterial Malformations in the Normal Heart and in Congenital Heart Disease. *New York: Academic Press, 1975:171.*
5. Neufeld HN, Schneeweiss A. Coronary Artery Disease in Infants and Children. *Philadelphia: Lea & Febiger, 1983:189.*
6. Alexander R, Griffith GC. Anomalies of the coronary arteries and their clinical significance. *Circulation 1956;14:800–805.*

Retroaortic Epicardial Course of the Left Circumflex Coronary Artery and Anteroaortic Intramyocardial (Ventricular Septum) Course of the Left Anterior Descending Coronary Artery: An Unusual Coronary Anomaly and a Proposed Classification Based on the Number of Coronary Ostia in the Aorta

Allen L. Dollar, MD, and William C. Roberts, MD

In recent years a number of articles and books have focused on various coronary anomalies.[1-4] One of the least frequent coronary anomalies is the combination of retroaortic epicardial course of the left circumflex (LC) coronary artery and anteroaortic intramyocardial course of the left anterior descending (LAD) coronary artery. Herein, we describe another such case and provide a classification for such cases based on the present and previously published cases.

A.S., an 87-year-old man, who during life never had evidence of myocardial ischemia or cardiac dysfunction, died from complications of gastrointestinal bleeding. At necropsy, the heart weighed 405 g. None of the 4 chambers was dilated. No grossly visible foci of myocardial fibrosis or necrosis were present. The 4 cardiac valves were normal. The origins and courses of the coronary arteries are shown in Figure 1.

There have been at least 6 previously reported necropsy patients[5-9] with combined retroaortic epicardial course of the LC and anteroaortic intramyocardial course of the LAD coronary arteries (Table I). None of the 6 previously reported patients had symptoms of cardiac dysfunction or myocardial ischemia. One[9] of the 6 patients, however, was found dead

From the Pathology Branch, National Heart, Lung, and Blood Institute, National Institutes of Health, Bethesda, Maryland 20892. Manuscript received April 18, 1989, and accepted June 26.

TABLE I Clinical Findings and Anomaly Class of Six Previously Reported Necropsy Patients with Retroaortic Epicardial Course of the Left Circumflex and Anteroaortic Intramyocardial Course of the Left Anterior Descending Coronary Artery

Study (Reference)	Year	Pt Age (yrs), Sex	Cardiac Cause of Death	Anomaly Class*
Bachdalek[5]	1867	60, F	—	I
Sanes[6]	1937	4, M	0	I
White[7]	1948	39, M	0	I
Schulte[8]	1985	71, F	0	I
Virmani†[9]	1989	64, M	+	III
Virmani[9]	1989	62, M	0	IIa

* See Figure 2. † This patient died suddenly in bed at home and at necropsy had extensive coronary atherosclerosis with severe luminal narrowing.
\+ = present; 0 = absent; — = no information available.

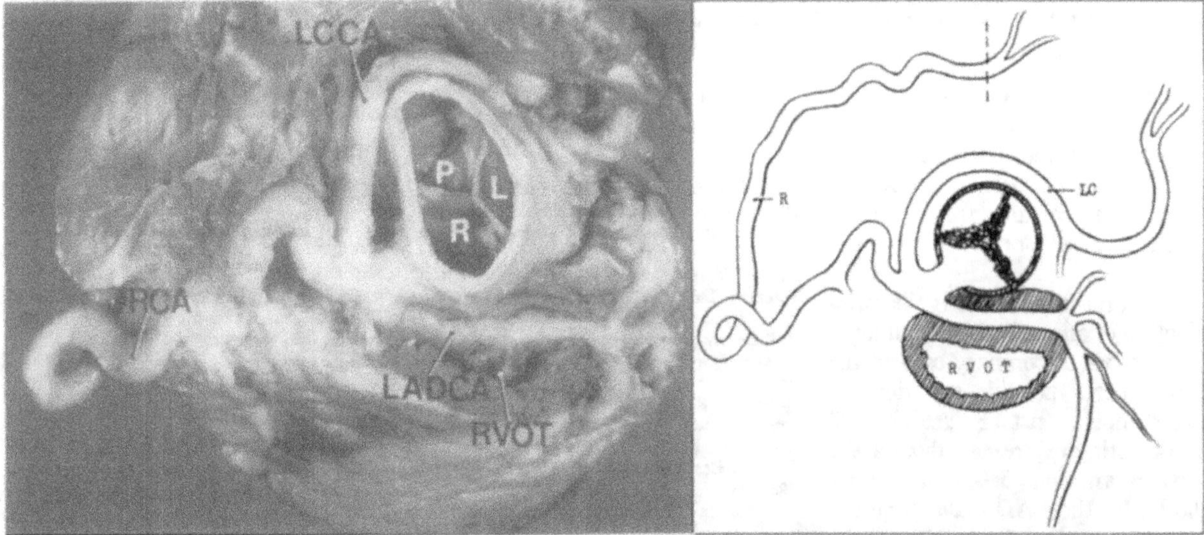

FIGURE 1. Heart from above in the 87-year-old man. The right coronary artery (RCA) arises from the right (R) sinus of Valsalva and within a centimeter of its origin, it gives rise to the left circumflex coronary artery (LCCA) and the left anterior descending coronary artery (LADCA). The latter artery courses caudally to penetrate into the ventricular septum located posteriorly to the right ventricular outflow tract (RVOT). The LADCA enters epicardium again anterior to the ventricular septum and quickly divides into 3 branches, one of which courses in the usual location of the LADCA. The initial portion of the RCA is very large and after origin of the LCCA and the LADCA, the RCA is very tortuous, so tortuous that it loops around itself. In contrast, neither the retroaortic LCCA nor the intramyocardial portion of the LADCA is tortuous. P = posterior and L = left sinus of Valsalva.

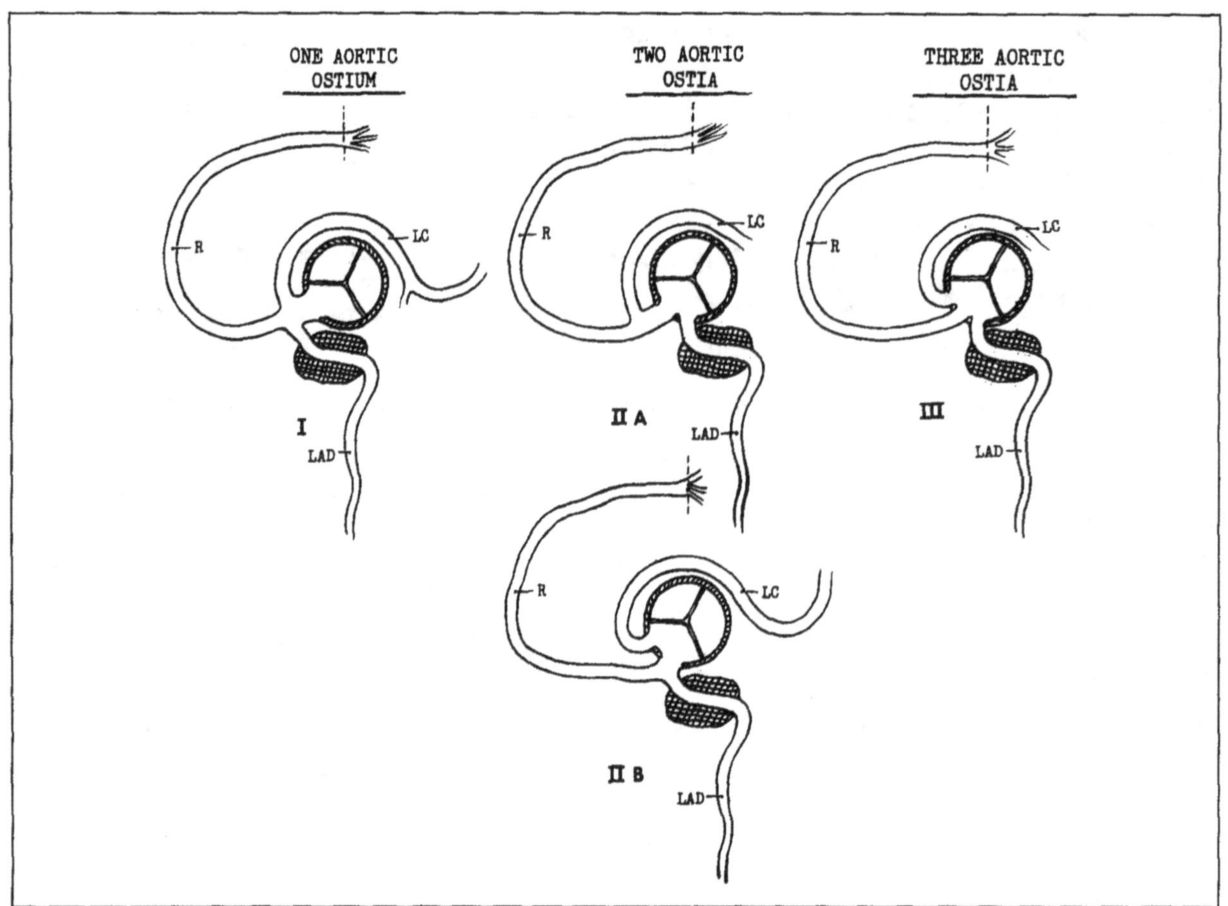

FIGURE 2. Four drawings of the complex of retroaortic epicardial left circumflex (LC) and anteroaortic intramyocardial left anterior descending (LAD) coronary arteries showing the possible origins of the LC and LAD from either the aorta or from the right (R) coronary artery. In type I (*left*) only a single coronary artery arises from the aorta and both LC and LAD coronary arteries arise from the right. In type II, there are 2 coronary ostia in the right sinus of Valsalva of the aorta, the right coronary artery and either the LAD (Type IIA) or the LC (Type IIB). No reports are available describing the type IIB variety. In type III, there are 3 coronary ostia in the aorta, LC, right and LAD coronary arteries.

in bed and necropsy disclosed severe atherosclerosis of all 3 major coronary arteries and a left ventricular scar. In these 6 patients, the LC and the LAD arose either from the right coronary artery or from the right aortic sinus.

A useful way to classify this combination of anomalies is according to the number of coronary ostia in the aorta. Three possible variations of this complex exist (Figure 2). If 2 aortic ostia are present, there are 2 further variations based on whether the LC or the LAD arises from the right coronary artery (Figure 2, IIa and IIb).

1. Voldaver Z, Neufeld HN, Edwards JE. Coronary Arterial Variations in the Normal Heart and in Congenital Heart Disease. *New York: Academic Press, 1975:171.*
2. Neufeld HN, Schneeweiss A. Coronary Artery Disease in Infants and Children. *Philadelphia: Lea and Febiger, 1983:189.*
3. Roberts WC. Major anomalies of coronary arterial origin seen in adulthood. *Am Heart J 1986;111: 941–963.*
4. Virmani R, Rogan K, Cheitlin MD. Congenital coronary artery anomalies: pathologic aspects. In: Virmani R, Forman MB, eds. Nonatherosclerotic Ischemic Heart Disease. *New York: Raven Press, 1989:153–183.*
5. Bachdalek H. Anomaler Verlauf der Kranzarterien des Herzens. *Virchow Arch Pathol Anat 1867; 41:260.*
6. Sanes S. Anomalous origin and course of the left coronary artery in a child: so-called congenital absence of the left coronary artery. *Am Heart J 1937;14:219–229.*
7. White NK, Edwards JE. Anomalies of the coronary arteries: report of four cases. *Arch Pathol Lab Med 1948;45:766–771.*
8. Schulte MA, Waller BF, Hull MT, Pless JE. Origin of the left anterior descending coronary artery from the right aortic sinus with intramyocardial tunneling to the left side of the heart via the ventricular septum: a case against clinical and morphologic significance of myocardial bridging. *Am Heart J 1985; 110:499–501.*
9. Virmani R, Chun PKC, Rogan K, Riddick L. Anomalous origin of four coronary ostia from the right sinus of Valsalva. *Am J Cardiol 1989;63:760–761.*

The Four Subtypes of Anomalous Origin of the Left Main Coronary Artery from the Right Aortic Sinus (or from the Right Coronary Artery)

William C. Roberts, MD, and Jamshid Shirani, MD

Most published reports of coronary arterial anomalies concern a single patient or only a small group of patients. Although much good and useful information, of course, can be derived from the study of a single patient, multiple cases of a major coronary anomaly are required to observe the various subgroups of a single major anomaly. We have studied at necropsy 17 patients in whom the left main coronary artery (LMCA) arose from either the right aortic sinus or the most proximal portion of the right coronary artery.[1-5] After its origin, the LMCA coursed to the left side of the heart by 1 of 4 routes, and the clinical consequences of such courses are described in this report.

Pertinent clinical and necropsy findings in the 17 patients are summarized in Table I, and the 4 subtypes are illustrated in Figure 1. In 2 patients (12%) (cases 1 and 2 [Table I]), the anomalously arising LMCA coursed anterior (group A) to the right ventricular outflow tract to reach the anterior sulcus (the anterior portion of the heart immediately anterior to the ventricular septum), where it then divided into the left anterior de-

From the Pathology Branch, National Heart, Lung, and Blood Institute, National Institutes of Health, Bethesda, Maryland 20892. Manuscript received February 21, 1992; revised manuscript received March 10, 1992, and accepted March 11.

scending and left circumflex coronary arteries.[5] In neither patient did the coronary anomaly appear to have caused cardiac dysfunction or myocardial ischemia.

In 9 patients (53%) (cases 3 to 11), the anomalously arising LMCA coursed in between (group B) the ascending aorta and pulmonary trunk before reaching the anterior sulcus.[2-4] The ostium of the LMCA was slit-like in 8 patients. In 7 of the 9 patients death was attributed to the coronary anomaly: sudden outside the hospital in 6, and secondary to severe intractable congestive heart failure (the result of a previous large acute myocardial infarct that had healed) in 1 (case 9).

In 2 patients (12%) (cases 12 and 13), the anomalous LMCA coursed within the crista supraventricularis muscle (group C) behind the right ventricular outflow cavity before reaching the anterior sulcus, and then dividing into the left anterior descending and left circumflex coronary arteries.[1] Neither patient ever had evidence of myocardial ischemia or cardiac dysfunction.

In 4 patients (23%) (cases 14 to 17), the anomalous LMCA coursed dorsal (group D) to the ascending aorta before reaching the usual area of bifurcation into the left anterior descending and left circumflex coronary arteries.[5,6] Although 2 of the 4 patients died from cardiovas-

TABLE I Clinical and Morphologic Findings in 17 Patients with Anomalous Origin of the Left Main Coronary Artery from the Right Coronary Artery or the Right Aortic Sinus

Case	Age (yr) & Sex	Origin of LMCA	Anomaly Group*	Length of LMCA (cm)	AP	SD	Death Outside Hospital	Cause of Death	Length of RCA > LCCA	Slit-Like Ostium	No. of Major CAs > 75% ↓ in CSA by Plaque	LV Scar (1 to 3+)	HW (g)
1	22 M	RAS	A	4.5	0	+	+	HC	+	0	0	0	870
2	44 F	RAS†	A	3.0	+	+	+	Trauma	+	0	0	0	255
3	13 F	RAS	B	1.1	0	+	+	Coronary anomaly	+	+	0	0	210
4	14 M	RAS	B	1.2	0	+	+	Coronary anomaly	+	+	0	0	370
5	14 M	RAS	B	—	0	+	+	Coronary anomaly	—	+	0	0	380
6	19 M	RAS	B	1.1	0	+	+	Coronary anomaly	+	+	0	0	325
7	29 M	RAS	B	—	+	+	+	Coronary anomaly	0	+	0	+	350
8	39 F	RAS	B	—	0	+	+	Coronary anomaly	0	+	0	0	220
9	64 F	RAS	B	2.4	+	0	0	Coronary anomaly	+	+	0	+++	510
10	81 M	RAS	B	2.0	0	+	+	Trauma	+	0	0	0	420
11	50 F	RAS†	B	—	0	+	+	Atherosclerotic CAD	+	0	3	+++	650
12	34 M	RAS	C	4.7	0	0	+	Trauma	+	0	0	0	330
13	48 M	RAS	C	4.5	0	+	+	Trauma	+	0	0	0	550
14	32 M	RAS	D	3.3	0	+	+	Trauma	0	0	0	0	325
15	45 M	RAS	D	4.5	+	+	+	Atherosclerotic CAD	+	0	1	+++	580
16	57 F	RAS	D	3.6	0	0	+	Opiate addiction‡	+	0	0	0	300
17	69 M	RCA	D	3.0	0	0	0	Forme fruste Marfan	+	0	0	0	685

*See Figure 1 for description.
†Common ostium of both RCA and LMCA.
‡Complications arising from the addiction.
AP = angina pectoris; CA = coronary artery; CAD = coronary artery disease; CSA = cross-sectional area; HC = hypertrophic cardiomyopathy; HW = heart weight; LCCA = left circumflex coronary artery; LMCA = left main coronary artery; LV = left ventricular; RAS = right aortic sinus; RCA = right coronary artery; SD = sudden death; + = present or positive; 0 = absent or negative; — = no information available.

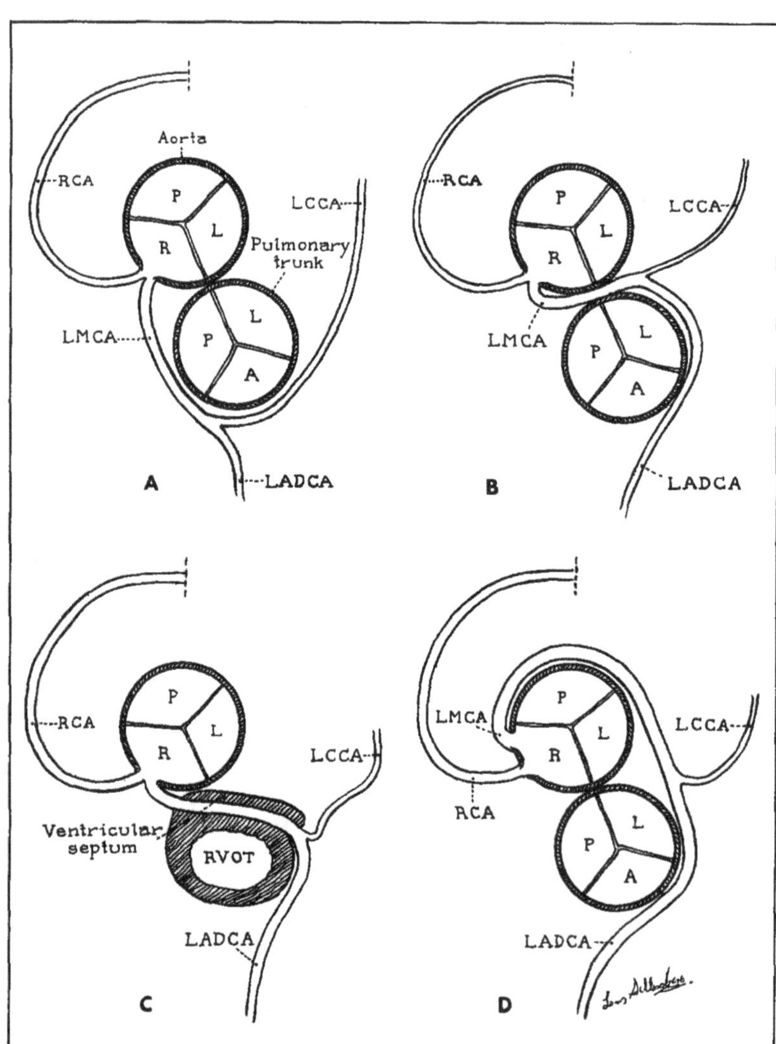

FIGURE 1. Diagram showing the 4 subtypes of anomalous origin of the left main coronary artery (LMCA) from the right aortic sinus. A = anterior; L = left; LADCA = left anterior descending coronary artery; LCCA = left circumflex coronary artery; P = posterior; R = right; RCA = right coronary artery; RVOT = right ventricular outflow tract.

cular disease (atherosclerosis in 1, and Marfan-type aortic disease in the other), in none could the cardiac problems be attributed to the coronary anomaly.

This brief report indicates that if an anomalously arising LMCA courses anterior (group A) to the right ventricular outflow tract, behind the right ventricular outflow tract (infracristal) (group C) or dorsal (group D) to the ascending aorta, symptoms of cardiac dysfunction or myocardial ischemia do not result. In contrast, if the anomalously arising LMCA courses between (group B) the pulmonary trunk and ascending aorta, symptoms of myocardial ischemia usually occur, and death is a frequent consequence.

1. Roberts WC, Dicicco BS, Waller BF, Kishel JC, McManus BM, Dawson SL, Hunsaker JC III, Luke JL. Origin of the left main from the right coronary or from the right aortic sinus with intramyocardial tunneling to the left side of the heart via the ventricular septum: the case against clinical significance of myocardial bridge or coronary tunnel. *Am Heart J* 1982;104:306–308.
2. Barth WC III, Roberts WC. Left main coronary artery originating from the right sinus of Valsalva and coursing between the aorta and pulmonary trunk. *J Am Coll Cardiol* 1986;7:366–373.
3. Roberts WC. Major anomalies of coronary arterial origin seen in adulthood. *Am Heart J* 1986;111:941–963.
4. Kragel AH, Roberts WC. Anomalous origin of either the right or left main coronary artery from the aorta with subsequent coursing between aorta and pulmonary trunk: analysis of 32 necropsy cases. *Am J Cardiol* 1988;62:771–777.
5. Roberts WC, Kragel AH. Anomalous origin of either the right or left main coronary artery from the aorta without coursing of the anomalistically arising artery between aorta and pulmonary trunk. *Am J Cardiol* 1988;62:1263–1267.
6. Waller BF, Reis RL, McIntosh CL, Epstein SE, Roberts WC. The Marfan cardiovascular disease without the Marfan syndrome. *Chest* 1980;77:533–540.

Congenital Hypoplasia of Both Right and Left Circumflex Coronary Arteries

William C. Roberts, MD, and Brian N. Glick, MD*

When the right coronary artery is dominant, i.e., it courses to the crux of the heart, the left circumflex coronary artery is usually quite small and therefore may

From the Pathology Branch, National Heart, Lung, and Blood Institute, National Institutes of Health, Bethesda, Maryland. Manuscript accepted March 1, 1992.

*Cardiology Fellow, Georgetown University Medical Center, Washington, D.C.

be considered hypoplastic (Figure 1). Conversely, when the left circumflex is the dominant coronary artery, i.e., it courses to the crux of the heart, the right coronary artery is usually small and therefore may be considered hypoplastic (Figure 1). Hypoplasia of both right and left circumflex coronary arteries in the same heart, however, is a rare occurrence (Figure 1). Examination of 3,400 hearts during the last 8 years disclosed at least 8 to have hypo-

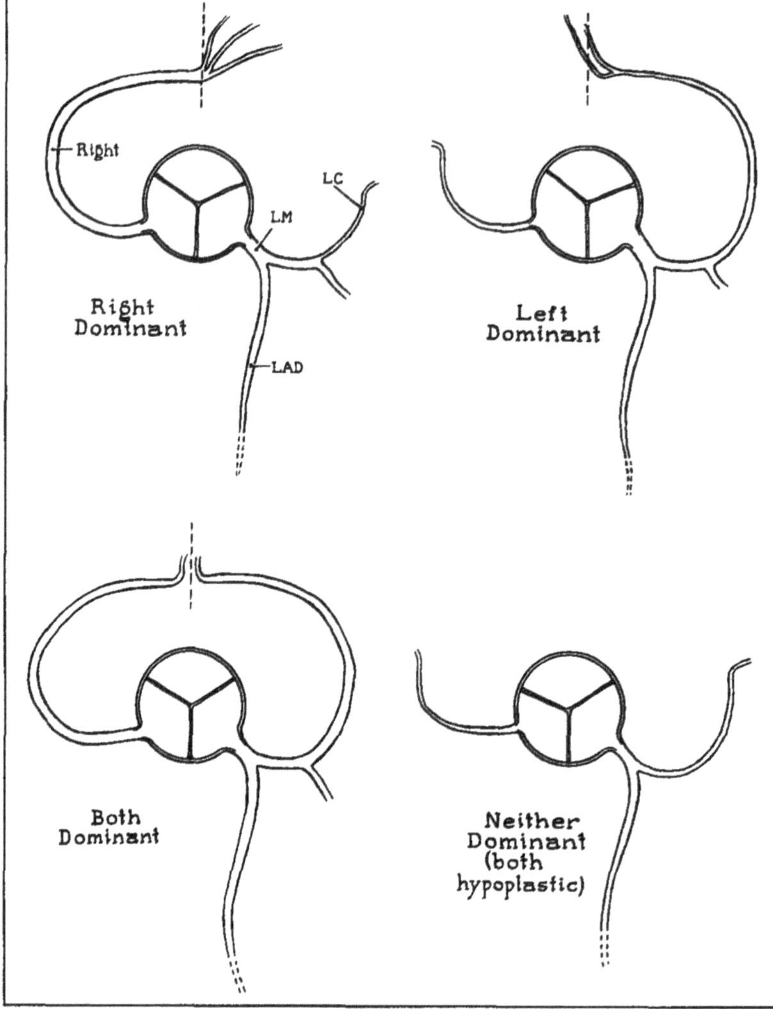

FIGURE 1. Diagram showing graphic definitions of *dominance* and *hypoplasia*. The 8 patients described had right and left circumflex (LC) coronary arteries similar to those depicted in the *bottom right diagram*. LAD = left anterior descending; LM = left main coronary artery.

BRIEF REPORTS **121**

TABLE I Clinical and Necropsy Findings in Eight Patients with Hypoplastic Right and Left Circumflex Coronary Arteries

Pt.	Necropsy Number	Age (yr)	Race	Sex	SD	SH	A	Associated Disorders	HW (g)	Number of CAs >75% ↓ in CSA	LV N	LV F	LADCA Past Apex (cm)	Actual Length/ Potential Length (cm) RCA	Actual Length/ Potential Length (cm) LCCA
1	DCMEO# 87-05-400	26	B	M	+	0	+	Stenotic unicuspid aortic valve	760	0	0	0	+(5)	6/12	9/12
2	DCMEO# 83-01-004	33	B	M	+	+	+	0	565	0	0	0	+(3)	9/12	7/12
3	DCMEO# 87-06-528	35	B	M	+	0	0	WPW syndrome	420	0	0	0	+(2)	7/11	9/12
4	DCMEO# 87-09-868	35	B	M	+	+	+	Morbid obesity	750	0	0	0	0	11/15	5/13
5	WHC# A91-91	41	B	M	+*	0	+	Atherosclerotic CAD	450	3	0	0	+(5)	11/13	3/11
6	WHC# A89-89	57	B	M	0	+	0	Chronic CHF	590	1	0	+	0	6/9	6/11
7	DCVAH# 87A-54	62	B	M	0	+	+	Chronic renal failure	525	0	0	+	+(3)	7/12	6/11
8	SH# A90-15	79	W	F	0	+	0	Chronic CHF	525	1	0	0	+(3)	8/11	5/10

*Died in cardiac catheterization laboratory shortly after angioplasty.
A = chronic alcoholism; CAD = coronary artery disease; CAs = coronary arteries; CHF = congestive heart failure; CSA = cross-sectional area; F = fibrosis; HW = heart weight; LADCA = left anterior descending coronary artery; LCCA = left circumflex coronary artery; LV = left ventricular; N = necrosis; RCA = right coronary artery; SD = sudden death; SH = systemic hypertension; WPW = Wolff-Parkinson-White.

plasia of both right and left circumflex coronary arteries. Certain findings in these 8 patients will be described here.

Pertinent findings in the 8 patients are summarized in Table I. The patients ranged in age from 26 to 79 years (mean 46). Seven were black men and 1, a white woman. At least 5 by history had had systemic hypertension. One (patient 1, Table I) had a severely stenotic unicuspid aortic valve. Patient 3 had an episode of supraventricular tachycardia 4 months before death, and electrocardiograms, after slowing of the heart rate, were typical of the Wolff-Parkinson-White syndrome. Patient 4 weighed 386 pounds (175 kg). Three patients had narrowing of 1 or more major epicardial coronary arteries >75% in cross-sectional area by atherosclerotic plaque: in patient 5 the right, left anterior descending, and left circumflex coronary arteries were severely narrowed; in patient 6, significant (>75%) luminal narrowing was limited to the distal portion of the left circumflex coronary artery and in patient 8, the left anterior descending was narrowed just over 75% in cross-sectional area by plaque. Two of the 3 patients underwent coronary balloon angioplasty. Grossly visible left ventricular scars were present in 2 patients: in patient 6 the healed myocardial infarct was large, transmural and posterior; in patient 7 the healed infarct was small, nontransmural (mainly subepicardial) and posterior. Thorough examination of the major epicardial coronary arteries in patient 7 disclosed insignificant (<50% cross-sectional area reduction) luminal narrowing. Five of the 8 patients died suddenly: 3 (patients 2, 3 and 4) were found dead at home, and when each was last seen alive they appeared in their usual state of health; 1 (patient 1), who had severe aortic valve stenosis, had fatal cardiac arrest while dancing in a disco; and 1 (patient 5) had fatal cardiac arrest in a cardiac catheterization laboratory shortly following insertion of a stent (after unsuccessful balloon angioplasty) for severe coronary arterial narrowing from atherosclerosis.

At necropsy, the heart weight was increased (>400 g) in all 8 patients (mean 573 g) (Table I). The left anterior descending coronary artery in all 8 patients appeared of a size expected for the weight of the heart. In 6 of the 8 patients the left anterior descending coronary artery coursed past the left ventricular apex to ascend on the posterior surface of the heart for distances ranging from 2 to 5 cm (Table I). The right and left circumflex coronary arteries, of course, were small and neither coursed to the crux posteriorly. The right coronary artery remained in the right atrioventricular sulcus for distances varying from 6 to 11 cm (mean 8) (Table I). These distances, compared with the total potential lengths of the right coronary artery from its ostium in the aorta to the crux posteriorly, indicate that this artery remained in the atrioventricular sulcus for 50 to 85% (mean 68%) of the potential distance within the atrioventricular sulcus from its aortic origin to the crux posteriorly. The left circumflex coronary artery remained in the left atrioventricular sulcus for distances varying from 3 to 9 cm (mean 6) (Table I), numbers indicating that the left circumflex coronary artery was located within the left atrioventricular sulcus for 27 to 75% (mean 54%) of the total potential length of the left atrioventricular sulcus from the origin of the left circumflex from the left main coronary artery to the crux posteriorly.

Hypoplasia of both right and left circumflex coronary arteries, to our knowledge, has never been reported angiographically. It was first reported at necropsy by Maron and associates[1] in a 17-year-old girl who died suddenly just after completing a 3-mile race. The only cardiac abnormality observed at necropsy was bilateral hypoplasia of the 2 major coronary arteries. Menke and colleagues[2] reported a 30-year-old man who died suddenly during a basketball game, and necropsy disclosed hypoplasia of both right and left circumflex coronary arteries. Each of these 2 arteries was described as being "half their normal length." No other potential functionally significant cardiac abnormalities were found at autopsy in the patient reported by Menke et al.

In the 8 patients reported herein only 3 (patients 5, 6 and 8) had had a coronary angiogram during life, and bilateral hypoplasia of the right and left circumflex coronary was not suspected from this study in any of them. Of the 8 necropsy patients, it appears likely that the bilateral coronary hypoplasia was of functional significance in 2 patients (nos. 2 and 7 [Table I]). Although 5 of the 8 patients died suddenly, a cause other than bilateral coronary hypoplasia was present in 4 of them. Patient 2, however, died suddenly and a cardiac condition other than bilateral coronary hypoplasia was absent. Two of the 8 patients had grossly visible left ventricular scars (healed myocardial infarcts): one of them (patient 6), however, had severe coronary atherosclerosis, but the other (patient 7) had no explanation for the left ventricular scar other than bilateral coronary hypoplasia.

Hypoplasia of a major epicardial coronary artery appears, with one exception, to be limited to the right and left circumflex coronary arteries. We have not observed or seen reported hypoplasia of the left anterior descending artery as long as it arose normally from the left main coronary artery, which in turn arose normally from the aorta. If, however, a single coronary artery arises from the aorta and if that single artery begins as a normally originating and coursing right coronary artery that continues past the crux as the left circumflex coronary artery, which when reaching the anterior surface of the heart continues as the left anterior descending coronary artery, the latter artery may become hypoplastic because this artery courses distally and approaches the cardiac apex (Figure 2).[3]

In the present study we defined hypoplasia to include 2 factors: (1) *small sized arteries*, and (2) *shorter courses so that neither reached the crux* (at the midportion of the atrioventricular groove posteriorly). We have observed at necropsy, however, at least 2 other patients with severe hypoplasia of both right and left circumflex coronary arteries, but 1 of the 2 arteries, despite their small sizes, nevertheless reached the cardiac crux. Although it could be argued that these type cases also constitute bilateral coronary hypoplasia, we believe it better to apply our more limited definition to this uncommon occurrence.

In summary, the hearts from 8 patients are described with hypoplasia of both right and left circumflex coronary arteries. It appeared that 2 of the 8 had evidence of myocardial ischemia as a direct consequence of the bilateral hypoplasia.

1. Maron BJ, Roberts WC, McAllister H, Rosing D, Epstein S. Sudden death in young athletes. *Circulation* 1980;62:218–229.
2. Menke DM, Waller BF, Pless JC. Hypoplastic coronary arteries and high take-off position of the right coronary ostium. A fatal combination of congenital coronary artery anomalies in an amateur athlete. *Chest* 1985;88:299–301.
3. Choi JH, Kornblum RN. Pete Maravich's Incredible Heart. *J Forensic Sci* 1990;35:981–986.

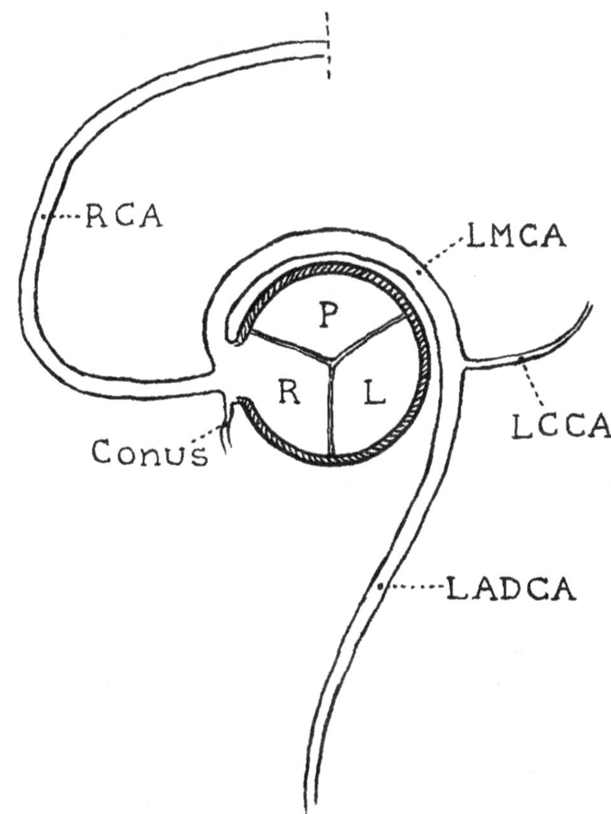

Fig. 1. Diagram showing anomalous origin of left main coronary artery from right aortic sinus with retroaortic coursing of anomalistically arising artery.

Origin of the left main coronary artery from the right aortic sinus with retroaortic course of the anomalistically arising artery

Jamshid Shirani, MD, and William C. Roberts, MD
Bethesda, Md.

Anomalous origin of the left circumflex coronary artery from the right aortic sinus or from the right coronary artery with retroaortic coursing of the anomalistically arising artery is the most common congenital coronary artery anomaly; it occurs in approximately one of every 300 human hearts.[1] In this laboratory we have studied 17 hearts with anomalously arising left circumflex coronary artery with retroaortic coursing. Anomalous origin of the left main coronary artery from the right aortic sinus or from the right coronary artery with retroaortic coursing of the anomalistically arising artery (Fig. 1), in contrast, is less common. In this laboratory we have studied four hearts with this latter anomaly. A description of the clinical and cardiac morphologic findings in these four patients is the purpose of this report.

From the Pathology Branch, National Heart, Lung, and Blood Institute, National Institutes of Health.

Reprint requests: Pathology Branch, NHLBI—Bldg. 10, Room 2N258, Bethesda, MD 20892.

4/4/39803

Certain findings in the four patients (three men and one woman) are summarized in Table I. The patients were 32, 45, 57, and 69 years of age (mean age 51 years) at the time of death. In none of the four patients did the coronary anomaly cause cardiac dysfunction or myocardial ischemia, and in none was it a factor in causing death. Three patients, one of whom has been reported previously,[2] died of noncardiac causes; the fourth died suddenly of consequences of atherosclerotic coronary artery disease. The left main and right coronary arteries each arose from a separate ostium, which was located in the right sinus of Valsalva in three patients; in the fourth patient a single ostium was present in the right aortic sinus, and the left main coronary artery arose as the first branch of the right coronary artery. In all four patients the left main coronary artery coursed posterior to the aorta and then branched at the usual site into the left anterior descending and left circumflex coronary arteries. The length of the left main coronary artery measured from the point of its origin in the right aortic sinus or from the right coronary artery to the site of its bifurcation into the left anterior descending and left circumflex coronary arteries was 3.3 to 4.5 cm (mean 3.6). The right coronary artery coursed to the crux and was much larger and longer than the left circumflex coronary artery

Table I. Clinical and morphologic findings in four patients with origin of the left main coronary artery from the right aortic sinus or right coronary artery with retroaortic course of the anomalistically arising artery

Patient number	Age (yr)	Sex	Mode of death	Heart weight (gm)	Number of ostia in right aortic sinus	Length of left main coronary artery (cm)	RCA > LCCA	No. of major coronary arteries >75% ↓ by plaque	LV scar
1	32	M	Trauma	325	2	3.3	0	0	0
2	45	M	Atherosclerotic CAD	580	2	4.5	+	1*	+
3	57	F	Infection	300	2	3.6	+	0	0
4	69	M	Forme fruste Marfan syndrome	685	1	3.0	+	0	0

CAD, Coronary artery disease; *LCCA*, left circumflex coronary artery; *LV*, left ventricular; *RCA*, right coronary artery.
*Left main coronary artery.

in three patients; in the fourth patient the left circumflex coronary artery coursed to the crux, and it was much larger and longer than the right coronary artery.

Origin of the left main coronary artery from the right aortic sinus or proximal portion of the right coronary artery was observed by Yamanaka and Hobbs[3] in 22 of 126,595 coronary angiograms performed at the Cleveland Clinic from 1960 to 1988. The course of the anomalistically arising coronary artery in these 22 patients, however, was not described.

Although none of our four patients had evidence of myocardial ischemia as a result of the coronary anomaly, Murphy et al.[4] reported a 12-year-old girl with a similar coronary anomaly who had acute dyspnea, central chest discomfort, and loss of consciousness on two occasions 7 months apart. The first episode occurred during a school soccer game and the second while she was competing in a one-mile race. During hospitalization after the second episode, she had evidence of an anterior wall acute myocardial infarction as determined by electrocardiogram and cardiac enzyme levels. A saphenous vein conduit was placed between the aorta and left anterior descending coronary artery.

REFERENCES

1. White NK, Edwards JE. Anomalies of the coronary arteries. Report of four cases. Arch Pathol 1984;45:766-71.
2. Waller BF, Reis RL, McIntosh CL, Epstein SE, Roberts WC. The Marfan cardiovascular disease without the Marfan syndrome. Chest 1980;77:533-40.
3. Yamanaka O, Hobbs RE. Coronary artery anomalies in 126,595 patients undergoing coronary arteriography. Cathet Cardiovasc Diagn 1990;21:28-40.
4. Murphy DA, Roy DL, Sohal M, Chandler BM. Anomalous origin of left main coronary artery from anterior sinus of valsalva with myocardial infarction. J Thorac Cardiovasc Surg 1978;75:282-5.

Solitary Coronary Ostium in the Aorta in the Absence of Other Major Congenital Cardiovascular Anomalies

JAMSHID SHIRANI, MD, WILLIAM C. ROBERTS, MD, FACC

Bethesda, Maryland

Objectives. This study examines the distribution patterns and the clinical significance of the "solitary coronary ostium" in the aorta in the absence of other major congenital cardiovascular anomalies.

Background. Ogden in 1970 classified "single coronary artery" into 14 basic distribution patterns. Since then, other patterns of distribution of single coronary artery have been recognized. Distinction has also been made between the cases with and without other major congenital cardiovascular anomalies or coronary artery atresia and those without these additional abnormalities. Single coronary artery has been generally considered to be a benign clinical entity.

Methods. This study describes 10 cases of single coronary artery at necropsy and reviews 87 previously reported cases, 35 diagnosed at necropsy and 52 by coronary angiography.

Results. We classified single coronary artery into 20 categories on the basis of the location of the solitary coronary ostium, the presence or absence of an aberrant-coursing coronary artery and the course taken by the aberrant-coursing coronary artery. When atherosclerotic coronary artery disease was absent, 15% (8 of 53) of the patients reviewed with single coronary artery had myocardial ischemia as a direct consequence of the coronary anomaly.

Conclusions. The anatomic classification presented is useful from both clinical and surgical viewpoints. This comprehensive classification of this rare anomaly facilitates description of the various distribution patterns of single coronary artery and their clinical significance.

(*J Am Coll Cardiol 1993;21:137–43*)

Solitary coronary ostium in the aorta, in the absence of other major congenital cardiovascular anomalies, is rare. We found reports of only 35 patients with this cardiac anomaly at necropsy (Table 1) (1–28), and of only 52 with this anomaly at coronary angiography (Table 2) (21,29–62). The largest necropsy study of this anomaly (10) included only 10 cases; in 5 of these the patients had other major congenital cardiovascular anomalies, in 1 the patient had a solitary coronary ostium in the pulmonary trunk and in 1 the patient had atresia rather than absence of the right coronary artery. We have examined at necropsy, 10 patients with solitary coronary ostium in the aorta unassociated with origin of coronary artery from the pulmonary trunk and in the absence of other major congenital cardiovascular anomalies (Table 3). Using clinical and morphologic data from these 10 patients and from previously published reports (1–62), we developed a classification for single coronary ostium in the aorta unassociated with other major congenital cardiovascular anomalies (Table 4). This report presents the classification and summarizes findings in our own 10 patients and in the patients previously reported on by others.

From the Pathology Branch, National Heart, Lung, and Blood Institute, National Institutes of Health, Bethesda, Maryland.

Manuscript received May 15, 1992, accepted June 15, 1992.

Address for correspondence: Pathology Branch, National Heart, Lung, and Blood Institute, National Institutes of Health, Building 10, Room 2N258, Bethesda, Maryland 20892.

Methods

The records of the Pathology Branch, National Heart, Lung, and Blood Institute, National Institutes of Health were searched for all cases of "single coronary artery." Cases associated with other major congenital anomalies of the heart or great vessels including origin of the coronary arteries from pulmonary trunk were excluded. In addition, cases in which single coronary artery was associated with atresia of a coronary artery were excluded.

The clinical summaries, general autopsy findings, photographs, diagrams and hearts were reviewed in each case. All material had been examined initially by one of us (W.C.R.) and then reviewed by both of us. In each case the position of the single coronary ostium, the course and distribution of the coronary arteries and the presence of aberrant coursing branches were recorded. Whether the lumens of the major epicardial coronary arteries were narrowed by atherosclerotic plaque was noted as were the heart weight and the presence or absence of left ventricular necrosis or fibrosis.

Results

Certain clinical and necropsy findings in the 10 patients are summarized in Table 3. The patients were 5 to 78 years old; 7 were male and 3 were female. In none of the 10 patients did the coronary anomaly cause any symptoms or signs of myocardial ischemia. The types of coronary anom-

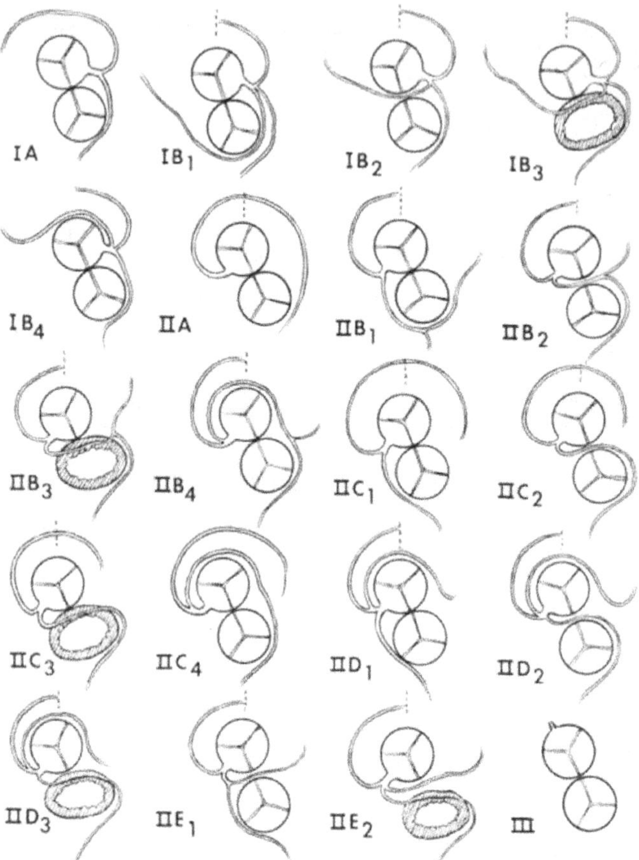

Figure 1. Diagram showing the origin and pattern of distribution of various types of solitary coronary ostium in the aorta.

aly observed in the 10 patients are delineated in Table 3. The solitary coronary ostium was located in the left aortic sinus in four patients (Patients 1 to 4) and in the right aortic sinus in six patients. When the solitary coronary ostium was located in the left aortic sinus, three of four patients had an "anatomic single coronary artery" in which the left main coronary artery divided normally into left anterior descending coronary artery and left circumflex coronary artery. The left circumflex coronary artery then coursed in the left atrioventricular (AV) groove to reach the crux and continued past this point in the AV groove to occupy the anatomic position normally occupied by the right coronary artery. In the remaining patient (Patient 4), the left main coronary artery trifurcated into the left anterior descending coronary artery, left circumflex coronary artery and an aberrant-coursing artery that coursed anterior to the right ventricle to reach the right AV groove and from there on continued as an otherwise normal right coronary artery.

An aberrant-coursing artery was present in all six patients whose solitary coronary ostium was located in the right aortic sinus. Of these aberrant coursing arteries, four were the left main and two were the left anterior descending coronary artery. The aberrant-coursing left main coronary artery reached the left side of the heart (to divide into the left anterior descending coronary artery and the left circumflex coronary artery) by coursing anterior to the right ventricle (Patient 5), in between the pulmonary trunk and the ascending aorta (Patient 6) or dorsal to the ascending aorta (Patients 7 and 8). In Patients 9 and 10, the aberrant-coursing coronary artery was the left anterior descending coronary artery, which reached the anterior ventricular groove by coursing beneath the right ventricular outflow tract within the superior portion of the ventricular septum.

A total of 87 patients with solitary coronary ostium in the aorta have been previously described by others. Certain clinical, morphologic or coronary angiographic findings in these patients are listed in Tables 1 and 2. The diagnosis was made at necropsy in 35 of these patients and by angiography in 52.

On the basis of morphologic and angiographic findings in

Table 1. Solitary Coronary Ostium in the Aorta: Clinical and Morphologic Findings in 35 Cases Diagnosed at Necropsy

Case No.	Anomaly Type*	Ref. No.	Age (yr)/ Gender	AP	AMI	SD	CAD	Cause of Death	HW (g)	Ostial Dimple	LV Scar
1	IA	1	37/M	–	–	–	–	Infective endocarditis	–	RAS	–
2	IA	2	33/M	–	–	–	–	Stroke	520	0	–
3	IA	3	39/F	–	–	–	–	Pneumonia	–	0	–
4	IA	4	63/M	–	–	–	–	Cancer	150	0	0
5	IA	5	44/F	0	0	+	0	Pulmonary embolism	400	0	0
6	IA	6	80/F	0	0	0	+	Cancer	340	RAS	0
7	IA	7	77/M	0	+	0	+	Cancer	325	0	+
8	IA	8	27/F	0	0	0	0	Dilated cardiomyopathy	350	0	0
9	IA	9	83/F	0	0	+	+	Ruptured CA aneurysm	320	PAS	0
10	IA	10	68/M	–	–	–	–	–	–	RAS	–
11	IA	10	70/F	–	–	–	–	–	–	0	–
12	IA	11	50/F	0	0	0	0	Mitral stenosis	–	0	0
13	IB_1	6	66/F	0	0	0	0	Infection	250	0	0
14	IB_2	12	–	–	–	–	–	–	–	0	–
15	IB_3	13	65/M	0	0	0	0	Cancer	380	0	0
16	IIA	14	46/M	+	+	0	–	Myocardial infarct	–	–	–
17	IIA	15	70/M	–	–	0	–	Cancer	–	–	–
18	IIA	16	40/M	0	+	+	0	Coronary anomaly	560	0	+
19	IIB_1	17	82/F	0	0	0	0	Pulmonary embolism	320	0	+
20	IIB_2	18	45/F	0	0	0	0	Infective endocarditis	–	0	0
21	IIB_2	15	13/M	+	+	0	0	Myocardial infarct	–	–	+
22	IIB_3	19	54/M	0	+	0	+	Pneumonia	750	0	+
23	IIB_3	15	36/M	0	0	+	0	Ventricular arrhythmia	–	–	–
24	IIB_3	15	28/M	0	0	+	0	Pulmonary embolism	–	–	–
25	IIB_3	15	54/F	0	0	0	0	Gastrointestinal bleeding	–	–	–
26	IIB_3	20	48/M	0	0	+	0	Trauma	550	0	0
27	IIB_4	21	84/F	+	+	+	+	Myocardial infarct	530	LAS	+
28	IIB_4	11	51/F	0	0	0	0	Aortic valve disease	–	0	0
29	IIC_2	22	65/M	0	0	0	0	Pneumonia	–	0	0
30	IIC_2	23	76/F	0	0	0	0	Cancer	370	LAS	0
31	IIC_3	24	54/M	+	+	0	+	Myocardial infarct	520	0	+
32	IIC_3	25	73/M	0	0	0	0	Cancer	–	0	0
33	IID_2	26	60/F	–	–	–	–	Infective endocarditis	–	0	–
34	IID_3	27	4/M	0	0	0	0	Renal failure	60	0	–
35	IID_3	28	39/M	0	0	0	0	Cerebral glioma	–	0	0

*See Table 4 for description of the anomaly type. AMI = acute myocardial infarct; AP = angina pectoris; CA = coronary artery; CAD = atherosclerotic coronary artery disease; F = female; HW = heart weight; LAS = left aortic sinus; LV = left ventricular; M = male; PAS = posterior aortic sinus; RAS = right aortic sinus; Ref. = reference; SD = sudden death; – = information not available; + = present; 0 = absent.

the 87 reported patients and in our own 10 patients, a simple, practical classification (Table 4) was made. The location of the solitary coronary ostium in relation to aortic sinuses, the presence or absence of an aberrant-coursing coronary artery and the course taken by the aberrant coursing coronary artery, when present, form the basis of the classification. The most frequently seen anomaly type is type IA (anatomic single coronary artery), of which 28 cases have been reported (including our 3). The other anomaly types have each been reported in ≤10 patients. We have not seen or found any reported examples of types IIC_4, IID_1, IIE_1, IIE_2, or III.

Information regarding the presence or absence of significant lumen narrowing in the major epicardial coronary arteries by atherosclerotic plaque is available in 85 of the 97 cases reviewed here. Of the 85 patients, 32 (38%) had atherosclerotic coronary artery disease (9 at necropsy and 23 by angiography). Eight (15%) of the 85 patients had clinical evidence of myocardial ischemia attributable to the coronary anomaly (Table 5); these patients were 13 to 65 years old at death (Patients 1 and 2) or coronary angiography (Patients 3 to 8). Four of the eight had angina pectoris, 5 had acute myocardial infarction and 3 had a positive exercise stress test. Two patients (Patients 1 and 2) died as a direct result of the coronary anomaly. Patient 1, a 13-year old boy, had a solitary ostium in the right aortic sinus and an aberrant-coursing left main coronary artery that originated from the right coronary artery and crossed to the opposite side of the heart between the ascending aorta and the pulmonary artery. He died 4 months after a massive myocardial infarction. Patient 2 had an anatomic single right coronary artery. As a professional basketball player he had participated in competitive athletic activity for many years without symptoms of myocardial ischemia. He died suddenly on the basketball court at age 40 years. At necropsy, his heart weighed 560 g.

Table 2. Solitary Coronary Ostium in the Aorta: Clinical and Angiographic Findings in 52 Patients Diagnosed by Coronary Angiography

Case No.	Anomaly Type*	Ref. No.	Age (yr)/Gender	Presenting Symptoms	AP	AMI		Nonfatal Cardiac Arrest	ECG	Ischemia		CA >90% ↓ Diameter by Plaque				Left Ventricular Wall Motion Abnormality			CA Surgery	
						Symptomatic	Silent			By EST	On Thallium Scan	LM	LADCA	LCCA	R	Ant	Post	Septum	IMA	SVG
1	IA	21	35/M	RBBB	0	0	0	0	RBBB	0	−	0	0	0	−	0	0	0	0	0
2	IA	21	38/M	Chest pain	+	0	+	0	MI	0	−	0	+	0	−	0	0	0	0	0
3	IA	21	46/F	Dyspnea	0	0	0	0	−	0	−	0	0	0	−	0	0	0	0	0
4	IA	29	21/M	Dizziness	0	0	+	0	PRWP	0	−	0	0	0	−	+	0	0	0	0
5	IA	30	39/M	Chest pain	0	0	0	0	Normal	0	−	0	0	0	−	0	0	0	0	0
6	IA	31	42/M	Chest pain	+	0	0	+	ST↓, V_1-V_4	0	+	0	+	0	−	0	0	0	0	0
7	IA	32	40/M	Chest pain	0	0	0	0	RBBB, VPC	0	−	0	0	0	−	0	0	0	0	0
8	IA	33	57/M	Chest pain	+	0	0	0	RBBB	+	−	0	+	0	−	0	0	0	0	0
9	IA	34	60/M	Chest pain	0	0	0	0	Normal	0	0	0	0	0	−	0	0	0	0	0
10	IA	35	63/M	Chest pain	+	0	+	0	PRWP	+	−	0	+	+	−	0	+	0	0	+
11	IA	36	44/M	Chest pain	0	0	0	0	ST-TΔ	0	−	0	0	0	−	0	0	0	0	0
12	IA	37	55/M	Fatigue	0	0	0	0	ST-TΔ	+	−	0	0	0	−	0	0	0	0	0
13	IA	38	51/M	Chest pain	+	+	0	0	ST-TΔ	0	−	0	0	+	−	0	0	0	+	0
14	IB$_1$	39	46/F	Chest pain	+	0	0	0	−	−	+	0	+	+	+	0	0	0	−	−
15	IB$_1$	40	65/F	Chest pain	+	0	0	0	LBBB	−	−	0	+	0	0	+	+	+	+	0
16	IB$_1$	41	65/M	Chest pain	0	0	0	0	LAFB	−	−	0	0	0	0	0	0	0	0	0
17	IB$_1$	41	54/M	Jaw pain	+	0	0	0	ST↓, V_3-V_6	−	−	0	+	+	+	0	0	0	0	0
18	IB$_1$	42	33/M	Chest pain	+	−	0	0	Normal	0	+	0	+	0	0	+	0	0	+	0
19	IB$_2$	43	24/F	Chest pain	+	−	0	0	RBBB, AMI	−	−	0	0	0	0	−	−	−	−	−
20	IB$_2$	30	46/M	Chest pain	+	0	+	0	MI	−	−	0	0	+	0	0	+	0	−	0
21	IB$_2$	30	48/F	Chest pain	0	0	0	0	QT↑	0	−	0	0	0	0	0	0	0	0	0
22	IB$_2$	30	54/M	Chest pain	+	0	0	0	LVH	0	−	0	0	0	0	0	0	0	0	0
23	IB$_2$	44	52/M	Chest pain	0	0	0	0	PRWP	0	−	0	0	0	0	0	0	0	0	+
24	IB$_2$	45	65/M	Chest pain	+	0	0	0	Normal	+	+	0	0	0	0	0	0	0	0	+
25	IB$_2$	46	50/F	Chest pain	−	0	0	0	−	0	−	0	0	0	0	0	0	0	0	0
26	IB$_4$	30	47/M	Chest pain	0	0	0	0	PRWP	0	−	0	0	+	0	+	+	+	0	0
27	IB$_4$	47	60/M	Dyspnea	0	0	0	0	LVH	−	−	0	0	0	0	0	0	0	0	0
28	II$_a$	48	−	−	0	0	−	−	−	−	−	−	−	−	−	−	−	−	−	−
29	IIB$_1$	43	65/F	Chest pain	+	0	0	0	LBBB	−	−	0	0	+	0	0	+	0	−	0
30	IIB$_1$	49	54/M	Chest pain	+	0	0	0	LVH	−	−	0	0	0	0	0	0	0	0	0
31	IIB$_1$	30	48/F	Chest pain	+	0	0	0	Normal	+	−	0	0	0	+	0	0	0	0	0
32	IIB$_1$	50	58/M	Chest pain	+	0	0	0	Normal	+	+	0	+	+	+	0	0	0	+	+
33	IIB$_1$	51	46/F	Chest pain	+	0	0	0	Normal	+	+	0	0	0	0	0	0	0	0	+
34	IIB$_1$	52	63/F	Chest pain	+	0	0	0	ST↑	−	−	0	+	+	+	0	0	0	0	0
35	IIB$_2$	53	46/F	Dyspnea	0	0	0	0	−	0	−	0	0	+	+	0	+	0	0	0
36	IIB$_2$	54	49/F	Chest pain	0	0	0	0	−	−	−	0	0	0	0	0	0	0	0	0
37	IIB$_2$	54	39/M	Chest pain	+	−	0	0	−	−	−	0	+	+	+	+	0	−	−	−
38	IIB$_2$	54	70/F	Chest pain	+	0	0	0	LVH, ST-TΔ	+	−	0	+	+	+	+	0	0	+	−
39	IIB$_2$	30	64/M	Chest pain	+	0	+	0	ST-TΔ	−	−	0	+	+	+	0	0	0	0	0
40	IIB$_2$	30	49/M	Chest pain	+	0	0	0	−	+	−	0	0	+	+	0	0	0	0	0
41	IIB$_2$	55	47/M	Chest pain	+	0	0	0	−	−	−	+	+	0	+	0	0	0	0	+
42	IIB$_2$	56	58/M	Chest pain	+	0	0	0	−	−	−	−	0	0	−	0	0	0	−	−
43	IIB$_4$	54	43/M	Chest pain	0	0	0	0	−	−	0	0	0	0	0	0	0	0	0	0
44	IIB$_4$	54	43/F	−	0	0	0	0	−	−	0	0	0	0	0	0	0	0	0	0
45	IIB$_4$	57	−	−	−	−	−	−	−	−	−	−	−	−	−	−	−	−	−	−
46	IIB$_4$	30	61/M	Chest pain	+	0	0	0	LVH, ST-TΔ	−	−	0	+	0	+	+	+	+	+	−
47	IIB$_4$	58	65/M	Fatigue	0	0	0	0	Normal	+	+	0	0	+	+	0	0	0	0	0
48	IIB$_4$	59	67/M	Chest pain	+	0	0	0	−	−	−	+	+	0	0	0	0	0	0	+
49	IIB$_4$	60	66/F	−	0	0	+	0	−	−	−	0	0	0	+	0	0	0	0	+
50	IIC$_1$	61	47/M	Chest pain	+	−	0	0	ST↑	−	0	−	0	0	0	0	0	+	0	+
51	IID$_2$	54	25/F	Chest pain	+	−	0	0	RBBB	0	−	−	0	0	0	+	0	0	0	0
52	IID$_3$	62	71/F	Chest pain	+	+	0	0	AMI	−	−	−	+	+	+	0	+	0	0	+

*See Table 4 for description of the anomaly type. AMI = acute myocardial infarct; Ant = anterior; AP = angina pectoris; CA = coronary artery; ECG = electrocardiogram; EST = exercise stress test; F = female; IMA = internal mammary artery; LADCA = left anterior descending coronary artery; LAFB = left anterior fascicular block; LBBB = left bundle branch block; LCCA = left circumflex coronary artery; LM = left main; LVH = left ventricular hypertrophy; M = Male; MI = myocardial infarct; Post = posterior; PRWP = poor R-wave progression; QT↑ = QT interval increase; R = right; RBBB = right bundle branch block; ST↓ = ST segment depression; ST↑ = ST segment elevation; ST-TΔ = ST-T wave changes; SVG = saphenous vein graft; VPC = ventricular premature complex. − = information not available; + = present; 0 = absent.

Table 3. Clinical and Morphologic Findings in 10 Patients With Solitary Coronary Ostium in the Aorta (present series)

Case No.	Anomaly Group*	Age (yr)/ Gender	AP	SD	Cause of Death	Death Outside Hospital	Length of RCA>LCCA	≥1 Major CA >75% ↓ in CSA by Plaque	LV Scar (1–3+)	HW (g)
1	IA	5/M	0	0	Airway obstruction	0	0	0	0	280
2	IA	39/M	0	+	Trauma	+	0	0	0	440
3	IA	73/M	0	0	Pneumonia	0	0	0	0	370
4	IB$_2$	65/M	0	0	Cancer	0	0	0	0	380
5	IIB$_1$	44/F	0	+	Trauma	+	+	0	+	560
6	IIB$_2$	50/F	0	+	CAD	+	+	+	+++	650
7	IIB$_4$	45/M	+	+	CAD	+	+	+	+++	580
8	IIB$_4$	69/M	0	0	Forme fruste Marfan	0	+	0	0	685
9	IIC$_3$	57/M	0	+	CAD	+	+	+	+	705
10	IIC$_3$	78/F	0	0	Pneumonia	0	+	0	0	545

*See Table 4 for description. AP = angina pectoris; CA = coronary artery; CAD = atherosclerotic coronary artery disease; CSA = cross-sectional area; F = female; HW = heart weight; LCCA = left circumflex coronary artery; LV = left ventricular; M = male; RCA = right coronary artery; SD = sudden death.

All cardiac chambers were dilated. The myocardium of the anterior left ventricular wall was extensively scarred. The left anterior descending coronary artery in this patient orig-

Table 4. Solitary Coronary Ostium in the Aorta

I. Solitary ostium in (or immediately cephalad to) the *left* aortic sinus
  A. Unassociated with an aberrant-coursing coronary artery (anatomic single coronary artery) (1–11,21,29–38)
  B. Associated with an aberrant-coursing right coronary artery (RCA); RCA arising from the left main coronary artery (LMCA) or from the left anterior descending coronary artery (LADCA) and coursing to the right atrioventricular sulcus:
    1. *anterior* to the right ventricle (type *a*) (6,39–42)
    2. *between* the pulmonary trunk and the ascending aorta (type *b*) (12,30,43–45)
    3. in the *crista* supraventricularis (type *c*) (13,46)
    4. *dorsal* to the ascending aorta (type *d*) (30)
II. Solitary ostium in (or immediately cephalad to) the *right* aortic sinus
  A. Unassociated with an aberrant-coursing coronary artery (anatomic single coronary artery) (14–16,48)
  B. Associated with an aberrant-coursing LMCA. LMCA arising from the RCA and coursing to the left side (to divide into the LADCA and the left circumflex coronary artery [LCCA]):
    1. *anterior* to the right ventricle (type *a*) (17,30,43,49–52)
    2. *between* the pulmonary trunk and the ascending aorta (type *b*) (15,18,30,53–55)
    3. in the *crista* supraventricularis (type *c*) (15,19,20,56)
    4. *dorsal* to the ascending aorta (type *d*) (11,21,30,54,57–60)
  C. Associated with an aberrant-coursing LADCA. RCA courses in the atrioventricular groove, past the crux, to form the LCCA. LADCA arises from the RCA and courses to the left side:
    1. *anterior* to the right ventricle (type *a*) (61)
    2. *between* the pulmonary trunk and the ascending aorta (type *b*) (23)
    3. in the *crista* supraventricularis (type *c*) (24,25)
    4. *dorsal* to the ascending aorta (type *d*)*
  D. Associated with aberrant coursing of both the LADCA and the LCCA. LCCA arising from the RCA and coursing to the left side dorsal to ascending aorta. LADCA arising from the RCA and coursing to the left side:
    1. *anterior* to the right ventricle (type *a*)*
    2. *between* the pulmonary trunk and ascending aorta (type *b*) (54,62)
    3. in the *crista* supraventricularis (type *c*) (26–28)
  E. Associated with aberrant coursing of both the LADCA and LCCA. LCCA arising from the RCA and coursing to the left side between the pulmonary trunk and the ascending aorta. LADCA arising from the RCA and coursing to the left side:
    1. *anterior* to right ventricle (type *a*)*
    2. in the *crista* supraventricular (type *c*)*
III. Solitary ostium in (or immediately cephalad to) the *posterior* aortic sinus*

*No reported example of this anomaly.

inated from the left circumflex coronary artery and had a very small diameter. Patient 3 had an anatomic single left coronary artery. This 21-year old man took part in vigorous physical exercise during adolescence without having any symptoms of cardiac dysfunction; acute myocardial infarction was diagnosed after an episode of exertional dizziness. In four of the eight patients (Cases 1, 4, 5 and 8) an aberrant-coursing coronary artery originated from the right coronary artery (three patients) or the left main coronary artery (one patient) and crossed to the opposite side between the ascending aorta and the pulmonary trunk. In one of the four (Patient 5), the diameter of the aberrant-coursing artery was narrowed at the site where it passed between the ascending aorta and the pulmonary trunk. This narrowing was believed to represent extrinsic compression of the artery. This 65-year old man had severe exertional angina pectoris and pacing-induced electrocardiographic changes of myocardial ischemia. After a saphenous vein bypass graft was inserted into the left anterior descending coronary artery, the symptoms subsided and no myocardial ischemia could be produced by pacing. In Patient 6, an aberrant-coursing right coronary artery originated from the left anterior descending coronary artery and coursed in the superior portion of the ventricular septum to reach the right side of the heart. Angina pectoris and myocardial ischemia (by thallium-201 myocardial imaging) were present in this 50-year old woman. In Patient 7, the left main coronary artery originated from the right coronary artery and coursed to the left side of the heart anterior to the right ventricular wall. Acute myocardial infarction (anterior left ventricular wall) occurred in this 25-year old woman despite the absence of narrowing in the coronary arteries by angiography.

Discussion

Solitary coronary ostium in the aorta was first reported by Hyrtl (63) in 1841. According to Hyrtl's postulate, a single coronary artery is present when the entire heart is supplied by one of the two coronary arteries (left main or right coronary artery) in the absence of any aberrant coursing

Table 5. Clinically Significant End Points in 8 of 97 Patients With Solitary Coronary Ostium in the Aorta*

Case No.	Ref. No.	Anomaly Type	Age (yr)/ Gender	Clinical End Point Attributable to Coronary Anomaly					
							Myocardial Ischemia		
				AP	AMI	SD	By EST	On Thallium Scan	Death
1	15	IIB$_2$	13/M	−	+	−	−	−	+
2	16	IIA	40/M	−	+	+	−	−	+
3	29	IA	21/M	−	+	0	−	−	0
4	43	IB$_2$	24/F	+	+	0	−	−	0
5	45	IB$_2$	65/M	+	0	0	+	−	0
6	46	IB$_3$	50/F	+	0	0	0	+	0
7	51	IIB$_1$	46/F	+	0	0	+	0	0
8	54	IID$_2$	25/F	0	+	0	0	−	0

*Pacing-induced electrocardiographic changes. Atherosclerotic coronary artery disease was absent in all eight cases. All abbreviations as in Tables 1 and 2.

branches. Three further attempts at classification were made as various types of single coronary artery were recognized (6,10,30). In 1950, Smith (6) recognized three different types of single coronary artery: type I or anatomic single coronary artery; type II, in which an aberrant-coursing coronary artery followed the usual distribution of the "missing" coronary artery after originating from a solitary coronary ostium located in the opposite aortic sinus; and type III, which included atypical cases that could not be classified as type I or II. Recognizing the inadequacy of such broad categories, Ogden and Goodyer (10) in 1970 proposed a more complete classification of single coronary artery. They classified the single coronary artery into 14 basic distribution patterns. Our type C category (aberrant-coursing coronary artery crossing to the other side of the heart in the crista supraventricularis) was not included in their classification. Moreover, patients with associated major anomalies of the heart and great vessels and those with coronary atresia were not separated. In 1979, Lipton and associates (30) described nine angiographic patterns of an isolated single coronary artery. Type C anomalies again were not included. One of the 10 patients reported in our study (Patient 5) was not classifiable by the angiographic patterns described (type IID$_2$ by our classification).

The presence or absence of significant coronary artery narrowing was described in 85 of the 97 cases reviewed. Among the 45 patients studied at necropsy, the presence or absence of significant coronary atherosclerosis was described in 35: 9 (26%) had significant coronary lumen narrowing and 7 of these 9 had associated foci of left ventricular fibrosis or necrosis. Of the 52 patients studied by coronary angiography, the presence or absence of coronary narrowing was described in 50: 23 (46%) had significant narrowing of 1 or more major epicardial coronary arteries and all 23 had angina pectoris or myocardial infarction. Thus, 32 (38%) of 85 patients had significant coronary artery narrowing by presumed atherosclerotic plaque; therefore, the myocardial ischemia, which occurred in 30 (94%), could not be attrib-

uted to the presence of the coronary anomaly. Of the remaining 53 patients who had insignificant or absent coronary artery narrowing, 8 (2 of the 26 necropsy cases and 6 of 27 angiographic cases) (15%) had clinical or morphologic evidence of myocardial ischemia that could be directly attributed to the presence of the coronary anomaly.

References

1. Plaut A. Versorgung des Herzens durch nur eine Kranzarterie. Frankf Z Pathol 1922;27:84–90.
2. Petren T. Ein Fall von Mangel der A. coronaria cordis dextra. Virch Arch 1930;278:158–64.
3. Kockel H. Eigenartige Kranzschlagadermissbildungen. Ziegl Beitr 1934–35;94:220–6.
4. Richter O. Überdas Fehlen einer Kranzarterie. Virch Arch 1937;299:637–42.
5. Krumbhaar EB, Ehrich WE. Varieties of single coronary artery in man, occurring as isolated cardiac anomalies. Am J Med Sci 1938;196:407–13.
6. Smith C. Review of single coronary artery with report of 2 cases. Circulation 1950;1:1168–75.
7. Stapley LA, Edwards JE. Single coronary artery. Arch Pathol 1951;52:470–2.
8. Halperin IC, Penny JL, Kennedy RJ. Single coronary artery: antemortem diagnosis in a patient with congestive heart failure. Am J Cardiol 1967;19:424–7.
9. Causing WC, Shuster M, Pribor HC, Amboy P. Single coronary artery with ruptured coronary artery aneurysm. Arch Pathol 1967;83:419–21.
10. Ogden JA, Goodyer AVN. Pattern of distribution of the single coronary artery. Yale J Biol Med 1970;43:11–21.
11. Vlodaver, Amplatz K, Burchell HB, Edwards JE. Single coronary ostium in the aorta. In: Coronary Heart Disease: Clinical, Angiographic and Pathologic Profiles. New York: Springer-Verlag 1976:189–216.
12. Engleman G. Ein Fall von Mangel einer Coronararterie. Anat Anz 1898;14:348–50.
13. Barbour DJ, Roberts WC. Origin of the right from the left main coronary artery (single coronary ostium in aorta). Am J Cardiol 1985;55:609.
14. Smith FR, Fisher P. Congenital absence of the left coronary artery. Am Surg 1987;53:664–6.
15. Cheitlin MD, DeCastro CM, McAllister HA. Sudden death as a complication of anomalous left coronary origin from the anterior sinus of Valsalva: a not-so-minor congenital anomaly. Circulation 1974;50:780–7.
16. Choi JH, Kornblum RN. Pete Maravich's incredible heart. J Forensic Sci 1990;35:981–6.

17. Ho SY, Adams J, Treasure T, Thiene G. Single coronary artery from the right sinus. Am J Cardiol 1985;55:865–6.

18. Gallavardin L, Ravault P. Anomalie d'origine de la coronaire anterieure. Lyon Med 1920;136:270–2.

19. Born E. Über Missbildungen der Kranzarterien und ihre Beziehungen zu Zirkulationsstörungen und plötzlichem Tod. Virch Arch 1933;290:688–704.

20. Roberts WC, Kragel AH. Anomalous origin of either the right or left main coronary artery from the aorta without coursing of the anomalistically arising artery between aorta and pulmonary trunk. Am J Cardiol 1988;62:1263–7.

21. Sharbaugh AH, White RS. Single coronary artery: analysis of the anatomic variation, clinical importance, and report of five cases. JAMA 1974;230:243–6.

22. Kinter AR. Anomalous origin and course of the left coronary artery. Arch Pathol 1931;12:586–9.

23. Leivo IV, Laurila PK. Atresia of left coronary ostium and left main coronary artery. Arch Pathol Lab Med 1987;111:1173–5.

24. Allen GL, Snider TH. Myocardial infarction with a single coronary artery. Arch Intern Med 1966;117:261–4.

25. Saner HE, Saner BD, Dykoski RK, Edwards JE. Origin of anterior descending coronary artery from right aortic sinus: intramyocardial tunneling to left side of heart. Arch Pathol Lab Med 1984;108:642–3.

26. Pachdalek E. Anomaler Verlauf der Kranzarterien des Herzens. Virch Arch 1867;41:260.

27. Sanes S. Anomalous origin and course of the left coronary artery in a child: so-called congenital absence of the left coronary artery. Am Heart J 1937;14:219–9.

28. White NK, Edwards JE. Anomalies of the coronary arteries: report of four cases. Arch Pathol 1948;45:766–71.

29. Warren SE, Alpert JS, Vieweg WVR, Hagan AD. Normal single coronary artery and myocardial infarction. Chest 1977;72:540–3.

30. Lipton MJ, Barry WH, Obrez I, Silverman JF, Wexler L. Isolated single coronary artery: diagnosis, angiographic classification, and clinical significance. Radiology 1979;130:39–47.

31. Phaneuf DC, Waters DD, Dauwe F, Theroux P, Pelletier G, Mizgala HF. Refractory variant angina controlled with combined drug therapy in a patient with a single coronary artery. Cathet Cardiovasc Diagn 1980;6:413–21.

32. Misra M, Puri VK, Husan M. Single coronary artery as an isolated anomaly. Ind Heart J 1985;37:402–4.

33. Tavernarakis A, Voudris V, Ifantis G, Tsaganos N. Anomalous origin of the right coronary artery arising from the circumflex artery. Clin Cardiol 1986;9:230–2.

34. Sheth M, Dovnarsky M, Chas SD, Kini P, Maranhao V. Single coronary artery: right coronary artery originating from distal left circumflex. Cathet Cardiovasc Diagn 1988;14:180–1.

35. Vassanelli C, Turri M, Morando G, Menegatti G, Zardini P. Single coronary artery from the left sinus of Valsalva. Cathet Cardiovasc Diagn 1989;16:245–6.

36. Jingxuan G, Jieming M, Weidong Y, Changjiang L, Mingzhe C. Single coronary artery. Henry Ford Hosp Med J 1990;38:85–6.

37. Dazai Y, Katoh I, Hara Y, Hoshida R, Job T, Tomino T. A rare case of infective aneurysm involving all three sinuses of Valsalva complicated by left single coronary artery. Jpn Circ J 1991;55:159–64.

38. Vvrolix MC, Geboers M, Sionis D, DeGeest H, DeWerf V. Right coronary artery originating from distal left circumflex: an unusual feature of single coronary artery. Eur Heart J 1991;12:746–7.

39. Amsel BJ, VanDerMast M. Right coronary artery originating from the left anterior descending artery. Eur Heart J 1986;7:719–20.

40. Habbab MA, Senft AG, Haft JI. Origin of the right coronary artery from the left anterior descending coronary artery: a very rare anomaly of coronary arterial origin. Am Heart J 1987;114:169–70.

41. Nath A, Kennett JD, Politte LL, Sanfelippo JF, Alpert MA. Anomalous right coronary artery arising from the midportion of the left anterior descending coronary artery: case reports. Angiology 1987;38:142–6.

42. Molajo AO, Bray CL. Accelerated atherosclerosis and myocardial infarction complicating anomalous origin of the right from the left coronary artery. Int J Cardiol 1989;23:409–12.

43. Hillestad L, Eie H. Single coronary artery: a report of three cases. Acta Med Scand 1971;189:409–13.

44. Husaini SN, Reaver WL, Wilson IJ, Lach RD. Anomalous right coronary artery arising from left mainstem. Cathet Cardiovasc Diagn 1983;9:407–9.

45. Bloomfield P, Erhlich C, Folland ED, Bianco JA, Tow DE, Parisi AF. Anomalous right coronary artery: a surgically correctable cause of angina pectoris. Am J Cardiol 1983;51:1235–7.

46. Meyers DG, McManus BM, McCall D, Walsh RA, Quaife MA. Single coronary artery with the right coronary artery arising from the first septal perforator. Cathet Cardiovasc Diagn 1984;10:479–84.

47. Goto Y, Matsuno Y, Yoshikane H, et al. Ruptured aneurysm of the sinus of Valsalva with single coronary artery. Cathet Cardiovasc Diagn 1989;17:172–4.

48. Smith FM, Graber VC. Coronary thrombosis with congenital absence of the left coronary artery. Arch Int Med 1926;38:222–5.

49. Baltaxe HA, Wixson D. The incidence of congenital anomalies of the coronary arteries in the adult population. Radiology 1977;122:47–52.

50. Milo S, Kishon Y, Goor D, Neufeld HN. Aorto-coronary saphenous vein bypass grafting in a patient with a single coronary artery arising from the right aortic sinus. Thorax 1980;35:207–9.

51. Kafrouni G, Khan H, Wolfson JL. Single right coronary artery: clinical and angiographic findings with surgical management. Ann Thorac Surg 1980;32:80–4.

52. Stauffer JC, Sigwart U, Vogt P, Aymon D, Kappenberger L. Transluminal angioplasty of a single coronary artery. Am Heart J 1991;112:569–71.

53. Kelly MJ, Wolfson S, Marshall R. Single coronary artery from the right sinus of Valsalva: angiography, anatomy, and clinical significance. Am J Roentgenol 1977;128:257–62.

54. Chaitman BR, Lesperance J, Saltiel J, Bourassa MG. Clinical, angiographic, and hemodynamic findings in patients with anomalous origin of the coronary arteries. Circulation 1976;53:122–31.

55. Iskandrian AS, Hakki AH, Bemis CE. Myocardial ischemia in a patient with anomalous origin of the left main coronary artery. Cathet Cardiovasc Diagn 1986;12:48–50.

56. Ishikawa T, Brandt PWT. Anomalous origin of the left main coronary artery from the right anterior aortic sinus: angiographic definition of anomalous course. Am J Cardiol 1985;55:770–6.

57. Kimbiris D, Iskandrian AS, Segal BL, Bemis CE. Anomalous aortic origin of coronary artery. Circulation 1978;58:606–15.

58. Mahapatra RK, Sethi S, Mahapatra D. Single right coronary artery and atherosclerosis. Ind Heart J 1984;36:254–6.

59. Vega M, Hamby RI. Aberrant main left coronary artery in a patient with unstable angina. Cathet Cardiovasc Diagn 1985;11:501–4.

60. Teplitsky I, Wurzel M, Melamed R, Aygen M. Anomalous origin of the coronary arteries. Angiology 1987;38:128–32.

61. Stroobandt R, Piessens J, Suy R, DeGeest H. Unstable angina pectoris in single coronary artery. Acta Cardiol 1974;24:469–75.

62. Rocco TA, Gray D, Easley RM, Gangemi R, Sengupta A. Single coronary artery originating from the right sinus of Valsalva. N Y State J Med 1988;39:328–30.

63. Hyrtl J. Einige in chirurgischer Hinsicht wichtige Gefässvarietäten. Med Jahrb Österr Staats 1841;33:17–38.

Coronary Ostial Dimple (in the Posterior Aortic Sinus) in the Absence of Other Coronary Arterial Abnormalities

Jamshid Shirani, MD, and William C. Roberts, MD

Normally 2 coronary arteries arise from the aorta, 1 from the aortic wall enclosing the right aortic sinus and the other from the aortic wall enclosing the left aortic sinus; the wall enclosing the posterior, i.e., noncoronary sinus, is smooth and devoid of any "dimples" or "buds" or other suggestions of a residua of a potential coronary ostium. Recently, we examined a heart with 2 normally arising coronary ostia and a dimple of an undeveloped coronary ostium in the third aortic sinus. Such an occurrence has not been seen by us in approximately 10,000 other hearts examined in a similar manner. This report briefly describes the cardiac morphologic finding in this 1 patient.

A 20-year-old man died of gunshot wounds. There was no injury to the heart. At necropsy, the heart weighed 250 g. *The left and right ventricular cavities were normal and no grossly visible myocardial scars were seen. The left main and the right coronary arteries arose normally from the left and right aortic sinuses, respectively (Figure 1). The left main coronary artery then divided into the left anterior descending and left circumflex coronary arteries, both of which thereafter coursed normally. In addition to the left main and the right coronary ostia, a coronary ostial dimple was present in the wall of the aorta slightly above the posterior aortic sinus (Figures 1 and 2). It measured 4 mm in diameter and 3 mm in maximum depth.*

Coronary artery ostia arise from the wall of the aortopulmonary trunk at the time of embryonic division of

From the Pathology Branch, National Heart, Lung, and Blood Institute, National Institutes of Health, Building 10, Room 2N258, Bethesda, Maryland 20892. Dr. Robert's current address is: Baylor Cardiovascular Institute, Baylor University Medical Center, 3701 Junius Street, P.O. Box E010, Dallas, Texas 75246. Manuscript received December 7, 1992; revised manuscript received January 29, 1993, and accepted February 1.

TABLE I Reported Cases of Coronary Ostial Dimple in the Presence of "Single Coronary Artery"

Patient	Ref.	Age (yr) & Sex	Location of "Single Ostium"	Location of Ostial Dimple	AP	AMI	SD	CAD	HW (g)	LV Scar	Cause of Death
1	3	37M	LAS	RAS	—	—	—	—	—	—	Infective endocarditis
2	4	68M	LAS	RAS	—	—	—	—	—	—	Cancer
3	5	80F	LAS	RAS	0	0	0	+	340	0	Cancer
4	6	76F	RAS	LAS	0	0	0	0	370	0	Cancer
5	7	84F	RAS	LAS	+	+	+	+	530	+	AMI
6	8	83F	LAS	PAS	0	0	+	+	320	0	Ruptured CA aneurysm

AMI = acute myocardial infarct; AP = angina pectoris; CA = coronary artery; CAD = atherosclerotic coronary artery disease; F = female; HW = heart weight; LAS = left aortic sinus; LV = left ventricular; M = male; PAS = posterior aortic sinus; RAS = right aortic sinus; SD = sudden death; — = information not available; + = present; 0 = absent.

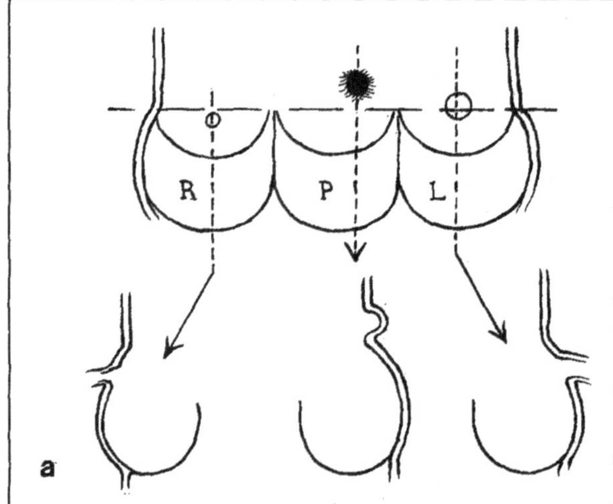

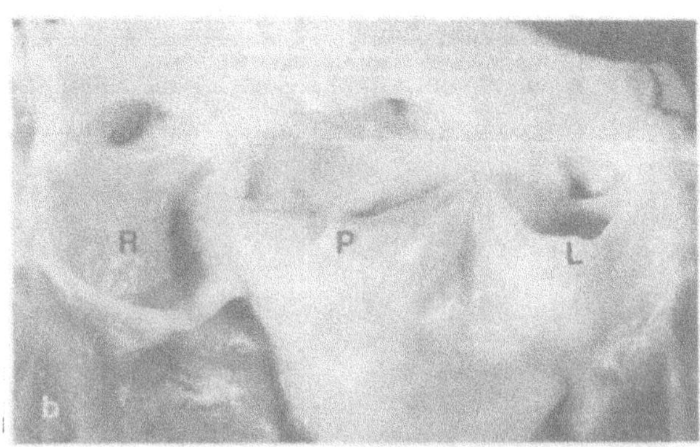

FIGURE 1. Diagram *(a)* and photograph *(b)* of the longitudinally opened aortic valve showing the positions of the 2 normal coronary ostia in the walls of the left (L) and the right (R) aortic sinuses and the coronary ostial dimple above the posterior (P) aortic sinus. The *horizontal broken line* separates the sinus and the tubular portions of the ascending aorta (sinotubular junction). The right and left coronary ostia are located in the wall of the aorta slightly below and at this sinotubular junction, respectively. The coronary ostial dimple is located slightly above the sinotubular junction.

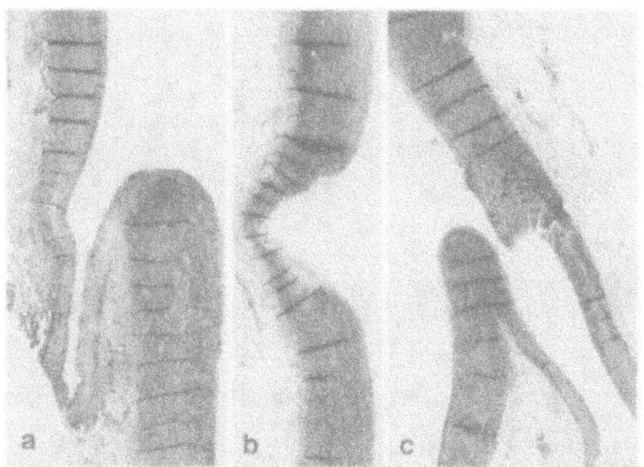

FIGURE 2. Photomicrograph of longitudinal sections of aorta through the right coronary ostium *(a)*, the coronary ostial dimple *(b)* and the left main coronary ostium *(c)*. The sections are taken as shown by the *broken vertical lines* through the coronary ostia in Figure 1a. The aortic media *(darker staining tissue)* continues through the wall of the ostial dimple. Movat stain ×13, reduced by 36%.

the trunk.[1] It is not known why the coronary arteries consistently arise from the left and right aortic sinuses, with only minor variations in their locations in most individuals. It has been suggested that the development of the coronary ostial dimples in the wall of the aortopulmonary trunk require the presence of a developing network of epicardial vessels in the heart.[2] This epicardial vascular network, then, induces the formation of the coronary ostial dimples as it approaches the aortopulmonary trunk. This hypothesis, however, would not explain the presence of coronary ostial dimples in the opposite aortic sinus in patients with "single coronary artery" and in the patient described here.

In addition to the heretofore described patient, at least 6 other cases of coronary ostial dimples or buds have been reported (Table I).[3–8] All 6 cases, however, differed from the present one in that the dimple was at a site where a coronary artery should have arisen but did not. In other words, all 6 previously reported cases of coronary dimple were in actuality examples of single coronary artery.[9] In our patient, on the other hand, a coronary dimple was present at a site where a coronary ostium is not normally present.

1. Angelini P. Normal and anomalous coronary arteries: definitions and classification. *Am Heart J* 1989;117: 418–434.
2. Conte G, Pellegrini A. On the development of the coronary arteries in human embryos, stage 14–19. *Anat Embryol* 1984;169:209–218.
3. Plaut A. Versorgung des Herzens durch nur eine Kranzarterie. *Frankf Z Pathol* 1922;27:84–90.
4. Ogden JA, Goodyer AVN. Patterns of distribution of the single coronary artery. *Yale J Biol Med* 1970;43: 11–21.
5. Smith JC. Review of single coronary artery with report of 2 cases. *Circulation* 1950;1:1168–1175.
6. Leivo IV, Laurila PK. Atresia of left coronary ostium and left main coronary artery. *Arch Pathol Lab Med* 1987;111:1173–1175.
7. Vlodaver Z, Amplatz K, Burchell HB, Edwards JE. Single coronary ostium in the aorta. In: Coronary Heart Disease: Clinical, Angiographic and Pathologic Profiles. New York: Springer-Verlag, 1976:189–216.
8. Causing WP, Shuster M, Pribor HC, Amboy P. Single coronary artery with ruptured coronary artery aneurysm. *Arch Pathol* 1967;83:419–421.
9. Shirani J, Roberts WC. Solitary coronary ostium in the aorta in the absence of other major congenital cardiovascular anomalies. *J Am Coll Cardiol* 1993;21: 137–143.